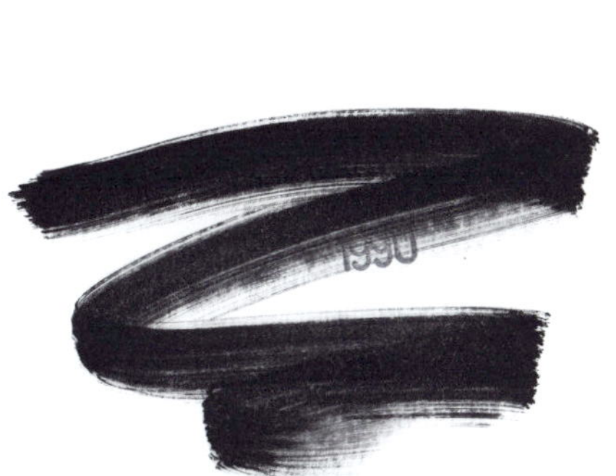

INFECTIONS IN PREGNANCY

INFECTIONS IN PREGNANCY

Edited by

Larry C. Gilstrap, III, M.D.
Department of Obstetrics and Gynecology
University of Texas Southwestern Medical Center
Dallas, Texas

and

Sebastian Faro, M.D., Ph.D.
Department of Obstetrics and Gynecology
Baylor College of Medicine
Houston, Texas

Wiley-Liss

Address all Inquiries to the Publisher
Alan R. Liss, Inc., 41 East 11th Street, New York, NY 10003

Copyright © 1990 Alan R. Liss, Inc.

Printed in United States of America

While the authors, editors, and publisher believe that drug selection and dosage and the specifications and usage of equipment and devices, as set forth in this book, are in accord with current recommendations and practice at the time of publication, they accept no legal responsibility for any errors or omissions, and make no warranty, express or implied, with respect to material contained herein. In view of ongoing research, equipment modifications, changes in governmental regulations and the constant flow of information relating to drug therapy, drug reactions and the use of equipment and devices, the reader is urged to review and evaluate the information provided in the package insert or instructions for each drug, piece of equipment or device for, among other things, any changes in the instructions or indications of dosage or usage and for added warnings and precautions.

Library of Congress Cataloging-in-Publication Data

Infections in pregnancy / editors, Larry C. Gilstrap, III, Sebastian
    Faro.
        p.   cm.
    ISBN 0-471-56221-1
    1. Communicable diseases in pregnancy.   I. Gilstrap, Larry C.
II. Faro, Sebastian.
    [DNLM: 1. Pregnancy Complications, Infectious.   WQ 256 I4343]
RG578.I53   1989
618.3—dc20
DNLM/DLC
for Library of Congress   89-12709
                                                                 CIP

Cover and Interior Design by Eytan Wronker

This book is dedicated to our wives and children:

JoEllen, Lori, Lisa, and Erin Gilstrap
and
Sharon, Christopher, Anne, Michael, and Jonathan Faro

Contents

Contributors

Joseph J. Apuzzio, M.D.
Department of Obstetrics and Gynecology,University of Medicine and Dentistry of New Jersey, Newark, NJ 07103-2757 [125, 133]

Susan M. Cox, M.D.
Department of Obstetrics and Gynecology, University of Texas Southwestern Medical Center, Dallas, TX 75235-9032 [247]

Patrick Duff, M.D.
Division of Maternal-Fetal Medicine, Madigan Army Medical Center, Tacoma, WA 98431-5418 [151]

Sebastian Faro, M.D., Ph.D.
Department of Obstetrics and Gynecology, Baylor College of Medicine, Houston, TX 77030 [1, 29, 45, 55, 75]

Larry C. Gilstrap, III, M.D.
Department of Obstetrics and Gynecology, University of Texas Southwestern Medical Center, Dallas, TX 75235-9032
[7, 15, 37, 115, 133, 185]

Hunter A. Hammill, M.D.
Department of Obstetrics and Gynecology, Baylor College of Medicine, Houston, TX 77030 [185]

Gary D.V. Hankins, M.D.
Department of Obstetrics and Gynecology, Wilford Hall United States Air Force Medical Center, Lackland Air Force Base, TX 78236-5300 [91, 193]

Frederick E. Harlass, M.D.
Division of Maternal-Fetal Medicine, Madigan Army Medical Center, Tacoma, WA 98431-5418 [151]

John C. Hauth, M.D.
Division of Maternal-Fetal Medicine, Department of Obstetrics and Gynecology, University of Alabama, Birmingham, AL 35294 [61]

Wesley Lee, M.D.
Department of Obstetrics and Gynecology, Baylor College of Medicine, Houston, TX 77030 [91]

Maurizio L. Maccato, M.D.
Department of Obstetrics and Gynecology, Baylor College of Medicine, Houston, TX 77030 [255]

The number in brackets is the opening page number of the contributor's article.

Mark G. Martens, M.D.
Department of Obstetrics and Gynecology, Baylor College of Medicine, Houston, TX 77030   [143, 177, 207]

John Owen, M.D.
Division of Maternal-Fetal Medicine, Department of Obstetrics and Gynecology, University of Alabama, Birmingham, AL 35294   [61]

Joseph G. Pastorek II, M.D.
Department of Obstetrics and Gynecology, Louisiana State University Medical Center, New Orleans, LA 70112-2822   [221]

Russell R. Snyder, M.D.
Department of Obstetrics and Gynecology, Wilford Hall United States Air Force Medical Center, Lackland Air Force Base, TX 78236-5300   [91, 193]

George D. Wendel, Jr., M.D.
Department of Obstetrics and Gynecology, University of Texas Southwestern Medical Center, Dallas, TX 75235-9032 [115, 125]

Edward R. Yeomans, M.D.
Department of Obstetrics and Gynecology, Wilford Hall United States Air Force Medical Center, Lackland Air Force Base, TX 78236-5300   [165]

Preface

Over the past few decades, there has been a significant proliferation of information regarding infectious diseases in the obstetric patient. This includes information regarding pathogenesis, diagnosis, adverse effects, and treatment options of the various infections encountered during pregnancy. Due to this "explosion" of information, there has been a gradual evolution towards the creation of a new subspecialty in infectious diseases in obstetrics and gynecology. Not only are infections a source of significant immediate morbidity to the mother, the fetus, and the newborn, but certain infectious agents may actually produce long-term or lasting effects on the unborn child in the form of malformations. There is little question that infectious complications result in a significant economic burden to the patients and society in general.

Although it is unrealistic to expect that every physician providing care for pregnant women become an "infectious disease expert," it is reasonable to expect that these physicians have at least a basic understanding of the pathogenesis, diagnosis, possible adverse fetal and newborn effects, and treatment of the more common infections encountered during pregnancy. These include bacterial, viral, fungal, and parasitic infections.

The major goal of this book is to provide the practicing clinician with recent information regarding the more common infections encountered in obstetrics as well as a few not so common but important infections. A special attempt has been made to provide guidelines, especially with regard to antimicrobial agents, for management of these infections in the pregnant or breast-feeding patient.

Larry C. Gilstrap, III, M.D.
Sebastian Faro, M.D., Ph.D.

1

Microflora of the Genital Tract

Sebastian Faro, M.D., Ph.D.

The female genital tract is divided into two major anatomical regions: the lower region includes the vulva, vagina, and cervix, and the upper region contains the uterus, fallopian tubes, and ovaries. The lower genital tract can be further subdivided into specific anatomical regions: the labia majora and minora, the prepuce of the clitoris, the glans clitoris, and vestibule that houses the urethral orifice, Skene's glands, the vaginal orifice, Bartholin's glands, the fourchette, and the hymenal ring or remnants. The vagina begins just beyond the hymen, or the remnants of the hymen, and the cervix lies at the apex. The perineal body separates the posterior fourchette and the rectum and maintains a physical separation between the vagina and the anus, thereby serving as a potential barrier to prevent a thorough mixing of the bacterial flora of the rectum with that of the vagina.

The lower genital tract, especially the vagina, represents a unique microsphere of microbiological life. The indigenous bacterial inhabitants consist of gram-positive and gram-negative aerobes and anaerobes.[1-4] The indigenous microflora of the lower genital tract most likely has evolved from the normal skin and fecal flora. The vaginal flora is subjected to both exogenous and endogenous pressures that have a direct influence on the bacterial population. There are major differences between the lower genital tract flora and the flora of the skin and rectum; these differences are more than likely due to the modifying effect of the environment of the vagina. The vulva and perineum are covered by skin that is composed of stratified squamous epithelium and contains numerous hair follicles as well as sebaceous, sweat, and apocrine glands.[5] Another unique characteristic of the lower genital tract environment is that the vulva is typically dry except for the folds between the labia majora and minora and the area medial to the labia minora, which are constantly moist. This environment is conducive to the growth of bacteria. Not unlike other parts of the body, the lower genital tract is colonized by typical skin flora (Table 1). The bacteria normally colonizing the skin are actually grouped into microcolonies and are not distributed evenly over the entire surface of the skin. These microcolonies are established at specific sites, e.g., hair follicles, sweat glands, etc. Bacteria found in the sebaceous area of a hair follicle are distributed according to depth, i.e., *Propionibacterium* is located deep in the follicle, whereas

Infections in Pregnancy, pages 1–5
© 1990 Alan R. Liss, Inc.

TABLE 1. Common Resident Bacteria of the Skin

Brevibacterium
Corynebacterium
Enterobacter
Escherichia
Klebsiella
Micrococcus
Peptostreptococcus
Propionibacterium
Proteus
Pseudomonas
Staphylococcus
Streptococcus

Staphylococcus and *Pityosporum* (a yeast) are located near the surface.[6] However, unlike other areas of the body, the vulva and perineum are constantly subjected to bacteria from the rectum and vagina. This constant invasion of bacteria from other regions creates a mixture within these microcolonies that differs from the typical bacteria found at other sites, e.g., axilla, scalp, etc. The perineum has adapted to colonization by fecal and vaginal flora, which is demonstrated by the resistance to infection by the numerous virulent bacteria present. This resistance to infection is exemplified following trauma and heavy contamination with feces, e.g., perineal laceration and/or incision at the time of delivery.

The lower genital tract is subjected to colonization by microorganisms through several different avenues. The hands act as major vectors of transporting a variety of bacteria from a variety of environments and thus bring a sample of these various microenvironments to the genital tract. Bacteria carried by the hands are gram-positive as well as gram-negative: *S. aureus*, *Proteus*, *Pseudomonas*, *Klebsiella*, *Enterobacter*, and *Escherichia*, to name a few.[7–10]

In addition to bacteria and yeast, other microorganisms of importance are the dermatophytes, the fungi. Although the fungi do not usually cause vulva infection, it is not uncommon to find these infections on the thorax, upper and lower abdomen, buttocks, and thighs. The two most common fungi that cause minor skin infections are *Microsporum* and *Trichophyton*; however, these organisms also can be recovered from asymptomatic healthy individuals.[11]

Sexual activity can affect the composition of vaginal microflora by transporting a variety of microorganisms to the genital tract. Oral-genital sex results in the deposition of indigenous oral cavity bacteria on the surface of the external genitalia and vestibule. Manual stimulation and intercourse introduce these organisms, as well as bacteria present on the perineum, into the vagina. The final effect of this mix of bacteria will depend on the inoculum size, as is demonstrated in those individuals who practice anal intercourse, who often develop vaginitis that is associated with a fetid odor. Bacterial studies of the vagina often reveal a high colonization of *Bacteroides fragilis* and *Peptostreptococcus*, bacteria not frequently recovered from healthy vaginas. Sexual intercourse also has the potential of transmitting bacteria such as *Neisseria gonorrhoeae*, *Chlamydia trachomatis*, *Mycoplasma hominis*, and *Ureaplasma urealyticum*, as well as other sexually transmitted organisms. Other significant bacteria include *Streptococcus agalactiae*, *Escherichia coli*, *Gardnerella vaginalis*, and *Haemophilus influenzae*; these can have significant consequences in the pregnant patient and the surgical patient.[12–15] In addition, the deposition of seminal fluid into the vagina results in a decrease in the hydrogen ion concentration, producing a more alkaline pH. The combination of a decrease in hydrogen ion concentration and an increase in abnormal microflora can produce an environment that is conducive to the establishment of bacterial vaginitis.

Hormones, primarily estrogen and progesterone, act physiologically to maintain the vaginal epithelium in a mature state, making it more resistant to infection. These hormones also facilitate the synthesis of glycogen, which is metabolized by the lactobacilli. The metabolic activity of the lactobacilli yields lactic acid, which maintains the vaginal pH between 3.8 and 4.2. This is extremely important because this pH range is unfavorable to the growth of the bacteria typically involved in bacterial vaginitis and favors the growth of the commensal bacteria.[16,17] The lactobacilli may have the primary role in the maintenance of a healthy vagina through the production of lactic acid and hydrogen peroxide. The production of hydrogen peroxide inhibits the growth of anaerobes.[18,19] This is an interesting observation, because the presence of lactobacilli is usually accompanied by other bacteria commonly seen in the healthy vagina, such as diphtheroids, corynebacteria, nondescript streptococci, etc. However, when an abnormal vaginal state is found, the lactobacilli as well as the other commensal bacteria are noticeably absent.[20–23]

Additional evidence of the influence of estrogen and progesterone on the bacteriology of the lower genital tract can be ascertained from examining the natural history of the microbiological changes associated with the changes in the hormonal status of the developing female. The neonatal vagina becomes colonized with bacteria during the first month of life, after which time the bacteria colonizing the vagina diminish rapidly. This alteration in indigenous bacterial colonization corresponds to the decreasing concentration of hormones, mainly estrogen, that initially originated from the mother. During the prepubertal period, the bacterial content of the vagina becomes sparse and this corresponds to a lack of estrogen and progesterone. The bacterial makeup of the vagina becomes increasingly complex during the reproductive phase, consisting of gram-positive and gram-negative aerobic as well as anaerobic bacteria. Lactobacilli are the predominant bacteria during the reproductive years and pregnancy. Coincident with the menopause there is a decrease in the estrogen and progesterone concentration, which results in a marked change in the types of bacteria inhabiting the vagina. The predominant bacteria are no longer the lactobacilli and other commensals, but the coliforms.[24,25]

Douching is not usually performed nor is it recommended for patients who are pregnant. However, when douching is performed, a variety of agents may be used, e.g., dilute acetic acid solutions, perfumed agents, antiseptic solutions, etc. Infrequent douching probably exerts no influence on the vaginal flora. Frequent douching, especially with antiseptic solutions, e.g., betadine, will decrease the commensal organisms, thus allowing the more aggressive bacteria to flourish. Some of these agents can also decrease the hydrogen ion concentration, establishing conditions more favorable for the growth of the more pathogenic bacteria.

Thus, the vagina serves as a natural incubator, providing the appropriate conditions, such as temperature, moisture, hydrogen ion concentration, and nutrients, for the growth of bacteria. This anatomical region is important because it provides a conduit to the upper genital tract and peritoneal cavity. Therefore, the vagina and cervix, with the indigenous microflora, become extremely important, along with the host's natural local and systemic defenses, in preventing infection. These factors become evident in those individuals whose vaginal flora is abnormal and who subsequently become pregnant or are to have pelvic surgery and are therefore at increased risk for infection.[26,27]

The indigenous microflora of the lower genital tract can be divided into two groups: commensal and pathogenic microorganisms (Table 2). The main commensal bacteria are the lactobacilli, diphtheroids, corynebacteria, and nondescript streptococci. The pathogenic bacteria are group B beta-hemolytic streptococci, staphylococci, enterococci, bacteroides, fusobacteria, *Gardnerella*, gram-negative facultative anaerobic bacteria, etc. In addition to the more commonly isolated bacteria listed in Table 2, the following bacterial isolates may be recovered: *Acinetobacter*, *Citrobacter*, *Providencia*, *Viellonella*, and *Clostridium*. The flora of the infected patient, as well as that of the healthy patient, can easily be altered by the addition

TABLE 2. Bacteria Indigenous to the Lower Genital Tract

Commensal
- *Bacillus* sp.
- *Corynebacterium* sp.
- Diphtheroids
- *Lactobacillus* sp.
- Streptococci not grouped

Pathogens
- Gram-positive aerobes
  - *Staphylococcus aureus*
  - *Staphylococcus epidermidis*
  - *Streptococcus agalactiae*
  - *Streptococcus faecalis*
- Gram-negative aerobes
  - *Escherichia coli*
  - *Enterobacter aerogenes*
  - *Enterobacter cloacae*
  - *Gardnerella vaginalis*
  - *Klebsiella pneumoniae*
  - *Morganella morganii*
  - *Proteus mirabilis*
- Gram-positive anaerobes
  - *Eubacterium*
  - *Peptostreptococcus*
- Gram-negative anaerobes
  - *Bacteroides bivius*
  - *Bacteroides disiens*
  - *Bacteroides fragilis*
  - *Bacteroides melaninogenicus*
  - *Bacteroides ovatus*
  - *Bacteroides thetaiotamicron*
  - *Bacteroides vulgatus*
  - *Fusobacterium necrophorum*

of antibiotics, even antibiotics administered for prophylaxis.[28–30] This change in microflora is significant because these patients become susceptible to infection by the dominant organism following an operative procedure.

It is not difficult to determine the status of the vagina and the microbial flora; that is, is it in a healthy or abnormal state. After inspecting the external genitalia, vagina, and cervix, the pH of the vaginal discharge should be determined. This is inexpensive and is accomplished by using litmus paper: the normal vagina pH is 3.8 to 4.5. A pH higher than 4.5 is indicative of abnormal bacterial growth. A positive "whiff" test, that is, the detection of a fishlike (amine) odor after the addition of KOH to a drop or two of vaginal discharge, also indicates the presence of abnormal vaginal flora.

Microscopic examination of vaginal discharge diluted with a drop of normal saline can also be used to determine the state of the vagina (see chapter 4). Knowing whether or not the vagina harbors an abnormal flora can lead to the prevention of vaginitis and, possibly, premature rupture of membranes, premature labor, neonatal infection, and postpartum endometritis. Determining whether or not bacterial vaginitis is present in the patient scheduled for hysterectomy may be the major factor in preventing postoperative infection. Simply treating vaginitis may lead to a decreased dependence on antibiotic prophylaxis.

Thus, by determining the bacteriological status of the vagina, the physician can have an impact on pregnancy outcome and on the postoperative course of the patient. Preliminary screening of the patient for vaginitis is practicing prophylaxis that is specifically directed on a potential focus of infection.

REFERENCES

1. Levison ME, Corman LC, Carrington ER, Kaye D: Quantitative microflora of the vagina. Am J Obstet Gynecol 127:80–85, 1977.
2. Bartlett JG, Moon NE, Goldstein PR, Goren B, Oonderdonk AB, Polk BF: Cervical and vaginal flora: Ecologic niches in the lower female genital tract. Am J Obstet Gynecol 130:658–661, 1978.
3. Gorbach SL, Menda KB, Thadepalli H, Keith L: Anaerobic microflora of the cervix in healthy women. Am J Obstet Gynecol 117:1053–1055, 1973.
4. Tashjian JH, Coulan CB, Washington JA II: Vaginal flora in asymptomatic women. Mayo Clin Proc 51:557–561, 1976.
5. Kaufman RH: Anatomy of the vulva and vagina. In Gardner HC, Kaufman RH (eds): "Benign Diseases of the Vulva and Vagina." Boston: G.K. Hall, 1981, pp 1–12.
6. Noble WC: Microbial skin disease: Its epidemiology. In: "Microbiology of Normal Skin." Current Topics in Infection Series. London: Edward Arnold, 1983, pp 5–23.
7. Casewell M: The role of the hands in nosocomial gram-negative infection. In Maibach HI, Aly R

(eds): "Skin Microbiology: Relevance to Infection." New York: Springer, 1981, p 192.

8. Casewell M, Phillips I: Hands as a route of transmission of Klebsiella species. Br Med J 2:1315, 1977.

9. Adams BG, Marrie TJ: Hand carriage of aerobic gram-negative rods may not be transient. J Hyg 89:33, 1982.

10. Haverkorn ML, Michel MF: Nosocomial Klebsiella. J Hyg 82:177, 1979.

11. Davis CM, Garcia RL, Riordan JM: Dermatophytes in military recruits. Arch Dermatol 105:558, 1972.

12. Lee W, Phillips LE, Carpenter RJ, Martens MG, Faro S: *Gardnerella vaginalis* chorioamnionitis. A report of two cases and a review of the pathogenic role of G. *vaginalis* in obstetrics. Diagn Microbiol Infect Dis 8:107–111, 1987.

13. Gravett MG, Hummel D, Eschenbach DA, Holmes KK: Preterm labor associated with subclinical amniotic fluid infection and with bacterial vaginosis. Obstet Gynecol 67:229–231, 1986.

14. Phillips LE, Faro S, Martens MG, Baker JL, Goodrich KH, Turner RM, Riddle G: Postcesarean microbiology of high-risk patients treated for endometritis. Curr Ther Res 42:1157–1165, 1987.

15. Pastorek J II, Bellow P, Faro S: Haemophilus influenzae implicated in puerperal infection. South Med J 75:734–736, 1982.

16. Larsen B, Galask RP: Vaginal microbial flora: Composition and influences of host physiology. Ann Intern Med 96:926–930, 1982.

17. Preti G, Huggins GR: Organic constituents of vaginal secretions. In Hafez ESE, Evans TN (eds): "The Human Vagina." Amsterdam: North Holland, 1978, pp 151–166.

18. Gilliland SE, Speck ML: Antagonistic action of *Lactobacillus acidophilus* toward intestinal and foodborn pathogens in associated culture. J Food Prot 40:820–823, 1977.

19. Tramer J: Inhibitory effect of *Lactobacillus acidophilus*. Nature 211:204–205, 1966.

20. Levison ME, Trestman I, Quich R, Sladowski C, Floro CN: Quantitative bacteriology of the vaginal flora in vaginitis. Am J Obstet Gynecol 133:139–144, 1979.

21. Keith L, England D, Bartizal F, Brown E, Fields C: Microbial flora of the external os of the premenopausal cervix. Br J Vener Dis 48:51–56, 1972.

22. Ohm MJ, Galask PP: Bacterial flora of the cervix from 100 prehysterectomy patients. Am J Obstet Gynecol 122:683–687, 1975.

23. Larsen B, Goplerud CP, Petzold CR, Ohm-Smith MJ, Galask RP: Postmenopausal genital tract cultures of women treated with estrogen compared to non-treated women. Obstet Gynecol 59:20–24, 1982.

24. Cruickshank R, Sharman A: The biology of the vagina in human subject. II. The bacterial flora and secretion of the vagina of various age periods and their relation to glycogen in the vaginal epithelium. J Obstet Gynaecol Br Emp 41:208–226, 1934.

25. Hunter CA, Long KR: A study of the microbiological flora of the vagina. Am J Obstet Gynecol 75:865–871, 1958.

26. Peterson EE: Disturbed vaginal flora as a risk factor in pregnancy. J Obstet Gynecol 6(1):516–518, 1986.

27. Rosene K, Eschenbach DA, Tompkins LS, Kenny GE, Watkins H: Polymicrobial early postpartum endometritis with facultative and anaerobic bacteria genital mycoplasmas and C. *trachomatis*. Treatment with piperacillin or cefoxitin. J Infect Dis 153:1028–1037, 1986.

28. Stiver HG, Forward KR, Tyrrell DL, et al.: Comparative cervical miroflora shifts after cefoxitin and cefazolin prophylaxis against infection following cesarean section. Am J Obstet Gynecol 149:718–721, 1986.

29. Moellering RC Jr: Enterococcal infection in patients treated with moxalactam. Rev Infect Dis 4:S708–S711, 1982.

30. Faro S, Phillips LE, Martens MG: Perspectives on the bacteriology of postoperative obstetric-gynecologic infections. Am J Obstet Gynecol 158(Suppl 3):694–700, 1988.

2

Antimicrobial Agents During Pregnancy

Larry C. Gilstrap, III, M.D.

Infections are relatively common during pregnancy. For example, urinary tract infections occur in 2–12% of all pregnant women, while acute chorioamnionitis occurs in 1–3% of such women. In addition, fungal, viral, and parasitic infections may also occur. Thus, the clinician is often faced with the dilemma of not only what antimicrobial agent to use, but also whether it is safe for the fetus or newborn. Moreover, the clinician must also be concerned with the ever-escalating number of personal injury suits, many of which are related to drugs and medications taken during pregnancy. Unfortunately, there is little available scientific data regarding both the efficacy and safety of the majority of these agents during pregnancy. However, with a few notable exceptions, these agents have been used in a relatively large number of pregnant women without any apparent adverse effects. The information that is available is mostly empiric and anecdotal.

When prescribing antimicrobial agents for the pregnant woman, there are several special considerations that must be taken into account. First, there are two patients involved, the mother and her unborn fetus, and it is fairly well documented that virtually all antimicrobial agents cross the placenta and are detectable in the fetus. Second, there are several physiological changes that occur in the mother secondary to pregnancy, such as increase blood volume, increased creatinine clearance, decreased serum-binding proteins, and decreased gastrointestinal motility, that may affect the absorption, maternal serum level, metabolism, and placental transfer of various antimicrobial agents. It is well documented that the maternal serum levels of ampicillin and certain aminoglycosides are decreased during pregnancy.[1] It is reasonable to assume that the serum levels of many other antimicrobial agents are also lower in pregnant women, especially during the latter half of pregnancy.

TERATOGENICITY

Obviously the greatest concern regarding antimicrobial therapy during pregnancy is whether a particular agent is teratogenic or causes adverse fetal effects. There are several crucial factors that must be taken into account. First and most important, is the fetus exposed to a specific antimicrobial agent from maternal ingestion and to what degree? As noted above, probably all such agents cross the placenta to some extent. Some

Infections in Pregnancy, pages 7–13
© 1990 Alan R. Liss, Inc.

agents, such as ampicillin, result in a significant fetal serum level, whereas other agents, such as erythromycin, are significantly bound to proteins in maternal serum and only a very small amount actually reaches the fetus. Another crucial factor is the gestational age at the time of drug exposure. With regard to teratogenicity, the most critical time period is the embryonic period of the first 8 weeks of pregnancy—the period of major organogenesis. However, agents such as tetracyclines may actually cause other adverse fetal effects (yellow discoloration of the diciduous teeth) if given during the latter half of pregnancy.

Another factor is susceptibility of the human species to the teratogenicity of a particular antimicrobial agent. Many drugs and medications may be teratogenic in various animal species, but not in humans. For example, the sulfonamides have been shown to be teratogenic in rats and mice,[2] but after 15 years of use there is little or no scientific evidence that they are teratogenic in humans.[3]

Yet another factor is the magnitude of the dose given. Almost any drug, including antimicrobial agents, may cause adverse effects and possibly fetal abnormalities if given in excessive amounts; therefore, the smallest possible effective dose of an antimicrobial agent should be used. Unfortunately, this is sometimes difficult to gauge because of the changing blood volumes and renal excretion of various agents during pregnancy.

FDA DRUG CLASSIFICATION

In an attempt to better classify drugs and medications with regard to potential adverse fetal effects, the Food and Drug Administration in 1979 established five categories for drugs, including antimicrobial agents, which are summarized in Table 1.[4] Briefly, antimicrobials that demonstrate no fetal risk and that have been proved safe for pregnancy are category A drugs. Category X antimicrobials would be proven teratogens. Although less than a perfect system, this classification is at least a step in the right direction. At present

TABLE 1. FDA Classification of Drugs

Category	Description
A	No fetal risk; proven safe for use during pregnancy
B	Fetal risk not demonstrated in animal or human studies
C	Fetal risk unknown; no adequate human studies
D	Some evidence of fetal risk. May be necessary to use drug
X	Proven fetal risk. Contraindicated for use during pregnancy.

Adapted from the Federal Drug Administration.[4]

there are no category A ("safe") or category X ("contraindicated") antimicrobial agents. There are many category B and C antimicrobial agents and a few in category D. Category B agents are probably safe for use during pregnancy. Because little is known about the safety of category C antimicrobials, they should be used only when clearly indicated. Category D agents should be avoided when possible and used only in serious or life-threatening situations for which other agents are not effective. Briggs et al.[5] have published an extensive textbook categorizing commonly used drugs according to this classification.

BETA-LACTAM ANTIBIOTICS

All beta-lactam antibiotics contain a beta-lactam ring and are bactericidal by virtue of inhibiting bacterial cell wall synthesis. Antibiotics in this group include the penicillins, cephalosporins, monobactams, and carbapenams.

Penicillins

Although there are no large prospective controlled studies regarding the safety and efficacy of the various penicillins during pregnancy, especially the newer extended ones, penicillins have been used for many years to treat infections in pregnant women. To date there are no data that would suggest that these agents are teratogenic. In the Collab-

TABLE 2. The Penicillins*

Natural penicillins
    Penicillin G, benzylpenicillin
    Penicillin VK, phenoxymethyl penicillin

Penicillinase-resistant or antistaphylococcal
penicillins
    Methicillin
    Oxacillin
    Nafcillin
    Cloxacillin
    Dicloxacillin

Extended-spectrum penicillins
    Ampicillin
    Amoxicillin
    Carbenicillin
    Ticarcillin
    Mezlocillin
    Azlocillin
    Piperacillin

*Category grouping according to manufacturer, author's opinion, or Briggs et al.[5]

TABLE 3. Penicillins Combined With Beta-Lactamase Inhibitors (FDA Category B)

Ticarcillin (3 g) plus clavulanic acid (100–200 mg)[a]
Amoxicillin (250–500 mg) plus clavulanic acid
    (125 mg)[b]
Ampicillin (250–500 mg) plus sulbactam (125 mg)[c]

[a]Timentin.
[b]Augmentin.
[c]Unasyn.

orative Perinatal Project, over 3,000 pregnant women were exposed to a penicillin-type drug during the first trimester without evidence of an increase in congenital anomalies or adverse fetal effects.[6]

All penicillins appear to cross the placenta and reach measurable levels in the fetus.[1,7] The various penicillins available today are summarized in Table 2.[8] All of the penicillins currently are classified as FDA category B drugs. As with ampicillin, the serum level of all penicillins is probably reduced during pregnancy secondary to the expanded maternal blood volume and possible increased renal excretion.

Several of the penicillins have been combined with beta-lactamase inhibitors (Table 3) to broaden their spectrum of activity. Two currently available beta-lactamase inhibitors are clavulanic acid and sulbactam. There is no information regarding the safety of these agents during pregnancy; however, the penicillins containing these agents are listed as FDA category B drugs by their manufacturer.

Cephalosporins

The cephalosporins make up the largest group of antibiotics and are generally divided into first-, second-, and third-generation categories.[9] Although there are no large studies regarding the efficacy and safety of cephalosporins during pregnancy, the first-generation cephalosporins have been used for many years in pregnant women without apparent adverse fetal effects. There are no reports of the cephalosporins being teratogenic, and they are all classified as FDA category B drugs.

The serum levels of many of the cephalosporins in pregnant women appear to be lower and the serum half-life shorter than in nonpregnant women.[1] Some of the currently available cephalosporins are summarized in Table 4.

CARBAPENEM AND MONOBACTAM ANTIBIOTICS

The carbapenems and monobactams are new classes of antibiotics. Imipenem (Primaxin) in combination with a renal enzyme inhibitor, Cilastin sodium, is the only currently available carbapenem antibiotic.[9] This antibiotic has the broadest spectrum of activity against both aerobic and anaerobic bacteria than any other currently available antibiotic. However, there are no scientific data regarding the safety of this antibiotic for use during pregnancy and it is thus a category C drug.

Aztreonam (Azactam) is the only currently available monobactam antibiotic. It is resistant to most beta-lactamases and has a spectrum of activity similar to the aminoglycosides and thus provides coverage against a wide variety of gram-negative bacilli, includ-

TABLE 4. Commonly Used Cephalosporins

First generation[a]
   Cephalothin (Keflin)
   Cephapirin (Cefadyl)
   Cephradine (Anspor, Velosef)
   Cefazolin (Ancef, Kefzol)
   Cephalexin (Keflex)
   Cefadroxil (Duricef, Ultracel)
   Cefaclor (Ceclor)

Second generation[a]
   Cefamandole (Mandol)
   Cefoxitin (Mefoxin)
   Cefotetan (Cefotan)
   Cefuroxime (Zinacef, Kefurox)

Third generation[a]
   Cefotaxime (Claforan)
   Cefoperazone (Cefobid)
   Ceftrizoxime (Cefizox)
   Ceftriaxone (Rocephin)

Adapted from Thompson.[9]
[a]All are category B drugs.

TABLE 5. Aminoglycosides

Agent	Category[a]
Streptomycin	D
Kanamycin (Kantrex)	D
Gentamicin (Garamycin)	C
Tobramycin (Nebcin)	D
Amikacin (Amikin)	C
Netilmicin (Netromycin)	D

[a]Category according to manufacturer, author's opinion, or Briggs et al.[5]

ing *Pseudomonas aruginosas.*[9] According to its manufacturer, aztreonam did not cause malformations in common laboratory animals and is listed as a category B drug. There are no studies in human pregnancies.

AMINOGLYCOSIDES

The aminoglycosides are used during pregnancy to treat acute symptomatic upper urinary tract infections (i.e., pyelonephritis). The aminoglycosides interfere with protein synthesis and are bactericidal.[10] Currently available aminoglycosides are listed in Table 5. With the exception of gentamicin and amikacin, the aminoglycosides are generally listed as category D drugs because of the concern that these agents may cause irreversible deafness in the fetus. There are several reports of ototoxicity reported in the fetuses of mothers who were treated with streptomycin.[5,11] Kanamycin has also been reported to cause hearing loss.[12]

Amikacin and gentamicin are both category C drugs because there are no reports to date linking either to fetal malformations or ototoxicity, although there is no reason to doubt that these two aminoglycosides could also result in fetal hearing loss if given in large enough doses over a protracted period. The serum levels of all of the aminoglycosides, including gentamicin, are lower in pregnant women than in nonpregnant women.[1]

Particular caution should be exercised when using aminoglycosides to treat pregnant women with acute pyelonephritis, as a significant number of such patients will have transient renal dysfunction (see chapter 3).

CLINDAMYCIN, CHLORAMPHENICOL, AND METRONIDAZOLE

Clindamycin, chloramphenicol, and metronidazole are commonly used to treat serious anaerobic infections. Although these infections are uncommon in pregnant women, they are relatively common in postpartum women, especially following cesarean section. Clindamycin and metronidazole are both category B drugs (Table 6), whereas chloramphenicol is a category C drug.

Although metronidazole (Flagyl) is a category B drug, the manufacturer issues a stern warning about its use during the first trimester of pregnancy. Its primary use in pregnancy is actually not for anaerobic infections, but for trichomoniasis. Unfortunately, there is no other effective treatment for this infection. However, most patients can be treated with local agents until they are past the critical point of organogenesis and can then be started on metronidazole. Chloram-

TABLE 6. FDA Category of Various Other Antibiotics

Agent	Category[a]
Clindamycin	B
Chloramphenicol	C
Metronidazole	B
Sulfonamides	B
Trimethoprim	C
Nitrofurantoin	B
Vancomycin	C
Tetracyclines	D
Erythromycin	B
Norfloxacin	C
Ciprofloxacin	C

[a]Category according to manufacturer, author's opinion, or Briggs et al.[5]

phenicol is rarely used today, even for serious anaerobic infections because of the fear of aplastic anemia. The "gray-baby syndrome" that was reported in premature infants given large doses of chloramphenicol has not been reported with maternal treatment.[13] There are no reports of fetal anomalies with either chloramphenicol or clindamycin.

SULFONAMIDES, TRIMETHOPRIM, AND NITROFURANTOIN

Sulfonamides, trimethoprim, and nitrofurantoin are commonly used to treat urinary tract infections. The sulfonamides are category B drugs and have not been reported to cause fetal malformations. However, it is well known that sulfonamides may compete for bilirubin binding sites, and there have been reports of newborn hyperbilirubinemia from maternal sulfonamide therapy near delivery.[1]

Trimethoprim is an antimicrobial that is used either alone or in combination with a sulfonamide, sulfamethoxazole (Bactrim or Septra). It is a category C drug. Although it was used to treat urinary tract infections in 120 pregnant women in one study without any apparent harmful fetal effects when compared with controls,[14] it is generally not recommended for use during pregnancy because it is a folic acid antagonist.

Nitrofurantoin is probably the most common antimicrobial used to treat lower urinary tract infections during pregnancy and for continuing suppressive therapy following acute pyelonephritis in pregnant women. It is a category B drug (Table 6), and there are no reports of associated fetal malformations. However, it has been reported to be associated with hemolytic anemia in pregnant women with glucose-6-phosphate dehydrogenase deficiency.[15]

ERYTHROMYCIN, VANCOMYCIN, AND TETRACYCLINE

Erythromycin is a category B drug and is probably very safe for use during pregnancy. Because of protein binding, very little erythromycin actually crosses the placenta.[1] In fact, if erythromycin is used as an alternative to treat syphilis in the penicillin-sensitive pregnant woman, the fetus may not be successfully treated[16] (see chapter 11).

Vancomycin is an antibiotic that is particularly effective against gram-positive organisms.[17] It is a category C drug (Table 6) and is used primarily during pregnancy for bacterial endocarditis prophylaxis in penicillin-allergic patients.

The tetracyclines, including the newer semisynthetic agents, are category D drugs. It is now well documented that tetracyclines may cause yellow-brown discoloration of the deciduous teeth.[18,19] Tetracycline has also been reported to result in acute fatty degeneration of the liver with azotemia, jaundice, and pancreatitis, especially in the presence of impaired renal function.[20]

QUINOLONES

The fluoroquinolones are relatively new antibiotics and thus are category C drugs. One such agent, norfloxacin, is a very effective antibiotic for the treatment of urinary tract infection. Ciprofloxacin is another new fluoroquinolone and is effective against a wide variety of gram-negative bacilli. How-

TABLE 7. Antifungals

Agent	Category[a]
Clotrimazole (Gyne-lotrimin, Lotrimin, Mycelex)	B
Miconazole (Monistat)	B
Nystatin (Mycostatin, Nilstat)	B
Butoconazole (Femstat)	C
Amphotericin (Fungizone)	B
Griseofulvin (Fulvicin, Grifulvin)	C

[a]Category according to manufacturer, author's opinion, or Briggs et al.[5]

TABLE 8. Antivirals

Agent	Category[a]
Amantadine (Symmetrel)	C
Idoxuridine (Stoxil)	C
Acyclovir (Zovirax)	C
Zidovudine (Retrovir, AZT)	C
Vidarabine (Vira-A)	C

[a]Category according to manufacturer, author's opinion, or Briggs et al.[5]

ever, because there is no information regarding the safety of these agents during pregnancy, they are not currently recommended for use during pregnancy.

ANTIFUNGALS

Candida vulvovaginitis is relatively common during pregnancy and may be treated with a variety of antifungals, which are listed in Table 7. Clotrimazole, miconazole, and nystatin are category B drugs, whereas butoconazole, the newest of the four, is a category C agent.[13]

Amphotericin B is a systemic antifungal used for the treatment of coccidiomycosis, cryptococcosis, and histoplasmosis. Although there is little information regarding its safety during pregnancy, it is listed as a category B drug.[13] Griseofulvin is an oral antifungal agent that is used for the treatment of various ringworm infections of the skin, nails, and hair; it is listed as category C by its manufacturer.[13]

ANTIVIRALS

The various antivirals are listed in Table 8; all are category C agents. Amantadine is an antiviral used for the treatment of influenza. There is probably little or no indication for the use of this drug during pregnancy. Vidarabine is used either topically for herpetic keratitis or intravenously for disseminated herpes infection, although acyclovir has largely replaced this drug for the latter infection.[21] There is little information regarding the safety of acyclovir during pregnancy, and it should be reserved for life-threatening viral infections such as varicella pneumonia[22] or disseminated herpes. Idoxuridine is a topical agent used for superficial keratitis and it can be used during pregnancy if necessary.

Zidovudine (Retrovir or AZT) is the only agent to date that has been shown to be at least partially effective for the treatment of the human immunodeficiency virus, or AIDS. Although there are no large studies regarding either the efficacy or safety of this drug during pregnancy, it is logical to use the drug to treat pregnant women with AIDS.[13] Clearly, the potential benefits of this drug outweigh any theoretical risk.

SUMMARY

Fortunately, the majority of antimicrobial agents are not associated with fetal malformations and can be used if necessary to treat infections during pregnancy. As with all medications, antimicrobial agents should only be used when clearly indicated.

REFERENCES

1. Landers DV, Green JR, Sweet RL: Antibiotic use during pregnancy and the postpartum period. Clin Obstet Gynecol 26:391–406, 1983.
2. Kato T, Kitagawa S: Production of congenital malformations in fetuses of rats and mice with various sulphonamides. J Congen Abn 13:7–15, 1973.
3. Wise R: Prescribing in pregnancy: Antibiotics. Br Med J 294:42–46, 1987.
4. Federal Drug Administration: Pregnancy categories

for prescription drugs. FDA Drug Bull, September 1979.

5. Briggs GG, Freeman RK, Yaffe SJ: "Drugs in Pregnancy and Lactation," 2nd edition. Baltimore: Williams & Wilkins, 1986.

6. Heinonen OP, Slone D, Shapiro S: "Birth Defects and Drugs in Pregnancy." Littleton, MA: Publishing Sciences Group, 1977, pp 297–313.

7. Gilstrap LC, Bawdon RE, Burris J: Antibiotic concentration in maternal blood, cord blood and placental membranes in chorioamniontis. Obstet Gynecol 72:124–125, 1988.

8. Wright AJ, Wilkowske CJ: The penicillins. Mayo Clin Proc 62:806–820, 1987.

9. Thompson RL: Cephalosporins, carbapenem and monobactam antibiotics. Mayo Clin Proc 62:821–834, 1987.

10. Edson RS, Terrell CL: The aminoglycosides: Streptomycin, kanamycin, gentamicin, tobramycin, amikacin, natilmicin and sisomicin. Mayo Clin Proc 62:916–920, 1987.

11. Donald PR, Sellars SL: Streptomycin ototoxicity in the unborn child. S Afr Med J 60:316–318, 1981.

12. Good R, Johnson G: The placental transfer of kanamycin during late pregnancy. Obstet Gynecol 38:60–62, 1971.

13. Gilstrap LC, Cunningham FG: Drugs and medications in pregnancy. Supplement 13, "Williams Obstetrics." Norwalk, CT: Appleton-Lange, 1987.

14. Brumfit W, Pursell R: Trimethoprim/sulfamethoxazole in the treatment of bacteriuria in women. J Infect Dis 128:S657–S663, 1973.

15. Powell RD, DeGowin RL, Alving AS: Nitrofurantoin induced hemolysis. J Lab Clin Med 62:1002–1003, 1963.

16. Fenton LJ, Light LJ: Congenital syphilis after maternal treatment with erythromycin. Obstet Gynecol 47:492–494, 1976.

17. Hermans PE, Wilhelm MP: Vancomycin. Mayo Clin Proc 62:901–905, 1987.

18. Rendle-Short TJ: Tetracycline and teeth and bone. Lancet 1:1188, 1962.

19. Kutscher AH, Zegarelli EV, Tovell HM, et al.: Discoloration of deciduous teeth induced by administration of tetracycline antepartum. Am J Obstet Gynecol 96:291–292, 1966.

20. Whalley PJ, Adams RH, Combs B: Tetracycline toxicity in pregnancy. JAMA 189:357–360, 1964.

21. Hermans PE, Cockerill FR: Antiviral agents. Mayo Clin Proc 62:1108–1115, 1987.

22. Hankins GDV, Gilstrap LC, Patterson A: Acyclovir treatment of varicella pneumonia in pregnancy. Crit Care Med 15:336–337, 1987.

3

Urinary Tract Infections in Pregnancy

Larry C. Gilstrap, III, M.D.

Urinary tract infections are relatively common in young women, and it has been estimated that approximately 15% of women will experience at least one episode of urinary tract infection during their lifetime.[1,2] There are several anatomical reasons for the increased frequency of urinary tract infections in women as compared to men. For example, the female urethra is relatively short (approximately 3–4 cm in length) and is in close proximity to the vaginal canal, which in turn borders the anus and rectum. The vagina is richly colonized with organisms from the lower gastrointestinal tract, such as *Escherichia coli*, *Klebsiella pneumoniae*, *Enterobacter*, and *Proteus* sp.—common pathogens isolated from women with urinary tract infections. Urethral trauma secondary to intercourse may also play a role in the colonization of the lower urinary tract, and acute cystitis has been reported to be associated with recent sexual intercourse.[3] Women acquire bacteriuria early in life; by way of example, 5% of girls at the time of high school[4] and 8% of nulliparous married women will have bacteriuria.[5]

It has been demonstrated that certain uropathogens have the unique ability to invade and attach themselves to the uroepithelium of the lower urinary tract. In particular, the p-fimbriated strains of *E. coli* are able to attach to specific receptors in the uroepithelium. This may be an explanation for why urinary tract infection is more common in women and why some women are more susceptible to persistent or recurrent bacteriuria and to the acquisition of upper tract infections such as acute pyelonephritis.[6,7] The exact role that bacterial adherence may play in the pathogenesis of urinary tract infections in pregnant women is unclear at this time.

During pregnancy, infections of the urinary tract may involve either the lower urinary tract or the upper urinary tract. Moreover, infections may be either symptomatic or asymptomatic. Infections that will be discussed in detail include asymptomatic bacteriuria, cystitis, and acute pyelonephritis.

ASYMPTOMATIC BACTERIURIA

As the name implies, asymptomatic bacteriuria (ASB) is the presence of a urinary tract infection in the absence of specific urinary tract symptoms. Pregnancy per se does not predispose an individual to the acquisition of bacteriuria, and the prevalence of bacteriuria in pregnant and nonpregnant women is es-

Infections in Pregnancy, pages 15–27

sentially the same. The prevalence of bacteriuria in pregnant women is approximately 5–6%, with rates as high as 10% in certain high-risk populations.[8] There are several predisposing factors associated with an increased frequency of bacteriuria during pregnancy. The most significant factor is socioeconomic status: indigent patients have a higher incidence of bacteriuria than nonindigent patients.[9] There is little or no evidence that race per se is significantly associated with bacteriuria; in fact, most studies found no significant difference in the prevalence of bacteriuria between black and white patients when controlled for socioeconomic status.[8,9] The association of either age or parity with bacteriuria during pregnancy is unclear. It has been established that pregnant women with sickle-cell trait have a twofold increase in the frequency of ASB when compared to pregnant women without sickle-cell trait.[10] Of significance is the fact that less than 1% of women will actually acquire bacteriuria during pregnancy if it is not present at the time of the initial screening culture.

Diagnosis

Because women with ASB have no symptoms, the diagnosis is based solely on demonstrating the presence of significant bacteriuria. From a bacteriology standpoint, the most commonly accepted definition of significant bacteriuria is the presence of $\geq 100,000$ organisms/ml of urine of a single uropathogen. The most common method of collection is by the clean-voided technique. Counts of less than 100,000 organisms/ml, unless obtained by catheterization, or specimens containing more than one organism generally represent contamination and not urinary tract infection. The accuracy of a single culture obtained by the clean-voided technique is approximately 85%; 96% accuracy is achieved with catheterization.[8,11] When bacteriuria is confirmed on a repeat specimen obtained by the clean-voided technique, the accuracy approaches that of catheterization. The presence of any bacteria obtained by su-

TABLE 1. Screening Techniques Used for the Detection of Bacteriuria During Pregnancy

Urinalysis
Leukocyte esterase activity
Drop of unspun urine
Nitrite (Griess) test
Urine culture
   Pour plate dilution
   Calibrated loop
Urine culture kits
   Testuria (Ayerst)
   Bactercult (Wampole)
   Uricult (Bristol)
   Microstix-3 (Ames)
   Bac-T-Screen (Marion)

prapubic aspiration is probably clinically significant and indicative of urinary tract infection. However, this latter technique is generally unacceptable to patients, unnecessary, and should be used only in very unusual circumstances. From a practical and cost-effective standpoint, a single specimen obtained by the clean-voided technique should be used for screening in the majority of pregnant women. Although there may be a 15% false-positive rate, false negatives are extremely uncommon.

Methods used to screen for the presence of bacteriuria during pregnancy are summarized in Table 1. Of these, the routine urinalysis is grossly inaccurate and should not be used as the sole screening tool to detect the presence or absence of bacteriuria. The presence of white blood cells or "pyuria" on urinalysis is not always indicative of urinary tract infection, especially ASB, and is often found in pregnant women without infection. However, the presence of bacteria in a drop of unspun urine has been shown to correlate with the presence of significant bacteriuria as demonstrated by urine culture.[12] The sensitivity and specificity of the other tests listed in Table 1 vary depending on the reference source. The urine culture remains the most accurate, albeit more expensive, screening method for detecting for the presence of bacteriuria during pregnancy. Most hospital laboratories use the pour plate or calibrated loop

TABLE 2. Microbiology of Urinary Tract Infections Encountered During Pregnancy

Escherichia coli[a]
Klebsiella-Enterobacter[a]
Enterococcus
Streptococcus
Staphylococcus
Proteus
Pseudomonas
Citrobacter

[a]Together for 85–90% of infections.

technique in performing quantitative urine cultures. Alternatively, several commercial kits that are easy to use, relatively inexpensive, and amazingly accurate, have been marketed for performing quantitative urine cultures.[13]

Microbiology of Urinary Tract Infections During Pregnancy

The most common bacterial isolates recovered in pregnant women with urinary tract infections, including ASB, are summarized in Table 2. The Enterobacteriaceae, especially *E. coli* and *Klebsiella-Enterobacter* sp. account for 85 to 90% of urinary tract infections during pregnancy. *Escherichia coli* is also responsible for the majority of recurrent urinary tract infections in young women, and it has been shown that these women are likely to have introital colonization with bacteria manifesting bacterial adherence.[14]

Importantly, group B streptococcus may be associated with ASB in a significant number of pregnant women.[15,16] *Staphylococcus saprophyticus* has also been reported to cause urinary tract infections in women.[17] Other organisms such as *Citrobacter, Proteus,* and *Pseudomonas* sp. are uncommon pathogens in urinary tract infections during pregnancy. Anaerobic bacteria probably play little or no role in the etiology of ASB during pregnancy.

Significance of Bacteriuria

It is neither necessary nor cost effective to perform routine screening for bacteriuria in asymptomatic nonpregnant young women. Asymptomatic bacteriuria in the nonpregnant patient probably carries little or no significant health risk. The same cannot be said for the pregnant patient in whom the presence of ASB clearly does carry a significant health risk. Although pregnancy does not predispose an individual to the acquisition of bacteriuria, it does predispose one to the acquisition of symptomatic urinary tract infection, i.e., acute pyelonephritis. It has now been well documented that as many as 28% of pregnant women with untreated bacteriuria will develop acute pyelonephritis.[8] Acute pyelonephritis in turn carries significant risk to both the mother and the fetus. In contrast, the incidence of acute pyelonephritis in women with bacteriuria who are treated is only approximately 3–4%.[8]

Other adverse effects that have been attributed to ASB in pregnancy include maternal anemia, maternal hypertension, increased frequency of prematurity, and an increased frequency of low-birth-weight infants.[18] Kass was the first to report an association between bacteriuria and prematurity and, more importantly, reported that eradication of bacteriuria during pregnancy would result in a decreased frequency of premature births.[19] While there have been additional studies supporting Kass's initial observation regarding bacteriuria and prematurity,[20,21] others report a lack of such association.[18,22] Thus, significant controversy remains regarding the possible association of bacteriuria and prematurity. One possible reason for the discrepancy is that the criteria used to define prematurity in the early reports was a birth weight of less than 2,500 g; many of these babies may actually have been growth retarded and not premature. As Cunningham and Whalley have pointed out, it is difficult if not impossible "to determine from early reports whether infants born to mothers with bacteriuria were premature, dysmature or both."[23] Another explanation for the diversity of opinion is the possibility that there may be a subgroup of pregnant women with bacteriuria, i.e., those who are at greater risk for complications. Also, it is now well established

TABLE 3. Association of Renal Bacteriuria With Hypertension, Anemia, Prematurity, and Low Birth Weight

	Renal bacteriuria (n = 114)	Controls (n = 114)
Mean gestational age at birth (weeks)	39.9	39.1
Mean birth weight (g)	3,254*	3,077*
Delivery before 37 weeks	4%	6%
Low birth weight	10%	14%
Hypertension	12%	15%
Anemia	2.6%	2.6%

Adapted from Gilstrap et al.[18]
*P < .05.

TABLE 4. Antimicrobial Regimens for the Treatment of Asymptomatic Bacteriuria During Pregnancy

Agent	Dosage[a]
Sulfonamides	500 mg to 1 g q.i.d.
Nitrofurantoin	50–100 mg q.i.d.
Cephalosporins	250 mg q.i.d.
Ampicillin	250 mg q.i.d.

[a]Oral dose given for 5 to 7 days.

that approximately 50% of women who have ASB have bacteriuria of renal origin,[18] and this group may be at increased risk for having premature or low-birth-weight infants.[24] In a study designed to test this hypothesis, Gilstrap and coworkers evaluated the antibody-coated bacteria test to localize the site of bacteriuria (i.e., renal or bladder) in 250 pregnant women with asymptomatic infection.[18] No association was found between the presence of bacteriuria and hypertension, anemia, prematurity, or an increase in low-birth-weight infants when compared to 250 pregnant women without bacteriuria. Moreover, these investigators were unable to identify a subgroup of pregnant women at higher risk, i.e., those with renal bacteriuria, for the various complications listed in Table 3. In fact, women with renal bacteriuria actually have significantly larger babies as compared to controls. A problem with this particular study was that for obvious reasons there was no control group of untreated bacteriuric patients. However, whether untreated bacteriuria is associated with prematurity or low birth-weight is probably a moot point, because all pregnant women should be treated to prevent this complication of acute pyelonephritis.

Treatment

Antimicrobial agents that can be used to successfully treat ASB during pregnancy are listed in Table 4. All of these are FDA category B drugs. Although no one regimen has proved satisfactory in all patients, a particular regimen that we have found to be especially successful in the majority of patients is nitrofurantoin macrocrystals 100 mg given once a day at bedtime for 10 days. Various single-dose regimens have also been used with reasonable success during pregnancy for the treatment of ASB[25–28]; these regimens are outlined in Table 5. For patients with frequent recurrent or persistent infections following therapy, continuous antimicrobial suppression for the remainder of pregnancy should be considered. A useful agent for continuous suppression is nitrofurantoin macrocrystals 100 mg given at bedtime for the remainder of pregnancy. The frequent use of antimicrobials such as ampicillin or cephalosporins either intermittently or for suppression may be associated with significant side effects such as the development of chronic vulvovaginitis secondary to an overgrowth of *Candida albicans.*

The combination of a sulfonamide and trimethoprim is a popular and efficacious regimen used to treat bacteriuria in the nonpregnant patient. Although this combination has been used in Europe successfully and without apparent adverse maternal or fetal effects, it is currently not recommended for use in pregnant women in the United States. The major reason for this is largely theoretical and based on the fact that trimethoprim is an antifolate. Other antifolates such as methotrexate and aminoptherin have been associated with fetal anomalies. However, according to

TABLE 5. Single-Dose Antimicrobial Therapy in Pregnant Women With Asymptomatic Bacteriuria

Reference	No. of patients	Antibiotic	Cure rate (%)
Bailey[25]	24	Cotrimoxazole	88
Jakobi et al.[26]	50	Amoxicillin or cephaloxin	84
Harris et al.[27]	86	Ampicillin or cephalexin plus probenecid	69
		Nitrofurantoin	
		Sulfisoxazole	
McFadyen et al.[28]	86	Cephalexin	65

available data it is unlikely that the combination of sulfonamide and trimethoprim results in fetal anomalies.

Recently a new group of antimicrobials, the quinolones, have proved especially successful in the treatment of urinary tract infections, and the FDA has approved one of these, norfloxacin, for the treatment of urinary tract infections. Although norfloxacin is effective against the majority of pathogens isolated from the urinary tract and is especially useful in resistant infections, there is little information available regarding its safety and efficacy during pregnancy. It is listed as a category C drug by its manufacturer and as such should not be used to treat ASB during pregnancy unless other antimicrobial agents have proved unsuccessful.

Amoxicillin has recently been combined with the beta-lactamase inhibitor clavulanic acid to provide better coverage against a variety of organisms. Although amoxicillin is an FDA category B drug, its combination with clavulanic acid should be reserved for patients who demonstrate resistant organisms or have persistent infections. Moreover, this combination is relatively expensive compared to ampicillin, sulfonamides, or nitrofurantoin.

Tetracycline has been reported to cause yellow-brown discoloration of the deciduous teeth of the fetus[29] and should generally be avoided during pregnancy. This is also true for the newer tetracyclines. As a group, the tetracyclines are listed as category D drugs.

Some antibiotics may cause adverse effects, such as hemolytic anemia or hyperbilirubinemia, in either the mother or fetus. These adverse effects are summarized in chapter 2.

Follow-up

Regardless of the antimicrobial agent selected or the duration of therapy, approximately one-third of women with ASB will experience either persistence or recurrence of infection during pregnancy. After the initial treatment of bacteriuria it is important to evaluate these patients with frequent surveillance urine cultures. For women with persistent or recurrent episodes of bacteriuria, suppressive therapy can be used as outlined above.

A significant number of women with bacteriuria during pregnancy will have bacteriuria when studied 10 to 14 years later.[30] In one study, approximately 38% of women who had bacteriuria during pregnancy also had bacteriuria many years later. On the other hand, only 5% of women without bacteriuria during pregnancy had bacteriuria 10 to 14 years later.[30] Although a significant number of women with bacteriuria during pregnancy will have urinary tract infections on subsequent follow-up, there is little evidence to suggest that this poses a significant risk to either their health or quality of life.[31]

CYSTITIS

Surprisingly, cystitis is not a commonly reported complication of pregnancy, and the exact incidence of this complication is not known. However, in one series it was re-

TABLE 6. Clinical and Laboratory Findings in Pregnant Women With Acute Cystitis

Urgency
Frequency
Suprapubic discomfort
Dysuria[a]
No fever or costovertebral angle tenderness
Positive urine culture
Occasional hematuria or pyuria

[a]Most reliable symptom.

TABLE 7. Localization of Site of Infection in 224 Women With Urinary Tract Infections During Pregnancy

	Site of infection	
	Renal	Bladder
Asymptomatic bacteriuria (n = 152)	45%	55%
Acute cystitis (n = 35)	5%	95%
Acute pyelonephritis (n = 37)	65%	35%

Adapted from Harris and Gilstrap.[32]

ported that cystitis occurred in approximately 1–2% of pregnant women.[32] Pregnancy per se does not appear to increase the risk of acquiring this particular infection, although one-third of the patients who develop cystitis have a positive screening culture for bacteriuria at their initial visit. The remaining two-thirds of the patients have either a negative screening culture or will present for the first time with cystitis during pregnancy.[32]

Diagnosis

Unlike pregnant women with ASB, pregnant women with cystitis usually present to the physician because of the symptoms listed in Table 6. Frequent complaints such as urgency, frequency, and nocturia are not particularly helpful during pregnancy, as many pregnant women without urinary tract infections also experience these symptoms. Suprapubic pressure or pain, a common symptom in nonpregnant women with cystitis, is also not helpful in making this diagnosis during pregnancy because many pregnant women will have this symptom secondary to pressure from the presenting fetal part, especially in the late second or third trimester of pregnancy. Burning on urination or dysuria is the most significant symptom in pregnant women with cystitis.

Common laboratory findings include a positive urine culture, pyuria, and occasionally gross hematuria. The presence of either pyuria or microscopic hematuria in the absence of a positive culture is usually not indicative of acute cystitis because as many as 10 to 15% of normal uninfected pregnant women can have these findings.[33]

Unlike patients with ASB, the majority (95%) of women with acute cystitis during pregnancy will have bacteria localized to the bladder (Table 7). The bacterial etiology of acute cystitis during pregnancy is similar to that for ASB and acute pyelonephritis, as summarized in Table 2.

Significance

The significance of acute cystitis during pregnancy is in the extreme discomfort it may cause the patient. Whether acute cystitis is associated with an increased risk of acute pyelonephritis or certain adverse pregnancy effects, such as hypertension, anemia, or prematurity, is unclear at this time. Although one might logically expect that the risk and complications (including pyelonephritis) of acute cystitis would be similar to that of ASB during pregnancy, this may not be true considering the fact that in 95% of the cases the infection is limited to the bladder, whereas in ASB 50% of the patients have been shown to have bacteriuria of renal origin.

Treatment

The treatment of pregnant women with acute cystitis is similar to that of pregnant women with ASB, except that single-dose regimens are generally ineffective and not recommended for use during pregnancy. Patients may be treated as outpatients with an oral preparation such as ampicillin or a cephalosporin (250–500 mg q.i.d.), a sulfonamide (1 g q.i.d.), or nitrofurantoin macrocrystals (100 mg q.i.d.) for 5 to 7 days. Because these patients are symptomatic, therapy is usually empiric and should be initiated before the results of the culture and sensitivity are known.

Follow-up

Approximately 25% of patients with acute cystitis during pregnancy will experience another infection of the urinary tract sometime during the pregnancy.[32] Thus it is important to follow these patients with frequent surveillance cultures coincident with their normal prenatal visits. There are no long-term follow-up studies of pregnant women with acute cystitis, but there is little reason to believe that their course would be any different than those with ASB.

ACUTE PYELONEPHRITIS

Acute pyelonephritis is one of the most common serious medical complications of pregnancy and occurs in approximately 1–2% of all pregnant women.[31] About two-thirds of the cases arise in women with preexisting bacteriuria, while approximately one-third occur in women who have not had bacteriuria documented during pregnancy.[31] Unlike bacteriuria or acute cystitis, pregnancy significantly increases the risk of acquiring acute pyelonephritis. The major reason for this is that pregnancy results in a relative "obstruction" of the urinary tract with resultant stasis of urine and bacteriuria as outlined in Figure 1. The reason for this relative obstruction is twofold. First, there is dilatation of the ureters secondary to the hormonal influences of pregnancy, especially that of progesterone. Progesterone has been shown to be a smooth muscle relaxant. Second, there is actual mechanical obstruction from the pregnant uterus and its contents, which results in a pressure gradient of approximately 15 ml of water between the lower and upper ureters.[34] In addition, there is an increased finding for both glucosuria and aminoaciduria that favors the proliferation of bacteria. Acute pyelonephritis during pregnancy is associated with several predisposing factors identical to those for ASB. Bacterial adherence may also play a role in the acquisition of acute pyelonephritis during pregnancy. Although the precise mechanism is unclear, Stenquist and associates did report a preponderance of p-fimbriated E. coli strains in pregnant patients with acute pyelonephritis as compared to pregnant women with ASB.[35]

The majority of cases of acute pyelonephritis occur in the second and third trimesters. In one review of 656 women with acute pyelonephritis, 482 cases, or 73%, occurred during the antepartum period.[31] Of these, 9% occurred in the first trimester, 46% in the second trimester, and 45% in the third trimester. This no doubt is secondary to the increase in relative obstruction and stasis of urine as pregnancy progresses.

Diagnosis

The diagnosis of acute pyelonephritis is based primarily on the presence of systemic signs and symptoms in the presence of a positive urine culture. Specific signs and symptoms include fever, chills, nausea, vomiting, and costovertebral angle (CVA) or flank tenderness. The fever may be quite high, reaching 40°C in many patients, and is generally spiking in nature. In one series, 85% of 656 women had a temperature of ≥38°C (100.4°F), and 12% ≥40°C (104°F).[31] One patient had a temperature of 107°F! Moreover, 54% had right CVA tenderness, 27% had bilateral CVA tenderness, and 16% had left CVA tenderness. Urinalysis reveals clumps of white blood cells and many bacteria and the urine culture will invariably be positive for one of the pathogens listed in Table 2. If the urine culture is negative, the patient should be questioned as to whether or not she is taking antibiotics. Many patients with pyelonephritis have had previous urinary tract infections and may have started antibiotics on their own. Even a single oral

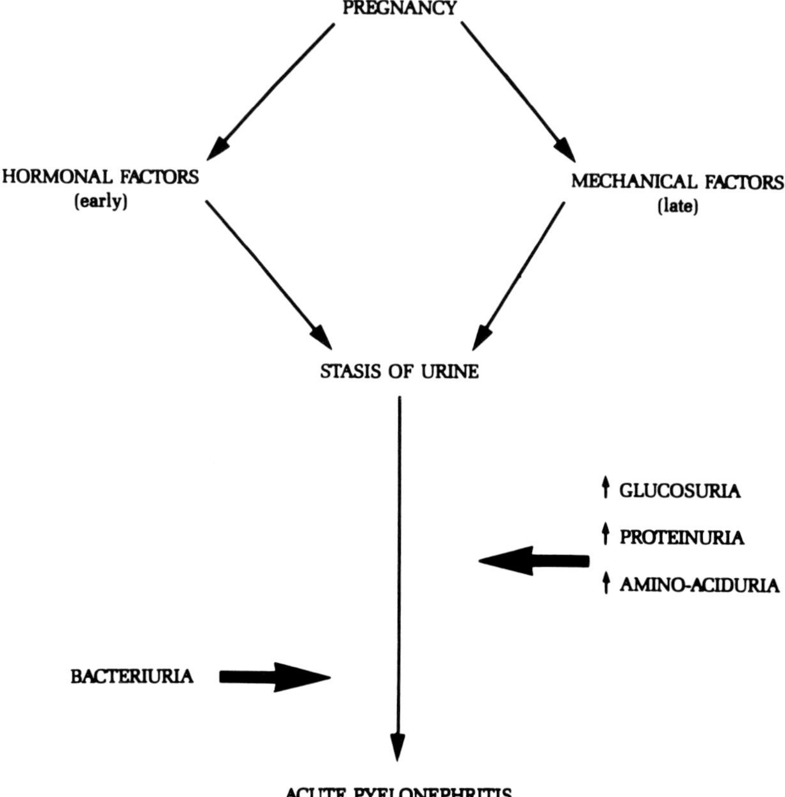

Fig. 1. Pathogenesis of acute pyelonephritis during pregnancy. Note: bacteriuria is present in two-thirds of cases on initial urine screen. (From Gilstrap et al.,[34] with permission of the publisher.)

dose of an antibiotic may render the urine sterile.

The peripheral blood white cell count may vary from normal to as high as 17,000 or greater. A number of patients will also exhibit a significant drop in their hematocrit. The serum creatinine may also be high in approximately 20% of the patients with a concomitant decrease in the 24-hour urine creatinine clearance.[36]

Adverse Maternal Effects

As outlined in Table 8, acute pyelonephritis may result in multisystem dysfunction.[34] Hypothalamic dysfunction is evident in many patients and is characterized by extremes of temperature ranging from high

TABLE 8. Multiple Organ System Dysfunction in Pregnant Women With Acute Pyelonephritis

Thermoregulatory instability
Hyperthermia
Hypothermia
Hematologic dysfunction
Anemia
Leukocytosis
Thrombocytopenia
Renal dysfunction
Elevated serum creatinine level
Decreased creatinine clearance
Pulmonary dysfunction
Adult respiratory distress syndrome (ARDS)

Adapted from Gilstrap et al.[34]

spiking temperatures ($\geq 40°C$) to very low temperatures or hypothermia ($\leq 35°C$).

Renal dysfunction is manifested by both an

elevated serum creatinine level and a significant decrease in the endogenous creatinine clearance. In a study by Gilstrap et al., 20% of pregnant women with acute pyelonephritis had a serum creatinine level greater than 1 mg/dl.[31] Approximately one-fourth of the patients will have a 24-hour creatinine clearance of less than 80 cc/minute corrected for body surface area.[36] This renal dysfunction is transient in nature and the creatinine clearance usually returns to normal within 3 to 6 weeks after an acute episode of pyelonephritis.

Hematologic abnormalities may also occur, and the most common manifestations are anemia (hematocrit < 30%) or a significant drop in the patient's hematocrit.[31,34] In extreme cases the patient may show drops in the hematocrit of 10 points or greater. Although dehydration followed by rehydration can certainly affect a patient's hematocrit, the drop in the majority of patients is not secondary to fluid changes, as evidenced by the fact that the hematocrit is generally still very low several days after the acute episode of pyelonephritis. In one study of pregnant women with acute pyelonephritis, 24 of 36 women, or 66%, had a hematocrit of <30 volumes percent and 36% had a decrease in the hematocrit of ≥6 volumes percent.[34] Although the platelets may be low in a few patients, overt thrombocytopenia is an uncommon manifestation; however, when it does occur, it is usually an ominous sign.[13]

Pulmonary dysfunction, ranging from a few infiltrates and mild respiratory distress to overt pulmonary failure and the adult respiratory distress syndrome (ARDS), may occur in one of every 50 pregnant women with acute pyelonephritis.[37] First described by Cunningham and associates in 1984,[38] respiratory insufficiency may be manifested by dyspnea, tachypnea, hypoxia, and x-ray findings of pulmonary infiltrates occurring in the first or second day following admission (Fig. 2).[37] These patients may also manifest renal dysfunction (serum creatinine > 1.2 mg/dl), evidence of red cell hemolysis, platelet counts less than 100,000/mm³, white blood cell counts greater than 14,000/mm³, and evidence of intravascular coagulation.[37] Scanning electron microscopy of the red cells of these patients has revealed evidence of red cell membrane damage and abnormal morphological forms such as schizocytes or echinocytes.[39]

It has been postulated that the multisystem dysfunction seen in pregnant women with acute pyelonephritis is secondary to the effects of endotoxin.[37] Considering ARDS, transient renal dysfunction, red cell hemolysis, thrombocytopenia, and intravascular coagulation, it makes sense that endotoxin or lipopolysaccharide is indeed the "common denominator."

Acute pyelonephritis may also result in overt septic shock in about 1–2% of women.[40] Obviously this is a life-threatening complication. Fortunately, the majority of pregnant women with acute pyelonephritis do not experience life-threatening complications or significant organ dysfunction; when the acute infection is appropriately treated, the organ dysfunction is generally transient in nature.

Adverse Fetal and Neonatal Effects

Acute pyelonephritis has been reported to be associated with an increase in both low-birth-weight and premature infants. This in turn is secondary to an increase in premature labor in patients with acute pyelonephritis. In one large series, approximately 15% of newborns of mothers with acute pyelonephritis were less than 2,500 g.[18] However, the mean birth weight in infants born to mothers with acute pyelonephritis was not significantly different from that of infants born to women without pyelonephritis (Table 9).

Treatment

General guidelines for the management of pregnant women with acute pyelonephritis are summarized in Table 10.[41] First, and of paramount importance, all pregnant women with acute pyelonephritis should be hospital-

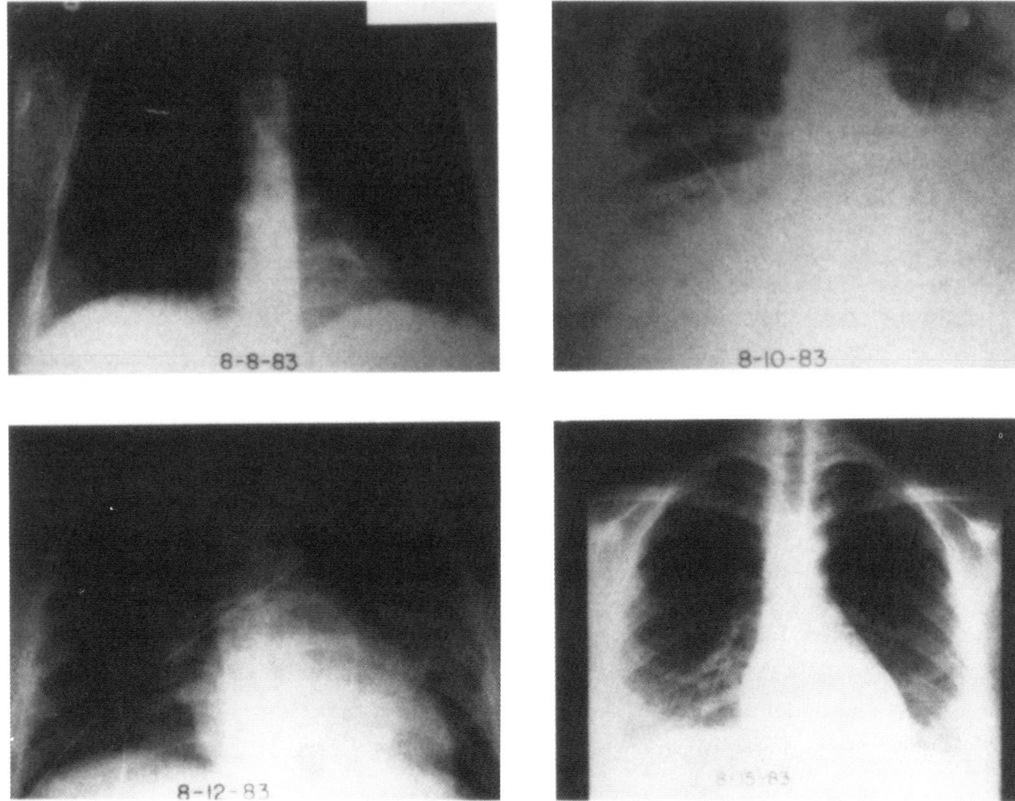

Fig. 2. Radiographic findings in pregnant women with acute pyelonephritis and ARDS. (From Cunningham et al.,[37] with permission of the publisher.)

TABLE 9. Neonatal Outcome in 487 Women With Acute Pyelonephritis vs. Controls

	Women with pyelonephritis	Controls
Birth weight < 2,500 g	71 (15%)	50 (10%)
Mean birth weight (g)	3,044	3,059
Perinatal losses	13 (2.7%)	12 (2.5%)
	+P 0.05	

Adapted from Gilstrap et al.[18]

TABLE 10. Guidelines for the Management of Acute Pyelonephritis in Pregnant Women

Hospitalization
Hydration
Intravenous antibiotics
Frequent monitoring of urine output and vital signs
Urine and blood cultures
Complete blood count and serum creatinine
Clinic follow-up with frequent surveillance cultures

Adapted from Gilstrap and Wendel.[41]

ized for close observation. Many of these women have nausea and vomiting, are dehydrated, and are unable to tolerate oral fluids or medications. These women should receive both parenteral hydration and antibiotics. Vital signs should be monitored frequently, as should urine output. Initial antimicrobial therapy is empiric because the results of the urine culture and sensitivity are not known and a wide variety of agents may be used (see Table 11).[41] Ampicillin alone is no longer recommended for acute pyelonephritis because in most hospitals many common uropathogens, such as *E. coli*, are resistant.

TABLE 11. Antimicrobial Regimens for the Treatment of Pregnant Women With Acute Pyelonephritis

Single-agent therapy
Ampicillin 500 mg to 1 g IV q 6 h
First-generation cephalosporin 500 mg to   1 g IV q 6 h
Cefoxitin 1–2 g IV q 6 h
Mezlocillin or piperacillin 3–4 g IV q 6 h
Combination therapy
(Aminoglycoside plus antibiotic listed above)
Gentamicin 3 mg/kg/day IV in divided doses
Tobramycin 3 mg/kg/day IV in divided doses

Adapted from Gilstrap and Wendel.[41]

Moreover, gentamicin or other aminoglycosides should be used with caution in these patients as a significant number will experience transient renal dysfunction, although the risk to the fetus appears to be very low. Therapy with a cephalosporin or one of the newer extended penicillins will generally result in a cure rate of 85 to 90%.[42] The majority of patients will be afebrile and asymptomatic within 24 to 48 hours after initiation of therapy. Other factors must be excluded in those patients who fail to respond during this time frame. Reasons for failure include resistant organisms, nephrolithiasis, segmental infection ("lobar nephronia"), or obstruction secondary to the pregnancy itself.

Follow-up

After discharge from the hospital, patients should be followed in the clinic with frequent urine culture surveillance. Recurrent infection is common and occurs in approximately 25% of patients following an initial episode.[31] In women for whom frequent clinic visits are not feasible, an alternative is to use continuous antibiotic suppressive therapy throughout pregnancy. In one review of suppressive therapy, the incidence of recurrence in women not receiving suppression was 60%, compared to approximately 3% in those receiving suppression.[43] Continuous suppression with nitrofurantoin macrocrystals, 100 mg orally every night, has proved to be a satisfactory regimen.[13]

Long-Term Prognosis

Women with either acute pyelonephritis or frequent urinary tract infections during pregnancy may ultimately be shown to have urinary tract abnormalities. As many as 27–37% of these women will have either recurrent infection or radiographic anomalies.[8,44] In an 8- to 13-year follow-up of 208 women with acute pyelonephritis, 41% were treated for one or more episodes of symptomatic urinary tract infections when not pregnant, and 38% of those with subsequent pregnancies had another episode of infection during pregnancy.[31] In spite of the risks of frequent recurrences and the presence of urinary tract abnormalities, it is uncommon for these women to have end-stage renal insufficiency.[45]

SUMMARY

Urinary tract infection is a common complication encountered during pregnancy, occurring in 2–10% of pregnant women. Detection and eradication of bacteriuria at the first prenatal visit is of paramount importance in preventing acute pyelonephritis and its attendant maternal and fetal risks. The majority of urinary tract infections are caused by gram-negative enteric bacteria, with *E. coli* being by far the most common single uropathogen. The urine culture remains the mainstay in diagnosis. Pregnant women with either ASB or cystitis can be treated as outpatients with oral antimicrobial agents. However, all pregnant women with acute pyelonephritis should be admitted to the hospital for close observation as well as parenteral hydration and antibiotics.

REFERENCES

1. Kass EH, Savage W, Santamarina BAG: The significance of bacteriuria in preventive medicine. In Kass EH (ed): "Progress in Pyelonephritis." Philadelphia: F.A. Davis, 1965, pp 3–10.
2. Schaeffer AJ: Recurrent urinary tract infections in

women: Pathogenesis and management. Postgrad Med 81:51–58, 1987.

3. Nicolle LE, Harding GK, Preiksaitis J, Ronald AR: The association of urinary tract infection with sexual intercourse. J Infect Dis 146:579–583, 1982.

4. Kunin CM: Urinary tract infections in children. Hosp Pract 11:91–98, 1976.

5. Sleigh JD, Robertson JG, Isdale MH: Asymptomatic bacteriuria in pregnancy. J Obstet Gynaecol Br Commonw 71:74, 1964.

6. Svanborg-Eden C, Eriksson B, Hason LA: Adhesion of *Escherichia coli* to human epithelial cells *in vitro*. Infect Immun 18:767–774, 1977.

7. Kallenius G, Winberg J: Bacterial adherence to periurethral epithelial cells in girls prone to urinary tract infection. Lancet iii:540–543, 1978.

8. Whalley P: Bacteriuria of pregnancy. Am J Obstet Gynecol 97:732, 1967.

9. Turck M, Goff BS, Petersdorf RG: Bacteriuria in pregnancy: Relation to socioeconomic factors. N Engl J Med 266:857, 1962.

10. Whalley PJ, Martin RG, Pritchard JA: Sickle cell trait and urinary tract infection during pregnancy. JAMA 189:903–906, 1964.

11. Kass EH: Asymptomatic infections of the urinary tract. Trans Assoc Am Physicians 69:56–60, 1956.

12. Kunin CM: Initial significance of bacteriuria visualized in the unstrained urinary sediment. N Engl J Med 265:589–590, 1961.

13. Hankins GDV, Whalley PJ: Acute urinary tract infection in pregnancy. Clin Obstet Gynecol 28:266–278, 1985.

14. Fowler JE, Stamey TA: Studies of introital colonization in women with recurrent infections. VII. The role of bacterial adherence. J Urol 117:472–473, 1977.

15. Wood EG, Dillon HC: A prospective study of group B streptococcal bacteriuria in pregnancy. Am J Obstet Gynecol 140:515–520, 1981.

16. Mead PJ, Harris RE: The incidence of group B beta hemolytic streptococcus in antepartum urinary tract infections. Obstet Gynecol 51:412–414, 1978.

17. Latham RH, Running K, Stamm WE: Urinary tract infections in young adult women caused by *Staphylococcus saprophyticus*. JAMA 250:3063–3066, 1983.

18. Gilstrap LC, Leveno KJ, Cunningham FG, Whalley PJ, Roark ML: Renal infection and pregnancy outcome. Am J Obstet Gynecol 141:709–716, 1981.

19. Kass EH: In Quinn EL, Kass EH (eds): "Biology of Pyelonephritis." Boston: Little, Brown, 1960, pp 399–400.

20. Stuart KL, Cummins GTM, Chin WA: Bacteriuria, prematurity and hypertensive disorders of pregnancy. Br Med J 1:554–558, 1965.

21. Brumfitt W: The effects of bacteriuria in pregnancy on maternal and fetal health. Kidney Int [Suppl] 8:113–119, 1975.

22. Whalley PJ, Cunningham FG: Short-term versus continuous antimicrobial therapy for asymptomatic bacteriuria in pregnancy. Obstet Gynecol 49:262–265, 1977.

23. Cunningham FG, Whalley PJ: Asymptomatic bacteriuria during pregnancy. In Buchsbaum HJ, Schmidt JD (eds): "Gynecologic and Obstetric Urology," 2nd edition. Philadelphia: W.B. Saunders, 1982, pp 519–537.

24. Zinner SH: Bacteriuria and babies revisited. N Engl J Med 300:853–855, 1979.

25. Bailey RR: Single-dose antibacterial treatment for bacteriuria in pregnancy. Drugs 27:183–186, 1984.

26. Jakobi P, Neiger R, Merzbach D, Paldi E: Single-dose antimicrobial therapy in the treatment of asymptomatic bacteriuria in pregnancy. Am J Obstet Gynecol 156:1148–1152, 1987.

27. Harris RE, Gilstrap LC, Pretty A: Single-dose antimicrobial therapy for asymptomatic bacteriuria during pregnancy. Obstet Gynecol 59:546–549, 1982.

28. McFadyen IR, Campbell-Brown M, Stephenson M, Seal DV: Single dose treatment of bacteriuria in pregnancy. Eur Urol 13:22–25, 1987.

29. Kutscher AH, Zegarelli EV, Tovell HM, Hochberg B, Hauptman J: Discoloration of deciduous teeth induced by administration of tetracycline antepartum. Am J Obstet Gynecol 96:291–292, 1966.

30. Zinner SH, Kass EH: Long-term (10 to 14 years) follow-up of bacteriuria of pregnancy. N Engl J Med 285:820–822, 1971.

31. Gilstrap LC, Cunningham FG, Whalley PJ: Acute pyelonephritis in pregnancy: An anterospective study. Obstet Gynecol 57:409–413, 1981.

32. Harris RE, Gilstrap LC: Cystitis during pregnancy: A distinct clinical entity. Obstet Gynecol 57:578–580, 1981.

33. Lacy SS: Urinary tract infections. In Buchsbaum HJ, Schmidt JD (eds): "Gynecologic and Obstetric Urology." Philadelphia: W.B. Saunders, 1978, pp. 301–323.

34. Gilstrap LC, Hankins GDV, Snyder RR, Greenberg RT: Acute pyelonephritis in pregnancy. Compr Ther 12:38–42, 1986.

35. Stenquist K, Standberl A, Lidin-Janson F, et al.: Virulence factors of *Escherichia coli* in urinary isolates from pregnant women. J Infec Dis 156:870–877, 1987.

36. Whalley PJ, Cunningham FG, Martin FG: Transient renal dysfunction associated with acute pyelo-

nephritis of pregnancy. Obstet Gynecol 46:174–177, 1974.
37. Cunningham FG, Lucas MJ, Hankins GDV: Pulmonary injury complicating antepartum pyelonephritis. Am J Obstet Gynecol 156:797–807, 1987.
38. Cunningham FG, Leveno KJ, Hankins GDV, Whalley PJ: Respiratory insufficiency associated with pyelonephritis during pregnancy. Obstet Gynecol 63:121–125, 1984.
39. Cox SM, Shelburne P, Mason RA, Cunningham FG: Erythrocyte morphology in women with acute antepartum pyelonephritis. Infectious Disease Society for Obstetrics & Gynecology, Snowmass, CO, August 1988 (abstract)
40. Cunningham FG, Morris GB, Mickal A: Acute pyelonephritis of pregnancy: A clinical review. Obstet Gynecol 42:112–117, 1973.
41. Gilstrap LC, Wendel GD: Urinary tract infections in pregnancy. Female Patient 13:57–60, 1988.
42. Cox SM, Cunningham FG: Ureidopenicillin therapy for acute antepartum pyelonephritis. Curr Ther Res 44:1029–1034, 1989.
43. Harris RE, Gilstrap LG: Prevention of recurrent pyelonephritis during pregnancy. Obstet Gynecol 44:637–641, 1974.
44. Leigh DA, Gruneberg RN, Brumfitt W: Long-term follow-up of bacteriuria of pregnancy. Lancet 1:603–605, 1968.
45. Freedman LR: Chronic pyelonephritis at autopsy. Ann Intern Med 66:697–710, 1967.

4

Vaginitis and Pregnancy

Sebastian Faro, M.D., Ph.D.

Vaginitis in nonpregnant and pregnant women is a major problem encountered in the treatment of the ambulatory patient. However, in the pregnant patient, the presence of vaginitis may take on significant importance, because it may have a bearing on whether or not a pregnancy will have a successful outcome. Vaginitis may also play a role in whether or not the pregnant patient will have an uncomplicated or complicated postpartum course. Vaginitis can be divided into four major categories: bacterial, fungal, viral, and protozoan. Since the sexually transmitted diseases will be dealt with formally in other chapters of this book, the present discussion will be limited to yeast vaginitis, bacterial vaginitis or vaginosis, and trichomonas vaginitis.

CANDIDA

The fungi are a diverse group of microorganisms that range from relatively simple organisms with simple life cycles to very complex organisms. The fungi grow as filamentous organisms or simple cellular organisms, or are dimorphic, that is, have the ability to grow as either filamentous or budding, typically yeast-like. The most common fungal vaginal infections are those caused by the genus *Candida*, with C. *albicans* being the most common species isolated. Other species of this genus, which are pathogenic for humans, are listed in Table 1. Yeast vaginitis is a frequent and often difficult infection to eradicate in the pregnant patient. The presence of yeast in sufficient numbers to cause symptoms of vaginal burning, itching, and burning with or after urination usually indicates that the vagina is acidic. This finding commonly implies that the vagina is colonized by an abnormal bacterial flora, because the bacteria, especially the more pathogenic aerobes, facultative anaerobes, and obligate anaerobes, do not flourish at the more acidic pH range, i.e., higher than pH 4.5. However, this is not always the case. It would be prudent for the physician to note on microscopic examination of the vaginal discharge whether or not there are "clue cells" present. The patient with yeast vaginitis is not particularly at risk to develop premature rupture of membranes or premature labor. The patient with recalcitrant yeast vaginitis or associated yeast esophagitis or oral thrush should be suspected of having immunosuppression.

Nonpregnant individuals with persistent

Infections in Pregnancy, pages 29–35
© 1990 Alan R. Liss, Inc.

TABLE 1. Pathogenic Yeasts

Candida albicans
Candida brumptii
Candida claussenii
Candida guilliermondii
Candida intermedia
Candida krusei
Candida lambica
Candida macedoniensis
Candida norvegensis
Candida parapsilosis
Candida pseudotropicalis
Candida slooffii
Candida stellatoidea
Candida tropicalis
Candida viswanathii
Candida zeylanoides
Torulopsis candida
Torulopsis glabrata

or recurring yeast vaginitis may have a transient and localized defect in cell-mediated immunity that prevents eradication of the yeast.[1] The defect appears to be a reduction in the in vitro proliferation of lymphocytes in response to *C. albicans*. Normally, there is a localized macrophage response, however *C. albicans* stimulates the production of prostaglandin E_2. This in turn inhibits the release of interleukin-2 and results in the blockage of lymphocyte proliferation. Cellular immunity is normally impaired in the pregnant patient.[2] Lymphocytes encountering microbial antigens usually respond by multiplying and differentiating. The B cells differentiate into plasma cells and produce antibodies, which bind to the microbes facilitating phagocytosis. T cells differentiate into lymphoblasts and produce lymphokines, which mediate both nonspecific and specific processes of resistance to infection.

The pregnant patient with candidiasis may not appear to have a decrease in localized cellular immunity, but there is an alteration in the vaginal microfloral environment that allows an overgrowth of *C. albicans*. Yeast may be found in up to 40% of asymptomatic women and can be regarded as part of the commensal vaginal microflora. These factors probably account for the fact that candidiasis is more frequent in pregnant than in nonpregnant patients. It is interesting to note that *Lactobacillus* and *C. albicans* may both flourish in the vaginas of pregnant women.[3] In the nonpregnant population, vulvovaginal candidial infection occurs in approximately 20% of the population, whereas in the pregnant population, the incidence is approximately 45%, in diabetics, 50%, and in women using oral contraceptive pills, 30%.[4,5] In a study examining the adherence of *C. albicans* to epithelial cells, it was found that the yeast was more likely to adhere to cells obtained from pregnant and diabetic women than those from controls.[6]

Several factors have been implicated as contributing to the development of yeast vulvovaginitis, including the availability of carbon sources, hormonal changes, alterations in the microflora, depression of localized cellular immunity, and adherence to vaginal epithelial cells. Horowitz et al. reported that individuals with excessive oral ingestion of foods rich in sugar, e.g., glucose, arabinose, and ribose, are more likely to develop candidiasis.[7] Patients who have an excessive dairy intake are subject to yeast infection and could reduce the incidence of infection by simply altering their diet. Lactose, a complex sugar, is common in dairy products and artificial sweeteners. Lactose can be reduced to ribose and arabinose, both of which can be utilized by yeast as a carbon source.

Progesterone has been found to enhance the adherence of *C. albicans* to vaginal epithelial cells. Intermediate vaginal cells have a greater affinity to bind yeast cells than do superficial epithelial cells.[8] Elevated levels of progesterone are seen during pregnancy, and therefore intermediate vaginal epithelial cells predominate.

Many different species of *Candida* exist (Table 1), but the predominant species responsible for vulvovaginitis are *C. albicans* and *C. glabrata*. Approximately 90% of the cases are due to *C. albicans*. *Candida (Toru-*

lopsis) glabrata is normally a saprophyte but can become virulent and cause infection, especially in the compromised patient. Risk factors for infection are prior antibiotic therapy, abdominal surgery, hyperalimentation, Foley catheterization, malignancy, diabetes, corticosteroid administration, alcoholism, urinary tract obstruction, malnutrition, and drug abuse.[9–13] Vaginitis due to infection with *C. glabrata* is uncommon, and when it occurs it is difficult to treat. Patients infected with *C. glabrata* do not respond to imidazoles, e.g., miconazole, clotrimazole, and ketoconazole. However, success has been achieved with irrigation with amphotericin B or nystatin.[14,15]

Successful treatment of vulvovaginal yeast infections has been difficult to achieve because of the lack of understanding of the pathophysiology of this infection. Yeasts are not virulent organisms, and therefore are not common pathogens of healthy individuals. The exception is vulvovaginitis, which commonly occurs in healthy women. Treatment of this infection has focused on the use of topical antifungal medications. However, because of the lack of success with topical agents in treating this infection, systemic agents have been developed. There are basically four groups of agents that are used to treat candidiasis, but not all are indicated for the pregnant patient. These four groups include the polyene macrolides, nystatin and amphotericin B, the imidazole derivatives, 5-fluorocytosine, and gentian violet.

The polyene antifungal agents bind to sterol components of the cell membranes and alter the permeability of the membranes, which results in leakage of cytoplasmic constituents, metabolic disruption, and eventually death of the cell. Nystatin has been used successfully in the treatment of vulvovaginitis and can be used in the pregnant patient. Amphotericin B should be used for systemic treatment and reserved for only the resistant mucocutaneous candidiasis. Amphotericin B should not be used in the pregnant patient unless systemic infection is present. Ampho-

tericin B is very toxic and may cause kidney damage, uremia, and hypokalemia. Similarly, 5-fluorocytosine should not be used during pregnancy. Once inside the cell, 5-fluorocytosine is deaminated to 5-fluorouracil and is phosphorylated prior to being incorporated into cellular RNA, which results in disruption of protein synthesis. Side effects of 5-fluorocytosine are blood dyscrasias, liver dysfunction, decrease in white blood cell count, elevated serum enzymes, nausea, vomiting, diarrhea, and skin rashes.[16–19]

Imidazoles are considered to be broad-spectrum antifungal agents, and the mainstays of treatment are butoconazole, clotrimazole, econazole, miconazole, terconazole, and ketoconazole. These agents function as inhibitors of ergosterol synthesis, which results in alteration of cell membrane permeability, alter nonsterol lipid composition of the plasma membrane, disrupt serbia metabolism, and probably have other deleterious effects on the cell wall.[20–22] Ketoconazole has been shown to block the synthesis of ergosterol and block electron transport in the mitochondrial cytochrome *c* oxidase step.[23] Ketoconazole is water soluble at pH 1–2 and is readily absorbed from the gastrointestinal tract. Ketoconazole may cause hepatotoxicity, and therefore should be used with care. The incidence of hepatitis is one in 12,000 to 15,000 patients receiving ketoconazole.[24] This agent has been found to inhibit cholesterol in mammalian cells and interferes with cytochrome P-450 enzyme systems in testis, ovary, adrenal gland, kidney, and liver.[25–28] Ketoconazole should generally not be used during pregnancy. The other imidazoles are best utilized as topical agents.

Treatment of *C. albicans* vaginitis during pregnancy should be focused on the symptomatic patient. A diagnosis should be established by observing the presence of budding yeast cells or pseudohyphae on microscopic examination of the vaginal discharge. Treatment should be instituted with miconazole or perhaps terconazole, which has been shown to be safe during pregnancy. The patient should be screened for diabetes, especially if she has recurrent or persistent candidiasis.

BACTERIAL VAGINITIS

The vagina harbors many different bacteria, both gram positive and gram negative, aerobic and anaerobic. However, the healthy vagina does not contain dense populations of these various types of bacteria, but on the contrary harbors only a relatively few different bacteria in large numbers. The predominant bacteria are commensal, with *Lactobacillus* making up the dominant flora. Several factors contribute to the alteration of the microenvironment of the vagina, which in turn causes shifts in the microbiological makeup of the lower genital tract. The major factor that determines which bacteria become dominant is the pH. A pH higher than 4.5 favors the growth of *Gardnerella vaginalis* and anaerobes. In addition, *Streptococcus agalactiae*, reported to colonize up to 25% of pregnant women, can also be found as a member of the vaginal flora.

Bacteria can interrupt a pregnancy by causing frank infection of the fetus, resulting in an intrauterine demise, or may cause premature rupture of membranes with or without labor or premature labor with intact membranes. Bacteria from the lower genital tract can ascend through the endocervical canal, penetrate the mucus, and colonize the amniotic membranes. The bacteria may cause a significant decrease in the tensile strength of the membranes, and the pressure exerted by the amniotic fluid may cause the weakened membranes to rupture. The bacteria can colonize and cause infection not only in the amniotic membranes, but also the amniotic fluid and the decidua. Several microorganisms have the ability to produce the enzyme phospholipase A_2, which is responsible for initiating the production of prostaglandin by cleaving arachidonic acid. This prostaglandin precursor is found in fetal membranes and decidual cells.[29] The bacteria capable of producing large amounts of phospholipase A_2, found in the vagina, are the anaerobes and *Gardnerella vaginalis*. Thus, a mechanism exists by which bacteria may indeed cause premature labor but not directly cause premature rupture of the membranes, mainly by inducing a subclinical infection of the amniotic membranes or decidua. Although the patient does not have the usual signs and symptoms of infection, she does have premature labor that is unresponsive to tocolytic therapy.

The vaginitis that is directly related to bacterial infection can be detected by performing two simple tasks. The vaginal discharge can be examined to determine the pH, and if the pH is greater than 4.5, this should be taken as being abnormal. Microscopic examination will reveal, usually, one of two pictures: the presence of clue cells with a noticeable absence of white blood cells and free-floating aggregates of bacteria or the presence of clue cells with numerous white blood cells and individual free-floating bacteria. The former presentation is characteristic of *Gardnerella vaginalis* vaginitis and the latter is characteristic of anaerobic bacterial vaginosis. Bacterial vaginosis, in one study, was found to be associated with preterm labor in 43% of the cases.[29,30]

An important question is whether all pregnant patients should be screened for an abnormal vaginal bacterial flora. An important consideration when attempting to answer this question is whether there are conclusive data to indicate that identifying and treating these patients does result in a decrease in the incidence of preterm rupture of membranes and preterm labor, with the ultimate reduction in preterm births. There is less than unanimity of opinion regarding which antibiotic regimen would be used in treating these patients.

It would seem simple enough to utilize the criteria for diagnosing bacterial vaginitis or vaginosis; however, not all patients with an abnormal vaginal pH will have an abnormal microflora consistent with that seen in bacterial vaginosis. The use of Gram's stain may be helpful. For example, if Gram's stain reveals a predominance of gram-positive rods (suggesting *Lactobacillus*), it could be interpreted as being normal. However, if Gram's stain reveals a large number of variable organisms, it probably means an abnormal flora. The next issue is which antibiotic should be administered. Metronidazole is not recommended for use in the first trimester of pregnancy, and in an ongoing study at the Baylor College of Medicine, metronidazole has not proved very effective in treating this disorder. The reason appears to be that when *Gardnerella vaginalis* is the predominant or sole cause of the infection, the strains isolated tend to be resistant. An acceptable protocol would be to evaluate only those patients who have a history of recurring vaginitis or sexually transmitted diseases or who have or complain of an abnormal discharge. The discharge should be diluted with normal saline, 1–2 cc, and examined microscopically for the characteristics described above. In addition, an attempt should be made to determine if *C. albicans* or *Trichomonas vaginalis* is present. The discharge should be analyzed for the detection of amines with and without the addition of concentrated sodium or potassium hydroxide ("whiff test"). A positive "whiff test" is another indication that the vaginal discharge is abnormal; however, a negative "whiff test" does not rule out the presence of vaginitis. Patients with bacterial vaginitis or vaginosis should also be screened for the presence of sexually transmitted diseases, e.g., *Chlamydia trachomatis*, *Neisseria gonorrhoeae*, and herpes simplex.

The treatment of bacterial vaginitis or vaginosis in the pregnant patient is as difficult as it is in the nonpregnant patient. Metronidazole, as stated earlier, should not be used in the pregnant patient, at least during the first trimester. It is an excellent anaerobic agent and functions through the reduction of its nitro group, which occurs inside the bacterial cell. During this metabolic process, cytotoxic intermediate products (free radicals) that disrupt the bacterial DNA are formed.[31–33] The

drug is almost completely absorbed from the gastrointestinal tract, and serum levels comparable to those achieved by the intravenous route are achieved by oral administration. The liver is the major site of metabolism, with the production of 2-hydroxymethyl oxamic acid, acetylmetronidazole, metronidazole glucuronide, glucuronide conjugate of hydroxymetronidazole, and a sulfate conjugate of hydroxymetronidazole.[34–36] The drug is extremely effective against anaerobes, especially *Bacteroides* sp. and *Fusobacterium*. The antibiotic is not active against *Actinomyces*, *Arachnia*, and *Propionibacterium*. Studies have shown that the metabolite of metronidazole may be active against a few aerobes, e.g., *Escherichia coli*.[37] The adverse effects of this drug are nausea, metallic taste, a disulfiram-like intolerance to alcohol, peripheral neuropathy, and potentiation of warfarin; it may be carcinogenic in animals. The evidence of carcinogenic action in humans is inconclusive, but the two published studies with a 10-year follow-up do not suggest an increased incidence of cancer in patients treated with metronidazole.[38,39] The antibiotic has also been shown to be mutagenic for bacteria.[40]

A possible agent for the treatment of bacterial vaginitis or vaginosis, although not tested nor approved by the FDA, is augmentin (amoxicillin plus clavulanic acid). This agent has an excellent spectrum of activity against gram-positive aerobes, gram-negative faculative anaerobes, and obligate anaerobes. Augmentin does not appear to possess any toxic activity to the fetus. Amoxicillin and ampicillin have been widely used to treat urinary tract infections as well as chorioamnionitis without any adverse congenital sequelae. A 1% clindamycin cream is presently under investigation for the treatment of bacterial vaginitis and should be promising.

TRICHOMONAS VAGINALIS

Trichomoniasis vaginalis is a protozoan that is a common cause of vaginitis. The disease is a particular problem in the pregnant patient because there is presently no substitute for metronidazole, which is the only effective drug against this parasite. The patient with a symptomatic infection generally complains of vaginal discomfort or even burning due to the severe inflammation and foul-smelling vaginal discharge. Examination often reveals the presence of petechial hemorrhages on the vaginal epithelium and portio of the cervix. The organism can usually be recognized on microscopic examination of the vaginal discharge. Patients in whom the diagnosis has not been established and who failed treatment with agents not effective against trichomoniasis should be strongly suspected of having *T. vaginalis* vaginitis. A specimen should be obtained from their vagina and used to inoculate Diamond's medium.

The finding of *T. vaginalis* may also be significant because there is an associated decrease in hydrogen ion concentration. The pH is usually higher than 4.5 and there is an increase in the anaerobic flora. This may be significant in that *T. vaginalis* may be associated with premature rupture of membranes and premature labor. The entity of vaginitis may also be potentially significant in those individuals who subsequently develop postpartum endometritis.

Treatment with metronidazole should be reserved for the symptomatic patient who is beyond the first trimester. It may be necessary, in rare instances, to treat a pregnant patient with metronidazole in the first trimester because of severe symptoms. Fortunately, metronidazole has been used for decades with apparent safety, and there are no human studies that would implicate it as a teratogen.[41] In one study of over 1,020 women given this drug during the first trimester of pregnancy, there was no increase in the frequency of congenital anomalies.[42] Although the single 2 g dose administered to women and their partners achieves cure rates of 85 to 90%, it is difficult for pregnant women to tolerate this dose. In a study comparing oral with intravaginal metronidazole,

no difference in cure was found.[39] However, the group assigned to receive oral metronidazole was administered a single 500 mg dose, once a day for 7 days, while the group receiving intravaginal metronidazole was administered 400 mg, twice daily for 7 days. The two groups did not receive the same dosage of medication, and it is unlikely that the two groups achieved similar concentrations of metronidazole in the vaginal fluid and epithelium.

REFERENCES

1. Witkin SS: Immunology of recurrent vaginitis. Am J Reprod Immunol Microbiol 15:34, 1987.
2. Purtilo DT, Hallgren HM, Yunis EJ: Depressed maternal lymphocyte response to phytohemagglutinin in human pregnancy. Lancet 1:767, 1976.
3. Goplerud CP, Ohm MJ, Galask RP: Aerobic and anaerobic flora of the cervix during pregnancy and in the puerperium. Am J Obstet Gynecol 126:852, 1976.
4. Kinsman OS, Collard AE: Hormonal factors in vaginal candidiasis rate. Infect Immun 315:1455, 1986.
5. Segal E, Lehrer N, Ofek I: Adherence of *Candida albicans* to human vaginal epithelial cells: Inhibition by amino sugar. Exp Cell Biol 50:13, 1982.
6. Segal E, Soroka A, Lehrer N: Attachment of Candida to mammalian tissues—Clinical and experimental studies. Abl Bakt Hyg 257:257, 1984.
7. Horowitz BJ, Edelstein SW, Lippman L: Sugar chromatography studies in recurrent candida vulvo vaginitis. J Reprod Med 29:441, 1984.
8. Sobel JD: Epidemiology and pathogenesis of recurrent vulvo-vaginal candidiasis. Am J Obstet Gynecol 152:924, 1985.
9. Sinnott JT, Cullison JP, Sweeny MP: Candida (Torulopsis) glabrata. Infect Control 8:334, 1985.
10. Valdivieso M, Lana M, Rodey GP, et al.: Fungemia due to *Torulopsis glabrata* in the compromised host. Cancer 38:1750, 1976.
11. Berkowitz ID, Robboy SJ, Karshmer AW, et al.: Torulopsis glabrata fungemia—A clinical pathological study. Medicine 58:430, 1979.
12. Kaufman CA, Tan JS: *Torulopsis glabrata* renal infection. Am J Med 57:217, 1974.
13. Sander LA, Young EJ, Musher DM, et al.: *Torulopsis glabrata* pneumonia in a malnourished woman. South Med J 72:1477, 1979.
14. Omer EE, Gumaa SA, El-Nacem HA, et al.: *Torulopsis glabrata* and *Candida albicans* in female genital

infections in the Sudan. Br J Vener Dis 57:165, 1981.

15. Clark JF, Faggett T, Peters B, et al.: Ulcerative vaginitis due to *Torulopsis glabrata:* A case report. J Natl Med Assoc 70:913, 1978.

16. Polak A: Effects of 5-fluorocytosive on protein synthesis and amino acid pool in *Candida albicans.* Sabouraudia 12:309, 1974.

17. Record CO, Skinner JM, Slight P, et al.: *Candida* endocarditis treated with 5-fluorocytosine. Br Med J 1:262, 1971.

18. Seligman SA: Treatment of vulval candidiasis with 5-fluorocytosine. Br Med J 3:173, 1974.

19. Steer PL, Marks MI, Klite PD, et al.: 5-fluorocytosine; an oral antifungal compound. Ann Intern Med 76:15, 1972.

20. Vanden Bossche H, Willemseus G, Cook W, et al.: Biochemical effects of miconazole on fungi II. Inhibition of ergosterol synthesis in *Candida albicans.* Chem Biol Interact 21:59, 1978.

21. Vanden Bossche H, Willemsens G, Cook W, et al.: In vitro and in vivo effects of the antimycotic drug ketoconazole on sterol synthesis. Antimicrob Agents Chemother 17:992, 1980.

22. Uno J, Shigematsu ML, Arai T: Primary site of action of ketoconazole on *Candida albicans.* Antimicrob Agents Chemother 21:912, 1982.

23. Shigematsu ML, Uno J, Arai T: Effect of ketoconazole on isolated mitochondria from *Candida albicans.* Antimicrob Agents Chemother 21:919, 1982.

24. Lewis JH, Zimmerman HJ, Benson GD, et al.: Hepatic injury associated with ketoconazole therapy: Analysis of 33 cases. Gastroenterology 86:503, 1984.

25. Sonino N: The use of ketoconazole as an inhibitor of steroid production. N Engl J Med 317:812, 1987.

26. Buttke TM, Chapman SW: Inhibition by ketoconazole of mutogens induced DNA synthesis and cholesterol biosynthesis in lymphocytes. Antimicrob Agents Chemother 24:278, 1983.

27. Soose DS, Kan PB, Hirst MA, et al.: Ketoconazole blocks adrenal steroidogenesis by inhibiting cytochrome P450 dependent enzymes. J Clin Invest 71:1495, 1983.

28. Santen RJ, Vanden Bossche H, Symoens J, et al.: Sites of action of low dose ketoconazole on androgen biosynthesis in men. J Clin Endocrinol Med 185A:187, 1985.

29. Bejar R, Curbelo V, Davis C, et al.: Premature labor II. Bacterial sources of phospholipase. Obstet Gynecol 57:459, 1981.

30. Gearett MG, Hummel D, Eschenbach DA, et al.: Preterm labor associated with subclinical amniotic fluid infection and with bacterial vaginosis. Obstet Gynecol 67:229, 1986.

31. Eggleston M: Metronidazole. Infect Control 7:514, 1986.

32. Larusso WJ, Tomasz M, Muller M, et al.: Interaction of metronidazole with nucleic acids in vitro. Mol Pharmacol 13:872, 1977.

33. Knight RC, Skohmowski IM, Edwards DI: The interaction of reduced metronidazole with DNA. Biochem Pharmacol 27:2089, 1978.

34. O'Keefe JP, Troc KA, Thompson KD: Activity of metronidazole and its hydroxy and acid metabolites against clinical isolates of anaerobic bacteria. Antimicrob Agents Chemother 22:426, 1982.

35. Tally FP, Sullivan CE: Metronidazole: In vitro activity pharmacology and efficacy in anaerobic bacterial infections. Pharmacotherapy 1:28, 1981.

36. Rosenblatt JE, Edson RS: Metronidazole. Mayo Clin Proc 62:103, 1987.

37. Onderdonk AB, Louie TJ, Tally FP, et al.: Activity of metronidazole against *Escherichia coli* in experimental intra-abdominal sepsis. Rev Infect Dis 3:535, 1981.

38. Beard CM, Noller KL, O'Fallon WM, et al.: Lack of evidence for cancer due to use of metronidazole. N Engl J Med 301:519, 1979.

39. Friedman GD: Cancer after metronidazole (letter to the editor). N Engl J Med 302:519, 1980.

40. McCann J, Ames BN: Detection of carcinogens and mutogens in Salmonella microsome test: Assay of 300 chemicals; discussion. Proc Natl Acad Sci USA 73:950, 1976.

41. Gilstrap LC, Cunningham FG: Drugs and medications in pregnancy. Supplement 13, "Williams Obstetrics." Norwalk, CT: Appleton-Lange, 1987, pp 1–10.

42. Rosa FW, Baum C, Shaw M: Pregnancy outcomes after first trimester vaginitis drug therapy. Obstet Gynecol 69:751, 1987.

5

Acute Chorioamnionitis

Larry C. Gilstrap, III, M.D.

Acute chorioamnionitis is an infection of the chorioamniotic membranes and the amniotic cavity. Microscopically, it is manifested by infiltration of bacteria and polymorphonuclear leukocytes between the layers of chorion and amnion. Clinically, it is manifested primarily by fever. Importantly, not all women with microscopic evidence of chorioamnionitis will have clinical evidence of disease or require antimicrobial therapy. Although "chorioamnionitis" is probably the most commonly used term, others include amnionitis, intraamniotic infection, and intrapartum infection. Intrauterine infection is less commonly used because it does not distinguish between intrapartum (chorioamnionitis) or postpartum (endometritis) infection.

The prognosis for these infections is generally good; however, acute chorioamnionitis may result in significant maternal, fetal, and neonatal morbidity. Moreover, despite the fact that the literature is replete with articles concerning both maternal and neonatal morbidity, there is actually a paucity of information regarding the bacterial etiology and the most ideal management protocol for women with acute chorioamnionitis.

INCIDENCE AND EPIDEMIOLOGY

The exact incidence of acute chorioamnionitis is not known, especially if the diagnosis is based on microscopic findings instead of clinical criteria. However, it has been reported that acute chorioamnionitis based on clinical criteria occurs in 0.5 to 1.0% of all pregnancies.[1–3]

Factors that appear to be associated with an increased risk of acute chorioamnionitis include premature rupture of membranes and/or premature labor,[3] protracted labor and ruptured membranes in term pregnancies,[1,4] colonization with certain bacteria such as *Neisseria gonorrhoeae*[5] or group B streptococcus,[6] or invasive procedure such as amniocentesis. Surprisingly, socioeconomic status does not appear to be associated with a significant increase in the risk of acute chorioamnionitis as it does with other pelvic infections such as endometritis. For example, Hauth and colleagues reported a frequency of 1.3% chorioamnionitis in a predominantly military

Infections in Pregnancy, pages 37–44
© 1990 Alan R. Liss, Inc.

TABLE 1. High-Virulence Organisms Isolated From Women With Acute Chorioamnionitis

Aerobes
Group B streptococcus[a]
Enterococcus
Streptococcus, other
Staphylococcus aureus
Escherichia coli[a]
Gram-negative bacilli, other
Anaerobes
Bacteroides bivius[a]
Bacteroides, other
Peptococcus, sp.
Peptostreptococcus sp.
Clostridia sp.
Fusobacterium sp.

Adapted from Gibbs et al.,[8] Yoder et al.,[9] and Sperling et al.[10]

[a]Most common isolates.

TABLE 2. Clinical Findings in Women With Acute Chorioamnionitis

Maternal fever	85–100%
Uterine tenderness	13–25%
Foul-smelling amniotic fluid	7–19%
Maternal tachycardia	19–84%
Fetal tachycardia	37–82%

Data from Gibbs et al.,[1] Hauth et al.,[2] Gilstrap et al.,[7] and Yoder et al.[9]

population,[2] while Gilstrap and colleagues reported an incidence of 1.5% in a predominantly indigent population.[7] Moreover, Looff and Hager reported an incidence of chorioamnionitis of approximately 0.7% in women predominantly of lower socioeconomic status.[3]

ETIOLOGY AND PATHOGENESIS

Acute chorioamnionitis is an infection involving the chorioamniotic membranes, the amniotic cavity, and amniotic fluid. Although the exact pathogenesis is not known, the majority of cases result from an ascending infection in the presence of ruptured membranes. It is well established that bacteria commonly found in the lower genital tract are commonly isolated from the amniotic cavity in women with acute chorioamnionitis, and that in the majority of cases, the infection is polymicrobial in nature.[8–10] In one study of 52 women with acute chorioamnionitis, a mean of 2.2 organisms per patient was found, with both aerobic and anaerobic organisms isolated from the majority of patients.[8] Common high-virulence organisms isolated from women with acute chorioamnionitis are summarized in Table 1. The three most commonly isolated organisms in one series were group B streptococcus, *Escherichia coli*, and *Bacteroides bivius*.[9] Some uncommon pathogens, such as *Listeria monocytogenes*,[11] *Lactobacillus* sp.,[12,13] *Haemophilus influenzae*,[14] *Ureaplasma urealyticum*,[15] and *Fusobacterium* sp.,[16,17] have also been implicated as etiologic in some women with acute chorioamnionitis.

Of interest is that two of the most commonly isolated bacterial pathogens in women with amnionitis, *E. coli* and group B streptococci, demonstrate both in vitro bacterial attachment and invasion of human chorioamnionitic membrane.[18] This may help explain how these pathogens gain access to the amniotic cavity in the presence of intact membranes.

DIAGNOSIS

The diagnosis of acute chorioamnionitis is primarily a clinical one and is based on the presence of maternal fever in the absence of other causes. Other clinical criteria that have classically been used to diagnose amnionitis include uterine tenderness, foul-smelling amniotic fluid, maternal tachycardia, and fetal tachycardia. These other clinical findings are somewhat variable, and indeed maternal fever remains the most significant and constant finding (Table 2).[1,2,7,9]

Various laboratory tests have been used as an aid in the attempt to confirm the diagnosis of chorioamnionitis; these tests are summarized in Table 3. From a practical standpoint, most of the laboratory tests that have been suggested provide little immediately useful clinical information. The most used laboratory test is no doubt the peripheral maternal leukocyte count. Although leukocytosis will

TABLE 3. Laboratory Tests That Have Been Proposed as an Aid in Confirming the Diagnosis of Amnionitis

Peripheral leukocyte count
Direct examination of amniotic fluid
  Leukocytes
  Bacteria
Amniotic fluid culture
Blood cultures
Gas-liquid chromatography
C-reactive protein
Leukocyte esterase
Microscopic examination of placenta and membranes

be found in the majority of women with amnionitis, many pregnant women without infection will demonstrate significant elevations in leukocytes, especially if in labor. Moreover, different authors have used different leukocyte levels to define "normal," and by utilizing different levels the frequency of leukocytosis in women with amnionitis has been reported to be as low as 3% and as high as 86%.[1,19,20]

One laboratory test that might provide immediately useful information is the direct examination of the amniotic fluid obtained through a transcervical intrauterine catheter. Gibbs and colleagues were able to obtain sufficient amniotic fluid in the majority of their patients by using this technique and recommended discarding the first 5–10 ml to minimize contamination from lower genital tract organisms.[8] Fluid thus obtained may be cultured and examined with Gram's stain to detect bacteria. The presence of bacteria on a Gram stain is supportive but not confirmatory of the diagnosis of acute chorioamnionitis.[8,20–22] Direct plating of amniotic fluid for quantitative bacterial studies would appear to be more accurate than Gram staining of unspun amniotic fluid for detection of bacteria.[8]

Examination of amniotic fluid for the presence of leukocytes as a marker for chorioamnionitis has also been reported, but the results have been contradictory.[8,20,22–25] This test has proved to have little clinical utility.

Amniocentesis may also be used to obtain fluid for either Gram staining or culture. However, this procedure is not without risk, and the risk must be weighed against the cost and clinical usefulness of the information obtained. Because there is little conclusive data to date supporting intervention solely on the basis of Gram stain results, there is probably little justification for performing amniocentesis in all women with a clinical diagnosis of amnionitis. Moreover, fluid cannot be obtained in more than 50% of the patients with ruptured membranes. Amniocentesis may be helpful from a clinical standpoint in the patient with intact membranes, fever, and suspected amnionitis, especially if remote from term (i.e., less than 30–32 weeks' gestational age).

Amniotic fluid and blood cultures may occasionally provide clinically useful information, especially in the patient who develops further complications. Such a patient is one who continues to be febrile following delivery.

Gas-liquid chromatography (GLC) for the identification of organic acid metabolites of various pathogenic bacteria has been reported to correlate with both clinical infection and positive amniotic fluid culture.[26,27] In one study, GLC was reported to be 94% sensitive and 95% specific.[26]

C-reactive protein (CRP), an abnormal protein produced by the liver in response to infection or inflammation, has been reported to be a sensitive marker in the serum of women with chorioamnionitis.[28–30] In one study, CRP was reported to have a sensitivity and specificity of 88% and 96%, respectively.[30] However, in a more recent study, it was reported that elevated CRP predicted infection in only 8 to 29% of patients, and 18% of patients with significant infection had normal CRP.[31] Thus, this test had little clinical utility in actual practice.

A simple, relatively inexpensive screening test of amniotic fluid, the leukocyte esterase test strip, has been reported to have a 91% sensitivity and 95% specificity in the diagnosis of acute chorioamnionitis.[32] However, in another study, a positive leukocyte esterase test was not associated with clinical chorioamnionitis (sensitivity 19%).[33]

Finally, microscopic examination of the placental membranes for leukocyte infiltration has been suggested as a means of confirming clinical amnionitis. However, since this is obviously accomplished retrospectively, this technique has very little clinical utility. Moreover, there appears to be poor correlation between leukocyte infiltration of the fetal membranes and actual clinical amnionitis.[20]

ADVERSE MATERNAL EFFECTS

Obviously, the most serious adverse maternal effect is death. In a review of 501 consecutive maternal deaths in Texas for 1969 to 1973, 10 were attributed to chorioamnionitis.[34] Similarly, Gogoi reported 14 maternal deaths in women with acute chorioamnionitis, 13 of whom were delivered by cesarean section.[35] Fortunately, although infection is still a cause of maternal morbidity in this country, it is uncommon. For example, there were no maternal deaths in 555 women with acute chorioamnionitis compiled from three recent studies.[2,7,19]

Acute chorioamnionitis may also result in significant maternal morbidity such as pelvic infection. The frequency of pelvic infection appears to be related primarily to the route of delivery, specifically cesarean section,[36] and the rate of cesarean section is increased in women with chorioamnionitis.[1,19] Maternal bacteremia has been reported to occur in 2–6% of women with amnionitis.[1,19] Postpartum infectious morbidity is less common in women delivered vaginally, although it does appear to be increased over that found in women delivered vaginally without chorioamnionitis.[7] Chorioamnionitis also results in an increased risk of cesarean delivery. Duff and associates have reported data that would suggest that this increase in operative delivery is secondary to an increased frequency of dysfunctional labor in women with acute amni-

TABLE 4. Perinatal Mortality and Morbidity in 312 Newborns of Women With Acute Chorioamnionitis

	Term (≥35 weeks) (n = 273)	Preterm (<35 weeks) (n = 39)
Perinatal mortality		
Fetal	4 (1.5%)	0
Neonatal	0	9 (23%)
Perinatal morbidity		
Proven sepsis[a]	10 (3.7%)	4 (10.2%)
IVH[b]	0	7 (18%)
NEC[c]	0	3 (7.7%)
Ventilated	4 (1.5%)	13 (33%)
Seizures	2 (0.7%)	1 (2.6%)

Adapted from Gilstrap et al.[7]
[a]Positive blood cultures.
[b]Intracranial hemorrhage.
[c]Necrotizing enterocolitis.

onitis.[37] For example, three-fourths of 65 women with term pregnancies and acute chorioamnionitis had abnormal labors, and 34% required cesarean section for failure to progress.[37] These authors also reported that women with acute chorioamnionitis required larger doses of oxytocin to effect adequate contractions.

ADVERSE FETAL AND NEONATAL EFFECTS

Acute chorioamnionitis may result in increased perinatal mortality, especially in the premature infant. For example, Gilstrap et al. reported four stillbirths but no neonatal deaths in 273 term pregnancies for a perinatal mortality rate of 15/1,000 (Table 4).[7] In 39 preterm infants, however, there were nine neonatal deaths (and no stillbirths) for a perinatal mortality rate of 230/1,000. None of these nine deaths were from proven sepsis. Although premature infants born to mothers with amnionitis have a significantly higher perinatal mortality rate than similar premature infants born to mothers without chorioamnionitis, the increased mortality cannot be totally explained by fetal infection alone.[1,7,38] Fortunately, the perinatal outcome is surprisingly good in term infants born to mothers with acute amnionitis.

Neonates born to mothers with acute amnionitis are at increased risk of sepsis and pneumonia. The majority of these infants, however, subsequently do very well. In the series by Gilstrap et al. there were only four (1.5%) neonates of 273 term newborns with a diagnosis of congenital pneumonia based on x-ray findings and only one (0.7%) had a positive culture.[7] However, 10 newborns of 312 had sepsis defined as a positive blood culture.

MANAGEMENT

There is universal agreement that women with acute chorioamnionitis should receive antimicrobial therapy and be delivered. Beyond that there is little agreement and surprisingly little data regarding the specifics of therapy. For example, there is no unanimity of opinion regarding the most efficacious antibiotic regimen for treating women with acute chorioamnionitis. The reason for this is that to date there have been no large comparative studies of commonly used antibiotics, although the combination of penicillin or ampicillin with an aminoglycoside has generally produced satisfactory results in the past.[1,2,7] Recently, it has been suggested that an antibiotic with coverage against anaerobes such as *Bacteroides* sp. should also be used, especially in women undergoing operative delivery.[10,39] In one recent preliminary study comparing a dual therapy of ampicillin and gentamicin with a triple therapy of ampicillin, gentamicin, and clindamycin (for anaerobic coverage) for the treatment of acute chorioamnionitis, Maberry and colleagues were unable to demonstrate any significant difference in the frequency of endometritis following cesarean section.[40] In the absence of randomized prospective studies, one of several antibiotic regimens outlined in Table 5 may be used. However, neither the efficacy nor safety of these regimens for the treatment of acute chorioamnionitis has been clearly established in large studies, although they would logically appear to be acceptable for treatment of the majority of women with amnionitis.

TABLE 5. Recommended Antibiotic Regimens for Treatment of Acute Chorioamnionitis

Single agent
  Cefoxitin/cefotetan
  Third-generation cephalosporin
  Piperacillin/mezlocillin
  Timentin
Combination
  Ampicillin/penicillin plus gentamicin plus
Clindamycin
  Mezlocillin/piperacillin plus gentamicin

Until recently, there was also no unanimity of opinion regarding the most ideal time to initiate antibiotic therapy, i.e., before or after cord clamping. However, it has now been established that unless delivery is imminent, i.e., less than 1 hour, antibiotics should be administered as soon as the diagnosis is made. In one study comparing antibiotic administration before and after cord clamping, Sperling and associates reported that 17% of neonates whose mothers received antibiotics after cord clamping had proven sepsis, compared to 3% of those whose mothers received antibiotics prior to cord clamping (Table 6).[41] In another study, Gilstrap and associates reported a significantly higher incidence of positive blood cultures for group B streptococcus in mothers who received antibiotics after cord clamping compared to before cord clamping (6% vs. 0%).[7]

In the only randomized prospective study to date regarding the timing of the initiation of antibiotics, Gibbs and associates reported a significantly lower incidence of neonatal sepsis when maternal antibiotics were started prior to cord clamping as compared to postpartum (0 vs. 21%; $P < .05$) in 45 women with acute chorioamnionitis.[42] Neonatal hospital stay was also shorter when antibiotics were started prior to cord clamping.[42]

Another important reason for starting antibiotics soon after the diagnosis of amnionitis is made is to prevent serious morbidity in the mother. Thus there is little reason to withhold antibiotics from either a maternal

TABLE 6. Frequency of Neonatal Sepsis in Mothers Who Received Antibiotics Before or After Cord Clamping

	Before cord clamping	After cord clamping
Sperling et al.[41]	6/211 (3%)	8/46 (17%)
Gilstrap et al.[7]	0/133 (0%)	8/140 (6%)
Total	6/344 (2%)	16/186 (9%)

or fetal standpoint once the diagnosis of chorioamnionitis is made.

Generally the method of delivery should be dictated according to standard obstetric indications. In other words, there is little or no evidence to suggest that cesarean section offers any specific advantage over vaginal delivery for either the mother or infant with a diagnosis of chorioamnionitis. Moreover, cesarean section may actually carry significant risk for mothers, especially with regard to endometritis. However, the cesarean section rate is significantly higher in women with acute chorioamnionitis secondary to dysfunctional labor.

There is little data regarding the most appropriate interval from diagnosis of infection to delivery, although some have advocated delivery by 1 to 12 hours.[43-45]. Neither Gibbs and associates[1] nor Hauth and colleagues[2] were able to identify a critical interval up to 12 hours from diagnosis to delivery with regard to neonatal morbidity or mortality. Whether intervals longer than 12 hours have a significant impact on morbidity is unclear at this time.

SUMMARY

Acute chorioamnionitis is a common complication of pregnancy. The diagnosis is based primarily on the presence of maternal fever in the absence of other obvious causes. Amnionitis may result in significant morbidity to both mother and fetus. Perinatal mortality is primarily related to gestational age and is relatively uncommon in term infants. Maternal mortality is rare but may still occur.

It is generally efficacious from both a maternal and fetal standpoint to start antibiotics as soon as the diagnosis of amnionitis is made. Management of women with acute chorioamnionitis consists of antibiotics and delivery. The critical interval from diagnosis of amnionitis to delivery with regard to morbidity is unknown at this time, but the majority of patients seem to do well at 12 hours or less. Cesarean section offers no specific advantage over vaginal delivery and should be reserved for obstetric indications.

REFERENCES

1. Gibbs RS, Castillo MS, Rogers PJ: Management of acute chorioamnionitis. Obstet Gynecol 136:709–713, 1980.
2. Hauth JC, Gilstrap LC III, Hankins GDV, Connor KD: Term maternal and neonatal complications of acute chorioamniontis. Obstet Gynecol 66:59–62, 1985.
3. Looff JD, Hager WD: Management of chorioamnionitis. Surg Gynecol Obstet 158:161–166, 1984.
4. Guzick DS, Winn K: The association of chorioamnionitis with preterm delivery. Obstet Gynecol 65:11–16, 1985.
5. Edwards LA, Barrada MI, Hamann AA, Hakanson EY: Gonorrhea in pregnancy. Am J Obstet Gynecol 132:637–641, 1978.
6. Regan JA, Chao SJ, James SL: Premature rupture of the membranes, preterm delivery and group B streptococcal colonization of mother. Am J Obstet Gynecol 141:184–186, 1981.
7. Gilstrap LC III, Leveno KJ, Cox SM, Burris JS, Mashburn M, Rosenfeld CR: Intrapartum treatment of acute chorioamnionitis: Impact on neonatal sepsis. Am J Obstet Gynecol 159:579–583, 1988.
8. Gibbs RS, Blanco JD, St Clair PJ, Castaneda YS: Quantitative bacteriology of amniotic fluid from women with clinical intraamniotic infection. J Infect Dis 145:1–8, 1982.
9. Yoder PR, Gibbs RS, Blanco JD, Castaneda YS, St Clair PJ: A prospective, controlled study of maternal and perinatal outcome after intra-amniotic infection at term. Am J Obstet Gynecol 145:695–701, 1983.
10. Sperling RS, Newton E, Gibbs RS: Intraamniotic infection in low-birth-weight infants. J Infect Dis 157:113–117, 1988.
11. Petrilli ES, D'Ablaing G, Ledger WJ: *Listeria monocytogenes* chorioamnionitis: Diagnosis by transab-

dominal amniocentesis. Obstet Gynecol 55(S):5–8, 1980.

12. Lorenz RP, Applebaum PC, Ward RM, Botti JJ: Chorioamnionitis and possible neonatal infection associated with *Lactobacillus* species. J Clin Microbiol 16:558–561, 1982.

13. Cox SM, Phillips LE, Mercer LJ, Stager CE, Waller S, Faro S: Lactobacillemia of amniotic fluid origin. Obstet Gynecol 68:134–135, 1986.

14. Winn HN, Egley CC: Acute *Haemophilus influenzae* chorioamnionitis associated with intact amniotic membranes. Am J Obstet Gynecol 156:458–459, 1987.

15. Cassell GH, Waites KB, Gibbs RS, Davis JK: Role of *Ureaplasma urealyticum* in amnionitis. Pediatr Infect Dis 5(S):247–252, 1986.

16. Altschuler G, Hyde S: Fusobacteria: An important cause of chorioamnionitis. Arch Pathol Lab Med 109:739–743, 1985.

17. Easterling TH, Garite TJ: *Fusobacterium*: Anaerobic occult amnionitis and premature labor. Obstet Gynecol 66:825–828, 1985.

18. Galask RP, Varner MW, Petzold CR, Wilbur SL: Bacterial attachment to the chorioamniotic membranes. Am J Obstet Gynecol 148:915–928, 1984.

19. Koh KS, Chan FH, Monfared AH, Ledger WJ, Paul RH: The changing perinatal and maternal outcome in chorioamnionitis. Obstet Gynecol 53:730–734, 1979.

20. Hollander D: Diagnosis of chorioamnionitis. Clin Obstet Gynecol 29:816–825, 1986.

21. Garite T, Freeman R, Linzey F, Braley P: The use of amniocentesis in patients with premature rupture of the membranes. Obstet Gynecol 54:226–230, 1979.

22. Listwa H, Robek A, Carpenter J, Gibbs R: Predictability of intrauterine infection in analysis of amniotic fluid. Obstet Gynecol 48:31–34, 1976.

23. Larsen JW, Goldkrand JW, Hanson TM, Miller CR: Intrauterine infection on an obstetric service. Obstet Gynecol 43:838–843, 1974.

24. Larsen J, Weis K, Lenihan J, Crumbie M, Haggers J: Significance of neutrophils and bacteria in the amniotic fluid of patients in labor. Obstet Gynecol 47:143–147, 1976.

25. Bobitt J, Hayslip C, Damato J: Amniotic fluid infection as determined by transabdominal amniocentesis in patients with intact membranes in premature labor. Am J Obstet Gynecol 140:947–952, 1981.

26. Gravett MG, Eschenbach DA, Speigel-Brown CA, Holmes KK: Rapid diagnosis of amniotic-fluid infection by gas-liquid chromatography. N Engl J Med 306:725–728, 1982.

27. Iams JD, Clapp DH, Contos DA, Whitehurst R, Ayers LW, O'Shaughnessy RW: Does extra-amniotic infection cause preterm labor? Gas liquid chromatographic studies of amniotic fluid in amniocentesis, preterm labor and normal controls. Obstet Gynecol 70:365–368, 1987.

28. Evans MI, Hajj SN, Devoe LD, et al.: C-reactive protein as a predictor of infectious morbidity with premature rupture of membranes. Am J Obstet Gynecol 138:648–652, 1980.

29. Hawrylyshun P, Bernstein P, Milligan JE, Soldin S, Pollard A, Papsin FR: Premature rupture of membranes: The role of C-reactive protein in the prediction of chorioamnionitis. Am J Obstet Gynecol 147:240–246, 1983.

30. Romem Y, Artal R: C-reactive protein as a predictor for chorioamnionitis in cases of premature rupture of the membranes. Am J Obstet Gynecol 150:546–550, 1984.

31. Ernest JM, Swain M, Block SM, Nelson LH, Hatjis CG, Meis PJ: C-reactive protein: A limited test for managing patients with preterm labor or preterm rupture of membranes? Am J Obstet Gynecol 156:449–454, 1987.

32. Hoskins IA, Johnson TRB, Winkel CA: Leukocyte esterase activity in human amniotic fluid for the rapid detection of chorioamnionitis. Am J Obstet Gynecol 157:730–732, 1987.

33. Romero R, Emamian M, Wan M, Yarkoni S, McCormack W, Mazor M, Hobbins JC: The value of the leukocyte esterase in diagnosing intra-amniotic infection. Am J Perinatol 5:64–69, 1988.

34. Gibbs CE, Locke WE: Maternal deaths in Texas, 1969 to 1973: A report of 501 consecutive maternal deaths from the Texas Medical Association's Committee on Maternal Health. Am J Obstet Gynecol 126:687–692, 1976.

35. Gogoi MP: Maternal mortality from cesarean section in infected cases. Br J Obstet Gynaecol 78:373, 1971.

36. Gilstrap LC III, Cunningham FG: The bacterial pathogenesis of infection following cesarean section. Obstet Gynecol 53:545–549, 1979.

37. Duff P, Sanders R, Gibbs RS: The course of labor in term pregnancies with chorioamnionitis. Am J Obstet Gynecol 147:391–395, 1983.

38. Garite TJ, Freeman RK: Chorioamnionitis in the preterm gestation. Obstet Gynecol 59:539–545, 1982.

39. Sweet RL, Gibbs RS: "Infectious Disease of the Female Genital Tract." Baltimore: Williams & Wilkins, 1985, pp 263–276.

40. Maberry M, Gilstrap L, Burris J, Bawdon R, Leveno K: A randomized comparative study of triple antibiotic therapy in the management of acute chorioamnionitis. Society of Perinatal Obstetricians, 9th Annual Meeting, New Orleans, LA, February 2–4, 1989, abstract 453.

41. Sperling RS, Ramamurthy RS, Gibbs RS: A comparison of intrapartum versus immediate postpartum treatment of intraamniotic infection. Obstet Gynecol 70:861–865, 1987.
42. Gibbs RS, Dinsmoor MJ, Newton ER, Ramamurthy RS: A randomized trial of intrapartum versus postpartum treatment of women with intraamniotic infection. Obstet Gynecol 72:823–828, 1988.
43. Schwarz RH, Fruiterman JP: Life-threatening infections in pregnancy. Clin Obstet Gynecol 19:561–575, 1976.
44. MacVicar J: Chorioamnionitis. In Charles D, Finland M (eds): "Obstetric and Perinatal Infections." Philadelphia: Lea & Febiger, 1973, pp 479–499.
45. Friedman EA: Obstetric infection in labor. In Charles D, Finland M (eds): "Obstetric and Perinatal Infections." Philadelphia: Lea & Febiger, 1973, pp 501–517.

6

Postpartum Endometritis

Sebastian Faro, M.D., Ph.D.

Endometritis is a relatively common complication of the postpartum period. It is still a significant cause of maternal morbidity and, rarely, mortality. The term "endometritis" basically refers to infection of the endometrium or decidua with extension into the myometrium. Other terms that have been used to define this infection include metritis, myometritis, endomyometritis, and puerperal sepsis. Involvement of the parametrial tissue is termed parametritis.

INCIDENCE

The incidence of endometritis varies significantly depending on the population studied and, more importantly, on the method of delivery, i.e., vaginal vs. cesarean section. The risk of developing endometritis following vaginal delivery is estimated to be between 1 and 3%.[1,2] In contrast, the frequency of endometritis following operative delivery or cesarean section may be as high as 95% in certain high-risk populations.[3] Considering that the current cesarean section rate is approximately 20–25%,[4] clinicians providing care for pregnant women can expect to encounter this complication frequently.

MICROBIOLOGY

The bacteria most commonly isolated from the inner uterine surface of patients with acute postpartum endometritis are *Streptococcus agalactiae*, *Streptococcus faecalis*, *Escherichia coli*, *Bacteroides bivius*; these and other frequently isolated bacteria are listed in Table 1. Less frequently isolated bacteria are *Citrobacter*, *Acinetobacter*, and *Pseudomonas*. Organisms acquired from an exogenous source include *Neisseria gonorrhoeae*, *Chlamydia trachomatis*, and group A beta-hemolytic streptococci. The exact role of *C. trachomatis* as an etiologic agent responsible for postpartum endometritis is controversial. There have been several reports documenting the isolation of *C. trachomatis* from the uterus in patients with postpartum endometritis, but many of these patients were treated with an antibiotic not active against this bacterium; yet, the patients were cured of their acute infection.[5,6] The difficulty that arises is that these patients are usually infected with multiple bacteria and it is difficult to assign a priority to one of more of the bacteria isolated.

Antepartum screening has been in progress on the Baylor obstetric service for the past 3 years, over which time approximately 3,500

Infections in Pregnancy, pages 45–54
© 1990 Alan R. Liss, Inc.

TABLE 1. Common Bacteria Isolated From Patients With Postpartum Endometritis

Aerobes	
Gram positive	Gram negative
Staphylococcus aureus	*Enterobacter aerogenes*
Staphylococcus epidermidis	*Enterobacter agglomerans*
	Enterobacter cloaeae
Streptococcus agalactiae	*Escherichia coli*
Streptococcus faecalis	*Gardnerella vaginalis*
Streptococcus viridans	*Klebsiella pneumoniae*
Beta-hemolytic streptococci	*Morganella morgagnii*
	Proteus mirabilis
Anaerobes	
Gram positive	Gram negative
Clostridium sp.	*Bacteroides bivius*
Peptostreptococcus sp.	*Bacteroides disiens*
	Bacteroides fragilis
	Bacteroides melaninogenicus
	Fusobacterium necrophorum
	Fusobacterium nucleatum

to 4,000 cervical specimens have been processed. The incidence of C. *trachomatis* is 12 to 15%. None of these patients were treated for C. *trachomatis* during the antepartum period. However, C. *trachomatis* is not commonly isolated from the cervix of women with premature labor PROM or the cervix or endometrium of women with endometritis.

Postpartum endometritis is most frequently a polymicrobial mixed aerobic and anaerobic infection. Usually both gram-positive and gram-negative bacteria can be isolated from the inner surface of the uterus of infected individuals.[3,7] Unimicrobial postpartum endometritis has been reported and tends to occur within the first 24 hours of delivery.[8–10] Bacteria such as *Haemophilus influenzae* and *Lactobacillus* sp. have been recovered from patients with postpartum endometritis.[11,12] The cases of *Lactobacillus* infection demonstrate virtual transmission of an infecting agent that ascends from the lower genital tract and causes chorioamnionitis, an endometritis with bacteremia in the mother and fetus. Bacteria such as *Mycoplasma* and *Ureaplasma* are of particular interest, because these bacteria are frequently found in the lower genital tract of asymptomatic individuals and have been responsible for postoperative infection.[13,14]

The most common circumstance surrounding unimicrobial postpartum endometritis is found in patients receiving antibiotic prophylaxis. Three doses of a cephalosporin antibiotic administered for prophylaxis to patients delivered by cesarean section has been shown to exert a selective pressure on the vaginal microflora.[15–18] There is a selection for resistant bacteria, primarily *Streptococcus faecalis* and *Enterobacter cloacae*. However, when the new beta-lactam antibiotics, e.g., cefoxitin and cefotetan, are used for prophylaxis, there is also a noticeable decrease in the number of anaerobic bacteria colonizing the lower genital tract.[15] This is also partially noted when a first-generation cephalosporin, e.g., cefazolin, is used, as there is a marked absence of peptostreptococci.[15,16] One major difference noted between these two antibiotics was the effect on *Lactobacillus* sp. Cefoxitin appeared to reduce the number of lactobacilli present, whereas cefotetan did not. This may or may not be significant in the dynamic relationship between all bacteria present. Lactobacilli presence is considered to be a major factor in maintaining the "normal" environment and preventing the more virulent bacteria, especially the anaerobes, from becoming dominant. When penicillins are administered for prophylaxis there does not appear to be selection toward a predominant organism, but there is a tendency to select for resistant gram-negative facultative anaerobic bacteria, e.g., *E. coli*. Thus the use of antibiotic prophylaxis not only has been demonstrated to reduce the incidence of postpartum endometritis but also influences the types of predominant bacteria that inhabit the lower genital tract, which, in turn, will ultimately determine the type of bacterial infection that may ensue.

INDIGENOUS VAGINAL FLORA
- Ruptured membrane
- Vaginal exams
- Internal monitoring

↓

INOCULATION OF LOWER UTERINE SEGMENT
- Prolonged labor
- Surgery

↓

COLONIZATION OF LOWER UTERINE
SEGMENT AND INCISION
- Surgical trauma
- Foreign body (suture)
- Devitalized tissue

↓

FAVORABLE ANAEROBIC MILIEU
- Blood and serum
- Decreased O_2 under bladder flap

↓

"POLYMICROBIAL PROLIFERATION"

↓

ENDOMETRITIS

Fig. 1. Pathogenesis of endometritis following cesarean section. (Adapted from Gilstrap and Cunningham.[3])

TABLE 2. Factors Reported to Predispose Individuals to the Development of Puerperal Infection

Cesarean section
Labor
Ruptured membranes
Internal monitoring
Number of vaginal exams
Anemia
Obesity
Anesthesia
Socioeconimc status

PATHOGENESIS

The pathogenesis of endometritis following operative delivery is summarized in Figure 1. The principle factors include contamination of inoculation, colonization, surgical trauma, foreign body (suture), and a favorable anaerobic milieu.[3] Obviously the same mechanism does not apply for infection following vaginal delivery, although inoculation and colinization do occur. Why some women develop endometritis following vaginal delivery and some do not is not clear at this time.

There are several factors that have been reported to increase the risk of infection following cesarean section (Table 2). Of the various factors, the most important include cesarean section, labor, and ruptured membranes. The presence of these three factors have resulted in an infection rate as high as 85% in some populations.[8] It is unclear whether the other factors listed in Table 2 are truly risk factors or simply commonly associated with infection.

It is important that physicians become familiar with the types of bacteria that are commonly isolated from infected patients on the ward in which their patients will be placed postoperatively. This information can only be provided if the physicians obtain cultures from their infected patients. The infection control personnel and hospital pharmacy can provide current data on the antibiotics used for prophylaxis. The physician who is attentive to this information will be able to choose, empirically, appropriate antibiotics for the infected patient. This type of rationale eliminates the practice of polypharmacy and reduces the use of toxic adverse effects and cost. Utilization of the approach suggested above is dependent upon a thorough evaluation of the patient suspected of having postpartum endometritis. Initially, the patient's history should be reviewed, because certain factors will have a bearing on the infection, such as how long was the patient in the hospital preoperatively, did she receive antibiotics prior to her surgery, does she have underlying medical illness, and so forth. Patients maintained in hospital for 3 days or longer will become colonized by the hospital flora, and the gram-negative facultative bacteria that colonize the patient tend to be resistant to many of the more commonly used antimicrobial agents. It is important to determine if the patient has been taking any therapeutic or maintenance antibiotics, as these will influence the bacterial makeup of the endogenous vaginal flora. Does the patient have any underlying chronic or acute medical illness, such as insulin-dependent diabetes, hypertension, pregnancy-induced hypertension, collagen vascular disease, or renal disease? The operative procedure should be reviewed in detail, because details such as the duration of the procedure and blood loss may be significant factors. Did the patient experience any hypoxia and, if so, how long did it last and did it recur? Were there any difficulties encountered during the extraction of the infant, e.g., was assistance required to push the presenting part from the vagina? The patient's postoperative course should be reviewed. Was antibiotic prophylaxis administered? Specific agent and dosage are important. When did the patient become febrile in relationship to the surgery and the administration of the last does of antibiotic prophylaxis? The patient who develops signs of infection within the first 24 hours postoperatively should not be ignored, especially if the oral temperature is ≥1.01°F. Diagnoses such as atelectasis (unless the patient has pneumonia), breast engorgement, dehydration, or cystitis, do not cause oral temperatures of this degree. These patients should be examined. Bacteria such as *Streptococcus agalactiae* (group B beta-hemolytic streptococci) frequently are the cause of early postpartum endometritis These patients will often manifest signs and symptoms of infection within 12 hours of surgery. The infection may be reminiscent of group A beta-hemolytic streptococcal disease, in that it is fulminant and can present similar to a septic shocklike picture. The organisms multiply rapidly, cause a bacteremia, and may produce distant foci of infection.

DIAGNOSIS

The diagnosis of endometritis is based primarily on the presence of a fever (≥38°C) and the exclusion of other causes. Abdominal pain, "foul lochia," and leukocytosis are also frequently listed as features of endometritis. However, leukocytosis is a common finding in labor and the postpartum period even in the absence of overt infection. Moreover, most patients will have some degree of abdominal pain following cesarean section. The significance of so-called "first day" fever is unclear at this time, but there is evidence to suggest that in many cases such fever represents actual infection (especially if following cesarean section).[19]

MANAGEMENT

Antibiotics will not make a significant difference within 24 hours of their administration as far as the signs and symptoms of infection are concerned. They will prevent the infection from becoming more severe. It is important to remember that when a patient is infected, the number of bacteria at the site of infection probably exceeds 10^5 cfu/cc, the bacteria are not in a synchronous growth phase, and, therefore, the antibiotic will not exert an effect on all the bacteria present at the same time. There is a lag time from administration of the first dose of antibiotic to achievement of adequate serum and tissue levels and, finally, to the time the antibiotic begins to have a demonstrable effect on the bacteria.

Allowing more time for observation of the patient who is not overtly septic or whose condition is stable provides an opportunity for the antibiotic to demonstrate whether or not it will be effective. The bacteria present in the myometrium, especially deep in the myometrium, of the uterus are not growing in a synchronous fashion; therefore, if a single bactericidal agent were to be administered, only those bacteria in the active growth phase would be affected. However, if the patient's condition is deteriorating, this is an indication that the inoculum load, with its metabolic products, is too great for the patient's own immune system to handle. This is a situation that requires not only broad-spectrum antibiotics, but agents that will maintain adequate serum and tissue levels. The concentration achieved in both the serum and tissues should be well above the MIC_{90} of the offending bacteria. Thus two important aspects of antibiotic therapy become significant: dosage and time interval between administration. The half-life of an antibiotic becomes important because one would not want to administer an agent such as a semisynthetic penicillin, e.g., piperacillin, Timentin, or Unasyn, every 8 hours since the serum and tissue levels will fall to extremely low levels prior to instituting the next dose and a steady state will not be approached. The end result is that decreasing serum and tissue levels of antibiotic allows the bacteria to reproduce unabated and also permits the selection of resistant strains.

Prior to instituting antibiotic therapy, the patient should be examined thoroughly. The examination should rule out a focus of infection at a site other than the pelvis, e.g., dental abscess, pneumonia, pyelonephritis, etc. There are clues that can be ascertained from the physical exam that will enable the physician to focus on the site of infection and also determine the degree of severity. A patient with endometritis who also has a distended abdomen suggests that the inflammatory exudate has exited through the fallopian tubes and has caused an inflammatory reaction involving that portion of the bowel, large and small, located in the pelvis. This results in the bowel losing its peristaltic action: it becomes flaccid and easily distends. Thus, a distended abdomen, tenderness, or pain upon palpation of the upper abdomen (actually compressing and releasing dilated loops of bowel) indicates that there is a paralytic ileus that is secondary to infection. Auscultation of the abdomen should be performed prior to conducting palpation of the abdomen. The absence of bowel sounds or type of bowel sounds (high pitched, rushes, etc.) should be recorded.

The pelvic examination begins with inspection of the external genitalia. If lesions are present a record should be made of the location, characteristics, and whether the lesion is painful. Serum from the lesion should be obtained and a portion should be examined by dark-field microscopy. A Gram stain should also be performed, a Giemsa stain should be conducted, and an antibody fluorescent stain for *Chlamydia* should be performed. A speculum should be inserted and the lochia should be cleaned from the cervix and vagina. The lochia exiting from the endocervical canal should be characterized as to color, odor, and amount. Specimens should be obtained from the fundal region of the uterus, with an instrument such as a pipelle.[17,20] This will provide a biopsy of tissue that can be placed in an anaerobic transport vial. This specimen can be processed for the isolation of aerobes, anaerobes, *Mycoplasma*, *Ureaplasma*, and *Chlamydia*. Using a biopsy specimen reduces the amount of contamination and is less costly because the single specimen can be processed to fulfill all requirements. Bimanual examination is conducted to determine the extent of involvement of the infection. When palpating the uterus, it is advisable to place the abdominal hand above the umbilicus if a low transverse abdominal incision is present; if a verticle incision is present, palpation should be lateral. Specimens of venous blood should be obtained for blood cultures. A catheterized urine specimen should be obtained for culture of typical uropathogens.

The choice of antibiotic can be made in a simple fashion, by knowing the types of bacteria commonly isolated from patients with endometritis in the community and the effect of antibiotic prophylaxis on the bacterial flora of the lower genital tract. It is appropriate to initially choose a single agent such as mezlocillin, piperacillin, Timetin, Unasyn, cefoxitin, cefotetan, ceftizoxime or cefotaxime,

TABLE 3. Single-Agent Regimens for the Treatment of Post Cesarean Section Endometritis

Agent	Dosage
Mezlocillin	3–4 g IV q 4 h
Piperacillin	3–4 g IV q 4 h
Timetin	3.1 g IV q 6 h
Unasyn	1.5–3 g IV q 6 h
Cefoxitin	1–2 g IV q 6 h
Cefotetan	1–2 g IV q 12 h
Cefoperazone	2 g IV q 12 h
Ceftrizoxime	1–2 g IV q 8 h
Cefotaxime	1–2 g IV q 12 h

as outlined in Table 3. Many studies have been conducted that demonstrated that single-agent therapy with a beta-lactam antibiotic is as effective as combinations such as clindamycin and gentamicin. The antibiotic chosen should be allowed 48 hours to demonstrate an effect before intervening or considering an alternate therapy, unless the patient's condition is deteriorating. After 48 hours, if the patient has not improved, she should be reexamined, a specimen should be obtained for culture of aerobic and anaerobic bacteria, and an additional antibiotic should be added to the current therapy. It would also be prudent to perform an ultrasound to determine if 1) there is fluid collection in the abdominal incision, 2) a retrovesicle fluid collection, a hematoma, or abscess is present, 3) there is a parametrial mass, or 4) retained placental tissue is present in the uterus. Fluid collection in the abdominal wound retrovesicle between the bladder flap and uterus, overlying the uterine incision or in the parametrial tissue, is most likely to be a hematoma. However, if this is found on postoperative day 4 or 5 and was not seen earlier, an abscess should be suspected.

The presence of a hematoma is a significant finding because it is likely to turn into an abscess. A hematoma located in the abdominal incision will prevent healing, and if not detected in the hospital, the patient usually returns because the wound spontaneously dehisces. A hematoma in the parametrial tissue reflects difficulty encountered when suturing the uterine incision, especially at the angle. This is significant because it indicates that extra suture was placed in this area, establishing a nidus for infection. Last, a retrovesicle hematoma can lead to fistula formation, or if it becomes infected, can lead to abscess formation with necrosis of the lower uterine segment.

Reculturing is beneficial because the original cultures obtained at the initiation of therapy will be helpful in guiding subsequent therapy.

The laboratory should be able to report whether or not there is growth on the aerobic plates and the Gram stain characteristics of the growing bacteria. If the bacteria are gram positive, then ampicillin can be added. However, if the bacteria are gram positive and the patient is already on a penicillin such as piperacillin or mezlocillin, staphylococcus should be suspected and vancomycin can be added. If it is gram-negative bacteria, then an aminoglycoside can be added. The most common bacteria found in patients with postpartum endometritis and in patients not responding to the initial antibiotic are either *Streptococcus faecalis* or *Enterobacter cloacae*. The second specimen again will be growing on the culture media within 48 hours, and again, the laboratory can report the Gram stain characteristics. This will either confirm or refute the first culture growth, and within 72 hours the antibiotic sensitivities will be known.

It is not unusual to find a patient started on piperacillin who appears within 48 hours to be improving and the following day has a temperature spike. Reviewing bacteriology, one finds that the initial culture grew out *E. coli* apparently sensitive to piperacillin. However, that would not be known at the time of the secondary increase in temperature, but the Gram stain characteristics would be known. Because it is a gram-negative rod, an aminoglycoside would be added. The second culture confirms that a gram-negative rod is growing again, and over the next 24 to 48 hours it is determined that *E. coli* is still present but is resistant to piperacillin and sensitive to an aminoglycoside. Thus, by obtaining specimens for culture and knowing the Gram stain characteristics one can choose an antibiotic to supplement the initial antibiotic being administered. How would one interpret a Gram stain that reveals a mixed flora that is both gram-negative and gram-positive bacteria?

If the patient is receiving penicillin, it is more likely that the gram-negative organisms are significant. However, one has to consider that 1) a resistant anaerobe is rarely the reason for failure, 2) if the patient is receiving piperacillin or mezlocillin it is unlikely that *S. faecalis* (gram-positive cocci) is the reason for the patient not responding, and 3) if the patient is receiving Unasyn or Timentin, it is likely that a gram-negative bacteria, e.g., *Enterobacter cloacae*, is probably the main reason for failure. If the patient is receiving a broad-spectrum cephalosporin agent like cefoxitin (a cephamycin) or cefotetan, the same approach can be taken.

There are several conditions associated with postpartum endometritis that may develop that cause patients not to respond or to appear to be responding slowly to therapy. The individual may develop ligneous cellulitis, or a pelvic phlegmon, which is characterized by a low-grade, spiking temperature, with peak temperatures between 101°F and 103°F, and an elevated WBC count that ranges between 14,000 and 17,000. The diagnosis is made by performing a bimanual examination of the pelvis, which reveals the presence of an area of marked induration, sometimes referred to as woody induration. The induration is frequently bilateral and extends from the cervix out laterally to the pelvic walls, characterized as a ridge extending bilaterally from the cervix. These patients respond to antibiotic therapy, but usually require a longer period of time to show initial signs of improvement. These patients should not undergo procedures that attempt to aspirate or drain these areas, as there is no collection of fluid. Some individuals have suggested that the addition of steroids to reduce the degree of inflammation. This has not been necessary as there have been no control studies demonstrating that steroids offer any advantage over antibiotics without steroids. Time is required to allow for resolution of this condition with continuation of antibiotics until the patient is afebrile, the WBC returns to normal, and the induration is resolved.

In some instances, the patient develops a broad ligament or retrovesicle hematoma. These hematomas can become infected because they develop 1) over the uterine incision and are contained by the bladder flap and become contaminated during the operative procedure or 2) at the angle of the uterine incision and dissect into the broad ligament. These masses can be identified by ultrasound, and if the retrovesicle can be aspirated and drained transabdominally, there is no need to perform an exploratory laparotomy because these individuals will usually respond to antibiotic therapy. However, if the patient shows no change over 72 to 96 hours while receiving broad-spectrum antibiotics, consideration should be given to surgical intervention. Sometimes these individuals will develop a vesicle-uterine fistula. The patient will complain of a constant watery discharge. This condition can be diagnosed by either an intravenous pyelogram or placing a Foley catheter in the bladder and instilling saline containing indigo carmine. A tampon is placed in the vagina and if it stains blue, the diagnosis is established.

Another complication of a retrovesicle hematoma is the development of an abscess. This is an extremely serious complication that may be accompanied by overt signs and symptoms of sepsis, or the patient may appear relatively asymptomatic. The infected hematoma may develop into a frank abscess. The abscess is usually overlying the uterine incision and can result in a serious infection of the myometrium. This advances into myonecrosis along the uterine incision line. The telltale sign of this condition is frequently the

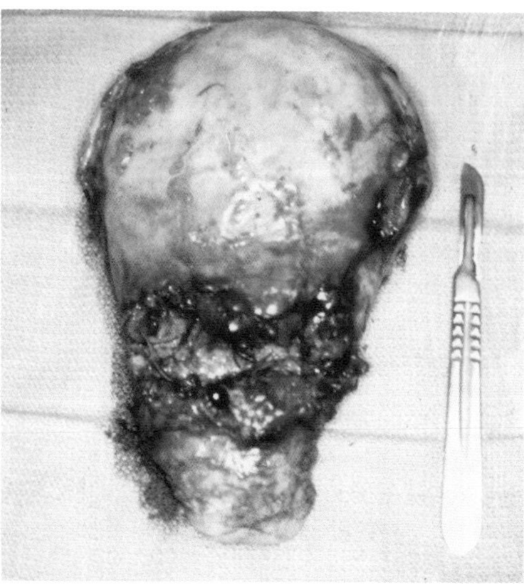

Fig. 2. Necrosis of the entire lower uterine segment, which was preceded by endometritis.

presence of a purulent exudate exiting from the abdominal incision and the vagina. Bimanual examination usually makes the diagnosis. The placement of one or two fingers into the uterus and palpation of the lower segment reveals that the fingers can be palpated with the abdominal hand or the fingers may just present in the abdominal wall. In some instances, the patient may just continue to have high spiking temperatures without the purulent drainage. The patient has localized peritonitis that does not extend above the umbilicus. These patients should be taken to surgery to undergo an exploratory laparotomy; they often require a hysterectomy. The lower uterine segment is often found to be necrotic. Frequently, the lower uterine segment is not present, the uterine vessels are thrombosed, and only the posterior uterine wall remains intact connecting the uterus to the cervix (Fig. 2). This is an important point to remember because in those patients who require hysterectomy and continue not to respond to antibiotic therapy, a diagnosis of septic pelvic thrombosis

should be considered. During the exploratory laparotomy, the vessels of the pelvis should be examined to determine if thrombosis is present.

Septic pelvic vein thrombosis can be diagnosed with the aid of computerized tomography of the pelvis; however, it can also be diagnosed by exclusion. The patient usually presents with high spiking temperatures and a CBC count in the range of 18,000 to 25,000. The patient is usually on triple antibiotics, e.g., clindamycin plus gentamicin plus ampicillin, and does not show any significant response. There have not been any well-controlled studies to determine if heparin therapy offers any real advantage or benefit over antibiotics administered for a prolonged period without it. The usual course of therapy is to add heparin, 10,000 units for a loading dose followed by infusing 1,000 units per hour intravenously. Most patients will show improvement within 72 hours, but it is not unusual for some patients not to improve until they have received 5 days of heparin and antibiotics.

Thus it is extremely important to evaluate the postcesarean section patients early, at the first sign of infection. There is no advantage to waiting 2 days or more, thereby allowing the infection to become well established. A thorough examination is required because not all fever reflects infection and not all infections are due to bacteria. Two other causes of febrile morbidity should be considered—viral illness and drug fever.

The patient with a viral illness may exhibit high spiking temperatures, but the physical is often unrewarding. No focus of infection is found. These patients are often given antibiotics because it is a difficult diagnosis to establish and it would be unwise to gamble, since a uterine bacterial infection can develop into a serious infection. The patient with drug fever is usually receiving a cephalosporin or penicillin. The temperature pattern is nonspecific, i.e., there is no particular pattern. The patient's pulse rate is not elevated and the WBC is usually within the normal range. The physical examination is normal, that is, there are no masses or areas of tenderness.

Early recognition of the infected patient, appropriate evaluation, and institution of appropriate antibiotics leads to quick resolution of infection.

PREVENTION

It is now well established that prophylactic antibiotics will significantly reduce the incidence of postpartum febrile morbidity following cesarean section. However, it is less than clear as to whether antibiotic prophylaxis will prevent serious infection.[17] In one study of over 1,000 patients, there was a twofold higher incidence of serious morbidity (i.e., abscess or septic thrombophlebitis) in women not receiving prophylaxis compared to those who did.[21] Although the incidence was statistically significant, it was not clinically significant (1% vs. 0.5%).[21]

A wide variety of antibiotics may be used for prophylaxis. General guidelines include the use of single agents, the use of first- or second-generation agents (such as ampicillin, cephradine, or cefoxitin), and the use of short-duration prophylaxis (i.e., one to three doses). The newer, broad-spectrum antibiotics such as the beta-lactamase inhibitors should be reserved for actual infections and not used for prophylaxis. Prophylactic antibiotics should not be given until after the umbilical cord is clamped. It is unclear if all women undergoing cesarean section should receive prophylaxis, especially those undergoing elective repeat operations. However, all women who have been in labor, have ruptured membranes, and who require cesarean section for failure to progress or have cephalopelvic disproportion are candidates for prophylactic antibiotics.

SUMMARY

Puerperal infection of endometritis is a relatively common complication encountered during the postpartum period. Well-established risk factors include operative delivery, ruptured membranes, and labor. The bacterial etiology is polymicrobial in the majority of cases. The diagnosis is based primarily on fever and exclusion of other causes. Treatment should be with a single agent that provides coverage against a broad spectrum of aerobic and anaerobic organisms. Antibiotic therapy should be continued until the patient has been afebrile for 24 to 48 hours. In uncomplicated patients it is not necessary to send the patient home on oral antibiotics as was done in the past.

REFERENCES

1. Gibbs RS: Clinical risk factors for puerperal infection. Obstet Gynecol 55:178–183, 1980.
2. Sweet RL, Ledger WJ: Cefoxitin: Single agent treatment of aerobic–anaerobic pelvic infections. Obstet Gynecol 54:193–198, 1979.
3. Gilstrap LC III, Cunningham FG: The bacterial pathogenesis of infection following cesarean section. Obstet Gynecol 53:545–549, 1979.
4. Gilstrap LC, Hauth JC, Toussaint S: Cesarean section: Changing incidence and indications. Obstet Gynecol 63:205–208, 1984.
5. Faro S, Sanders CV, Aldridge KE, et al.: Use of a single-agent antimicrobial therapy in the treatment of polymicrobial female pelvic infections. Obstet Gynecol 60:232–236, 1982.
6. Faro S, Phillips LE, Baker JL, et al.: Comparative efficacy and safety of mezlocillin versus cefoxitin versus clindamycin plus gentamicin in the treatment of patients with postpartum endometritis. Obstet Gynecol 69:760–766, 1987.
7. Phillips LE, Faro S, Martens MG, et al.: Postcesarean microbiology of high-risk patients treated for endometritis. Curr Ther Res 42:1157–1165, 1987.
8. Faro S: Group B, beta-hemolytic streptococci and puerperal infections. Am J Obstet Gynecol 139:686–689, 1981.
9. Faro S: Antibiotic prophylaxis. In Galask RP, Larsen B (eds): "Infectious Diseases in the Female Patient." New York: Springer-Verlag, 1986, pp 243–250.
10. Pastorek JG, Faro S. Aldridge KE, et al.: Moxalactam versus clindamycin plus tobramycin for the treatment of puerperal infections. South Med J 80:1116–1119, 1987.
11. Pastorek JG, Bellow PH, Faro S: Haemophilus influenza implicated in puerperal infection: A report

of two cases and review of the literature. South Med J 75:734–736, 1982.

12. Cox SM, Phillips LE, Mercer LJ, Sager CW, Waller S, Faro S: Lactobacillemia of amniotic fluid origin. Obstet Gynecol 68:134–135, 1986.

13. Phillips LE, Faro S, Pokorny SF, et al.: Postcesarean wound infection by *Mycoplasma hominis* in a patient with persistent postpartum fever. Diagn Microbiol Infect Dis 7:193–197, 1987.

14. Wallace RJ Jr, Browne AK, Lin JS, et al.: Isolation of *Mycoplasma hominis* from blood cultures in patients with postpartum fever. Obstet Gynecol 51:181–185, 1978.

15. Faro S, Cox SM, Phillips LE: Influence of antibiotic prophylaxis on vaginal microflora. J Obstet Gynecol 6(Suppl):54–56, 1986.

16. Stever HG, Forward KR, Tynell DC, et al.: Comparative cervical flora–microflora shift after cefoxitin or cefazolin prophylaxis against infection following cesarean section. Am J Obstet Gynecol 149:718–721, 1984.

17. Gilstrap LC III: Puerperal infection. In Faro S (ed): "Diagnosis and Management of Female Pelvic Infection in Primary Care Medicine." Baltimore: Williams & Wilkins, 1985, pp 151–167.

18. Gilstrap LC III: Prophylactic antibiotics for cesarean section and surgical procedures. J Reprod Med 33:588–590, 1988.

19. Filker R, Monif GRG: The significance of temperature during the first 24 hours postpartum. Obstet Gynecol 53:358–361, 1979.

20. Martens MG, Faro S, Hammill H, Riddle G, Smith D: Transcervical uterine cultures with a new endometrial suction curette: A comparison of three sampling methods in postpartum endometritis. Obstet Gynecol (in press).

21. Mead PB: Prophylactic antibiotics and antibiotic resistance. Semin Perinatol 1:101–111, 1977.

7

Group B Streptococcal Infection
(*Streptococcus agalactiae*)

Sebastian Faro, M.D., Ph.D.

In the early 1900s, streptococcal infections were attributed to group A or D or to the viridans group. In 1935 Lancefield and Hare isolated *Streptococcus agalactiae* from the vaginas of postpartum women.[1] Lancefield differentiated the streptococci into serogroups by detecting antigenic differences in the cell wall carbohydrates.[2] Group-specific antigens were extracted and identified using specific antisera. Groups A through H and K through U have been identified. The most common serogroups associated with humans are A, B, C, D, and G. The group B streptococci are subdivided into five serotypes based upon cell wall carbohydrates, specifically referred to as S-substances. The five serotypes are Ia, Ib, Ic, II, and III.

Group B streptococci are responsible for a variety of human infections such as prostatitis, pyelonephritis, pneumonia, septic arthritis, peritonitis, cellulitis, bacteremia, postpartum endometritis, and neonatal early- and late-onset disease. In adults the organism infects two groups of patients, young healthy women who undergo obstetric or gynecologic procedures and older patients in their sixties who have underlying disease. Eichoff and colleagues demonstrated a relationship be-

tween diabetes mellitus associated with severe peripheral vascular disease and *S. agalactiae* infection.[3]

EPIDEMIOLOGY

The female lower genital tract is the site of carriage of *S. agalactiae* responsible for postpartum endometritis and neonatal infection. The organism has also been implicated in preterm premature rupture of the membranes and preterm delivery.[4,5] The carriage rates of this organism vary with geographic area, and rates ranging from 5 to 25% have been reported. It appears that the main site of carriage is the rectum, and colonization of the vagina occurs by contamination via the perineum.[6–8] Carriage of the organism has been demonstrated in the urethra and subprepucial area in males. An association has been found between sexual activity and female carriage rates, but an actual connection between *S. agalactiae* and sexual transmission has not been established. Colonization rates were found to be highest in patients attending a venereal disease clinic, but there was no association with other sexually transmitted diseases.[9,10]

Infections in Pregnancy, pages 55–60
© 1990 Alan R. Liss, Inc.

MICROBIOLOGY

Streptococcus agalactiae has the ability to wax and wane within the lower genital tract of patients; however, it is unrealistic to think that the organism actually has this ability. First, the presence of the bacterium in the rectum (the reservoir) probably remains unchanged but is influenced by the other bacteria present. This is probably also true for the vagina. Colonization rates have been shown to vary depending upon the media used to transport and culture the organism.[11,12] One factor that seems to be important in the risk of fetal and neonatal infection is maternal bacteriuria. The presence of *S. agalactiae* in maternal urine in a concentration greater than 10,000 cfu/cc is more likely to be associated with the delivery of infants who are at greater risk for colonization and infection.[13–16] In one study of 858 pregnant women, 186 or 22% were found to be colonized by group B streptococci.[13] The rectum was found to be the most frequently colonized site, and 64 women were found to have bacteriuria with group B streptococci. Urine was obtained at the time of delivery from 1,786 women and *S. agalactiae* was isolated from 7%; 1% of these women harbored more than 10,000 cfu/cc of urine. Two other observations of importance are that maternal bacteriuria is more frequently associated with neonatal pneumonia and postpartum endometritis.[17,18]

Intrauterine infection with *S. agalactiae* has been reported to occur in the presence of ruptured amniotic membranes, but it has also been found to occur in women with intact membranes.[19,20] In one study, the records of 15 neonates who died secondary to group B streptococcus infection were reviewed.[20] Six infants were born to mothers whose membranes were intact; five of the 15 infants did not have any clinical signs of intrauterine infection. All the infants were born after 28 weeks of gestation and weighed under 1,000 g; six of the infants were stillborn. This study is significant in that it points out that intrauterine infection can occur in the presence of intact membranes and infection can also be silent. Thus, when an intrauterine demise occurs, infection should be suspected.

The strategy to combat *S. agalactiae* infection must be concerned with infection in two patients—the mother and fetus. Much has been written concerning the prevention of infection with regard to maternal carriage of *S. agalactiae*. The serotype that appears to be most prevalent in neonatal infection is type III. Pregnant women with low serum antibody to type III are more likely to deliver infants at risk for neonatal infection.[21,22] Sera obtained from pregnant women of lower socioeconomic groups were found to contain higher antibody titers to type III if they were colonized when compared to women who were not colonized.[22] Passive immunization of the fetus by maternal antibody may offer the infant protection from severe disseminated infection.

Maternal infection can be divided into two categories: antepartum infection (i.e., chorioamnionitis) and postpartum infection (i.e., endometritis). Both of these infections can have serious sequelae. For example, chorioamnionitis can result in premature rupture of the membranes and premature labor. The end result may be either intrauterine death or delivery of an infected premature infant who is likely to suffer significant morbidity. The patient who is colonized is also at risk to develop postpartum endometritis, especially if delivered by cesarean section. Infection in this setting is unlike polymicrobial endometritis in that onset of infection is abrupt and usually within 12 hours following delivery. Temperatures are usually markedly elevated ($>102°F$) and tachycardia is invariably present. Spill of infectious exudate may occur from the fallopian tubes resulting in a paralytic ileus and abdominal distention. Bacteriuria is common, and bacteremia and frequently wound infection may also occur.[23,24] Thus it is important that this infection be recognized early to prevent the sequelae that often follow severe sepsis. Specifically, patients with bacteremia are at risk for endocarditis and overt sepsis, which may in turn progress to the development of adult respiratory distress syndrome. Both of these complications are associated with a high degree of mortality.

Prophylaxis against neonatal infection has been proposed by administering antibiotics intrapartum. Women who are colonized and have perinatal risk factors (premature rupture of membranes, premature labor, prolonged rupture of membranes preceding delivery, and intrapartum fever) may represent approximately 5% of an obstetric population. The premature infant represents the group at greatest risk for infection (4%) and accounts for the largest group of infected infants with early-onset disease (and has approximately a 95% fatality rate).[25-27] The route of infection from mother to fetus by either an ascending infection or acquisition of the organism at birth justifies preventive measures. Early-onset infection usually appears within 12 hours of delivery and correlates with the appearance of maternal postpartum endometritis. The prevalence of pneumonia in infected infants, the association of amniotic fluid infection, the frequency of neonatal colonization, and bacteremia all support the concept of prevention.[28-34] Boyer and Gotoff reported a 9% neonatal colonization rate in women given ampicillin prophylaxis, compared to a 51% neonatal colonization rate in women who did not receive prophylaxis.[25] Early-onset infection did not occur in the ampicillin group but did occur in five cases in the control group. Four of the infants developed pneumonia, all had bacteremia, and two neonatal deaths occurred. Postpartum maternal febrile morbidity was more common among the control group, 21% vs. 8%. One postpartum case of endometritis and septicemia occurred in the control group.

Thus, *S. agalactiae* infection poses a significant problem to the mother, fetus, and neonate. Various strategies have been proposed in an attempt to prevent neonatal infection: antepartum screening of the obstetric patient beginning at the first antepartum visit or at 26 weeks, prophylactic administration of antibiotics to laboring women, and the prophylactic administration of antibiotics to the newborn. Boyer et al. randomized 576 intrapartum patients known to be colonized with group B streptococcus to either treatment with ampicillin or no treatment.[35] They found that in the group receiving ampicillin, there was a significant reduction in postpartum colonization with group B streptococcus. More importantly, there were no cases of neonatal early-onset infection in the treatment group, compared to six cases of neonatal infection in the nontreatment group.

It is estimated that the overall neonatal attack rate is approximately 4/1,000 live-births and the mortality rate is 20%. The infants with early-onset disease may develop signs and symptoms within the first few hours of life or may actually present with hypoxia, hypotonia, or respiratory distress at birth. Dillion et al. observed that over a 6-year period 20% of pregnant women in their population were colonized and that approximately 50% of their newborn infants were also colonized.[36] These authors reported that the number of sites colonized in the newborn was the major determinant of the incidence of infection. Infants colonized in three or four sites have an attack rate of 50/1,000, whereas infants colonized at one or two sites have an attack rate of approximately 5/1,000. It is estimated that more than $7 million per year is spent to provide care for women and children infected with group B streptococcus.

MANAGEMENT

Screening of all pregnant patients for colonization by group B streptococcus is not a simple procedure. If nonselective media are used, e.g., blood agar, colonization rates of 4 to 5% will be found. However, if selective broth medium is used, rates as high as 15 to 25% may be found. Thus the problem is identifying the colonized patient and the appropriate time to establish that the individual is colonized. In small private practices, it may be feasible to screen all obstetric patients. However, on large services, such as the Baylor obstetric service, which delivers between 15,000 and 18,000 patients per year, this is neither feasible nor economical. In this setting, patients presenting with premature rupture of membranes, premature labor, cervical bleeding, sexually transmitted disease, or any condition that may necessitate early delivery, should be screened for group B colonization. In those instances in which there is no time to wait for culture results, empiric therapy should be considered. To avoid unnecessary administration of ampicillin to all patients at risk for early delivery, several rapid tests have been evaluated but the results thus far have not been encouraging. An alternative is to perform Gram stains of the endocervical and (catheterized) urine specimens. Specimens for the isolation of group B streptococcus, *Neisseria gonorrhoeae*, *Chlamydia trachomatis*, and herpes simplex should also be sent. If gram-positive cocci are found on the Gram stain, a tentative diagnosis of group B colonization or bacteriuria can be made and the patients started on ampicillin, 2 g every 6 hours until delivery. At delivery, the neonatal service should culture the infant. The placenta may be cultured by obtaining tissue from the bed of the placenta, as well as separating the chorion from the amnion and obtaining a specimen from the opposing surfaces. In addition, blood should also be obtained from the fetal circulation after the umbilical cord has been clamped. This is accomplished by cleansing the cord that is attached to the placenta with betadine and after wiping the betadine off, aspirating 10 cc of umbilical vein blood. The blood is divided into two 5 ml aliquots: one portion is used to inoculate an aerobic and the other an anaerobic blood culture bottle. Maternal ampicillin is continued until the patient has received three postpartum doses, providing she remains afebrile.

Following the protocol outlined above, we have been successful in reducing the infection rate or allowing determination of those individuals at risk. In addition, it has permitted the rapid identification of those infants with infection. If intrauterine bacteremia has occurred, obtaining a large sample of fetal blood via the umbilical vein will yield a larger inoculum than aspirating a 1 or 2 cc sample from the fetus directly. Growth occurs and is detected much sooner. This scheme is not dissimilar to those that have been published by various authors.

Another approach to the prevention of group B beta-hemolytic neonatal infection is active immunization of pregnant women. Infection in the neonate correlates with the presence of type-specific antibodies: individuals with low levels of antibody are more susceptible to disseminated infection. Baker et al. vaccinated 35 pregnant women with a purified type III capsular polysaccharide vaccine.[37] Twenty (57%) developed antibody in response to the vaccine and persisted 3 months postpartum. Sixty-two percent of the induced antibody was IgG and crossed the placenta. Antibody to type III antigen within the infant correlated with that of the mother. Serum samples from neonates with ≥ 2 μg of antibody to type III uniformly promoted effective opsonization, phagocytosis, and bacterial killing in vitro type III strains. This small study presents an alternative to the use of antibiotic prophylaxis to prevent neonatal infection.

SUMMARY

Risk factors for group B streptococcal disease in the newborn include premature rupture of the membranes, premature labor or delivery, and group B streptococcal bacteriuria. Newborns born to mothers without these risk factors have an attack rate of less than 1/1,000 livebirths. In addition, colonized women without these risk factors have an increased risk of delivering an infected infant if they develop intrapartum fever, regardless of gestational age, and are at greater risk for delivering an infant with early-onset disease. The attack rate in this latter group is approximately 130/1,000 livebirths. Prior to embarking on a program to prevent group B streptococcal infection, it would be prudent for physicians to review the incidence of *S. agalactiae* infection in their own hospital. The intent of any preventive program is to decrease the attack rate, but it should not expose large numbers of patients to penicillin unnecessarily.

REFERENCES

1. Lancefield RC, Hare R: Serologic differentiation of pathogenic and nonpathogenic strains of hemolytic streptococci from parturient women. J Exp Med 61:335–349, 1935.
2. Lancefield RC: A serological differentiation of human and other groups of hemolytic streptococci. J Exp Med 57:571–595, 1933.
3. Eichoff TC, Klein JO, Daly A, et al.: Neonatal sepsis and other infections due to group B beta-hemolytic streptococci. N Engl J Med 271:1221–1228, 1964.
4. Regan JA, Chao S, James LS: Premature rupture of membranes, preterm delivery and group B streptococcal colonization of mothers. Am J Obstet Gynecol 141:184–186, 1981.
5. Desa DJ, Treveren CL: Intrauterine infections with group B, beta-hemolytic streptococci. Br J Obstet Gynaecol 91:237–239, 1984.
6. Persson KMS, Bjerre B, Elfstrom L, et al.: Fecal carriage of group B streptococci. Eur J Clin Microbiol 5:156–159, 1986.
7. Dellon HC, Gray E, Pass MA, et al.: Anorectal and vaginal carriage of group B streptococci during pregnancy. J Infect Dis 145:794–799, 1982.
8. Easmon CSF: Group B streptococcus. Infect Control 7:135–137, 1986.
9. Embil JA, Martin TR, Hansen NH, et al.: Group B beta-hemolytic streptococci in the genital tract: A study of foreign clinic populations. Br J Obstet Gynaecol 85:783–786, 1978.
10. Jackson DH, Hinder MS, Stringer J, et al.: Carriage and transmission of group B streptococci among STD clinic patients. Br J Vener Dis 58:334–337, 1982.
11. Badri MS, Azaaneh S, Cruz AC, et al.: Rectal colonization with group B streptococcus: Relation to vaginal colonization of pregnant women. J Infec Dis 135:308–312, 1977.
12. Persson K, Bjerre B, Hanson H, et al.: Several factors influencing the colonization of group B streptococci—rectum probably the main reservoir. Scand J Infect Dis 13:171–175, 1981.
13. Persson K, Bjerre B, Elfstrom L, et al.: Group B streptococci at delivery: High count in urine increases risk for neonatal colonization. Scand J Infect Dis 18:525–531, 1986.
14. Wood EJ, Dellon HC: A prospective study of group B streptococcal bacteriuria in pregnancy. Am J Obstet Gynecol 140:515–520, 1981.
15. Moller M, Borch K, Thomsen AC, et al.: Rupture of fetal membranes and premature delivery associated with group B streptococci in urine of pregnant women. Lancet 2:69–70, 1984.
16. White CP, Wilkins EGL, Roberts C, et al.: Premature delivery and group B streptococcal bacteriuria. Lancet 2:586, 1984.
17. Christensen K, Snenningsen N, Dahlander K, et al.: Relation between neonatal pneumonia and maternal carriage of group B streptococci. Scand J Infect Dis 14:261–266, 1982.
18. Christensen K, Dahlander K, Ingemarsson I, et al.: Relation between maternal urogenital carriage of group B streptococci and post-maturity and intrauterine asphyxia during delivery. Scand J Infect Dis 12:271–275, 1980.
19. Desa DJ, Trevenen CL: Intrauterine infections with group B beta-hemolytic streptococci. Br J Obstet Gynaecol 91:237–239, 1984.
20. Blanc WA: Pathways of fetal and early neonatal infection: Viral placentitis, bacterial and fungal chorioamnionitis. J Pediatr 59:473–496, 1961.
21. Baker CJ, Webb BJ, Kasper DL, et al.: The natural history of group B streptococcal colonization in the pregnant woman and her offspring. II. Determination of serum antibody to capsular polysaccharide from type III, group B streptococcus. Am J Obstet Gynecol 137:39–42, 1980.
22. Baker CJ, Baker DL: Correlation of maternal antibody deficiency with susceptibility to neonatal group B streptococcal infection. N Engl J Med 294:753–756, 1976.
23. Faro S: Group B streptococcus and puerperal sepsis. Am J Obstet Gynecol 138:1219–1220, 1980.
24. Faro S: Group B beta-hemolytic streptococci and puerperal infections. Am J Obstet Gynecol 139:686–689, 1981.
25. Boyer KM, Gotoff SP: Prevention of early onset neonatal group B streptococcal disease with selective intrapartum prophylaxis. N Engl J Med 314:1665–1669, 1986.
26. Boyer KM, Gadzala CA, Bud LI, et al.: Selective intrapartum chromoprophylaxis of neonatal group B streptococcal early onset disease. I. Epidemiologic rationale. J Infect Dis 148:795–801, 1983.
27. Yow MD, Mason EO, Leeds LJ, et al.: Ampicillin prevents intrapartum transmission of group B streptococcus. JAMA 241:1245–1247, 1979.

28. Blanc WA: Amniotic infection syndrome: Pathogenesis, morphology, and significance in circumnatal mortality. Clin Obstet Gynecol 2:705–734, 1959.

29. Benirschke K: Routes and types of infection in the fetus and newborn. Am J Dis Child 99:714–721, 1960.

30. Baker CJ: Early onset group B streptococcal disease. J Pediatr 93:124–125, 1978.

31. Ablow RC, Driscoll SG, Effman EL, et al.: A comparison of early onset group B streptococcal neonatal infection and respiratory distress syndrome of the newborn. N Engl J Med 294:65–70, 1976.

32. Courcol RJ, Roussel-Delvallez M, Puech F, et al.: Quantitative bacteriological analysis of amniotic fluid. Biol Neonate 42:166–175, 1982.

33. Pjati SP, Pildes RS, Jacobs NM, et al.: Penicillin in infants weighing two kilograms or less with early onset group B streptococcal disease. N Engl J Med 308:1383–1389, 1983.

34. Siegel JD, McCracken GH Jr, Threlkeld N, et al.: Single dose penicillin prophylaxis against neonatal group B streptococcal infections: A controlled trial in 18,738 newborn infants. N Engl J Med 303: 769–775, 1980.

35. Boyer KM, Gadzola CA, Kelly PD, et al.: Selective intrapartum chemoprophylaxis of neonatal group B streptococcal early onset disease, III. Interruption of mother-to-infant transmission. J Infect Dis 148: 810–816, 1983.

36. Dillion HC, Hastings MJG, Neill J, et al.: Group B streptococcal carriage and disease: A 6-year prospective study. J Pediatr 110:31–36, 1987.

37. Baker CJ, Rench MA, Edwards MS, et al.: Immunization of pregnant women with a polysaccharide vaccine of group B streptococcus. N Engl J Med 319:1180–1185, 1988.

8

Episiotomy Infection and Dehiscence

John Owen, M.D., and John C. Hauth, M.D.

Since its initial description in 1741 by Sir Fielding Ould, the episiotomy (or more appropriately the perineotomy) has been the subject of much debate, particularly concerning its indications and purported benefits.

The most commonly held opinions in favor of episiotomies are that their use prevents later pelvic relaxation, minimizes trauma to the fetal head, and decreases the incidence of severe perineal laceration. One of the most basic tenets about episiotomy is that it substitutes a clean incision for a ragged tear, thus permitting an easier repair and better healing.[1] Unfortunately, data to support these conjectures are lacking.[2-4] While the advantages of the median episiotomy compared to the mediolateral approach have been well described by Smith, Harris, Beynon, and Kaltreider and Dixon,[5-8] others have expressed concern over the incidence of median episiotomy extension through the external sphincter ani muscle and rectal mucosa.[2,9-11] Authors at institutions primarily using median episiotomies report between a 2 and 8% incidence of complete (third- and fourth-degree) perineal lacerations.[9] Most, however, report a very low incidence of serious complications from either complete perineal lac-

erations or from elective episioproctotomies, as shown in Table 1.[5-30]

The intent of this chapter is to explore the available literature concerning infection, dehiscence, and other related complications of episiotomies and spontaneous perineal lacerations.

ANATOMY OF THE PERINEUM

While a thorough knowledge of the perineal anatomy is needed for the understanding and proper management of episiotomy complications, a complete review is beyond the scope of this chapter. However, reference to a schematized diagram of the important structures may be useful (Fig. 1).

The anterior perineum is supported superficially by the bulbocavernosus muscles, which lie directly beneath the labia majora, and the superficial transverse perineal muscles, whose lateral attachments are the ischial tuberosities. These four muscles join at right angles between the vaginal introitus and anus and have a tendinous attachment to the exterior anal sphincter forming the perineal body. These structures and the overlying vaginal mucosa and perineal skin are usually incised when performing a median

Infections in Pregnancy, pages 61–74
© 1990 Alan R. Liss, Inc.

TABLE 1. Summary of the Incidence of Third- and Fourth-Degree Episiotomy Lacerations and the Resultant Complications

Date	Author	3°/4° incidence (%)	No. of cases	Percentage of complications	Type of complications
1948	Kaltreider and Dixon[8]	5.0	710	12.0	2.5%, Infection 2.1%, Partial dehiscence 4.3%, Fistula 3.0%, Skin separation
1949	Smith[5]	1.85	28	15.0	11.0%, Abscess 4.0%, Fistula
1949	Ingraham et al.[12]	3.1 (3°) 1.7 (4°)	159	1.2	0.6%, Poor healing 0.6%, Required reoperation
1951	D'Errico and Mckeogh[13]	10.5	16		None
1952	McNulty[14]	0.5	75		None
1952	Hofmeister[15]	2.6	60		None
1954	Dodek[16]	0.95	121		None
1955	Cunningham and Pilington[17]	10.75	31		None
1955	Fulshear and Fearl[18]	0.2	37		None
1960	Fleming[19]		130	0.8	Abscess
1960	Jacobs and Adams[20]	2.0	109	6.8	0.9%, Fistula 3.7%, Infection 0.9%, Incontinence
1960	Brantley and Burwell[21]	1.3	134	5.2	0.75%, Fistula
1960	Barter et al.[22]	1.8	272		None
1961	Sieber and Kroon[23]	23.1	410	2.2	0.2%, Fistula 2.0%, Abscess
1961	Wendt and Wolfgram[24]	4.4	22[a]		None
1961	Pilkington et al.[25]	2.2	123[a]	0.8	Abscess
1962	Norris[26]	23.9	225[a]	1.7	Fistula
1963	Taylor[27]		20		None
1964	O'Leary and O'Leary[28]	13.1 (3°) 13.8 (4°)	1,224	0.73	Simple infection No dehiscence, abscesses
1970	Harris[6]	8.4 (3°) 4.6 (4°)	870	3.9	3.7%, Reduced sphincter tone 0.1%, Infection 0.1%, Fistula
1974	Beynon[7]	5.5 (3°) 8.0 (4°)	157	0.6	Fistula
1974	Walker[29]	46.9	262[a]		None
1980	Coats et al.[30]	6.1 (3°)	19		None
1986	Gass et al.[9]	3.9	8		None
1987	Thorp et al.[11]	21.0	39		None
1988	Legino et al.[10]	17.0	743	<1	Rectovaginal fistulae

[a]Includes elective complete perineotomies.

episiotomy. Just superficial to and covering these muscle groups is Colles' fascia, which extends anteriorly and cephalad to become Scarpa's fascia on the abdominal wall. Later-ally, Colles' fascia reaches the ischiopubic rami and becomes contiguous with the fascia lata. Deep to Colles' fascia is the inferior fascia of the urogenital diaphragm. Posterior to

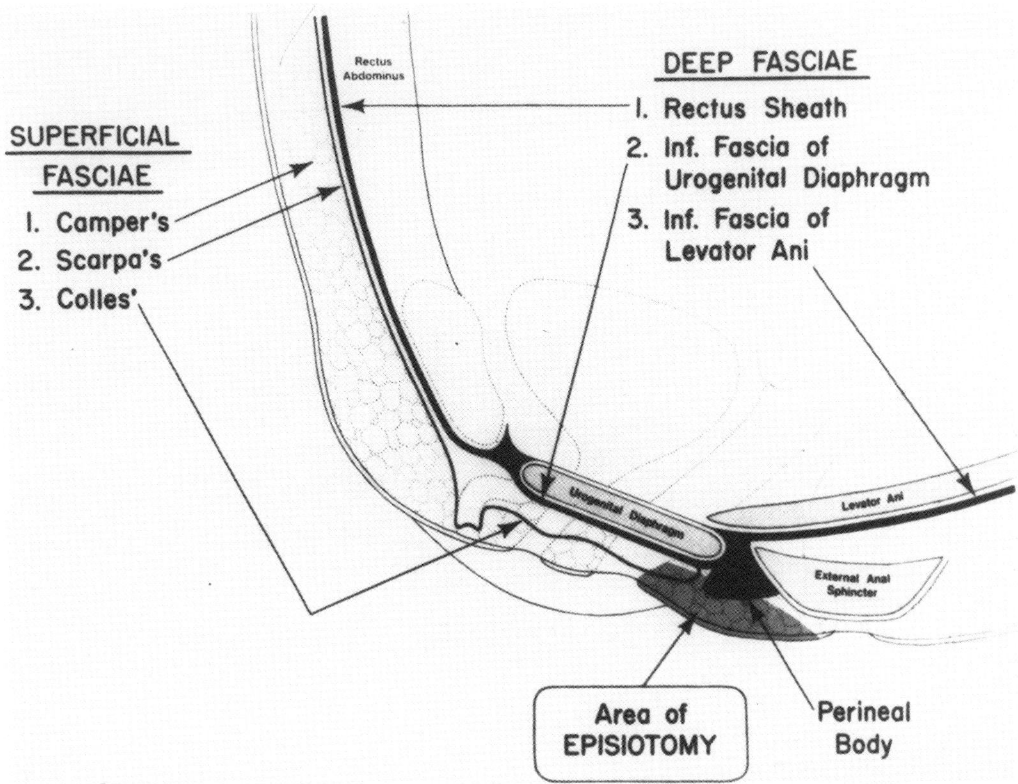

Fig. 1. Sagittal section of the perineum showing the significant muscle groups and fascial layers.(From Shy and Eschenbach,[32] with permission of the publisher.)

Colles' fascia is the fatty tissue in the is-chiorectal fossa that lies between the levator ani group and the gluteus maximus.

COMPLICATIONS

The more serious episiotomy complications include hematomas, cellulitis, abscess formation, and superficial or complete dehiscence. While it is realized that these complications are not infrequently interrelated, they will be discussed separately in the next sections.

Infections

A 1983 review of episiotomy by Thacker and Banta reported that the incidence of episiotomy infections, variously defined, including both median and mediolateral incisions, was between 0.5 and 3.0%.[4] In none of the studies reviewed were control data presented from gravidas with spontaneous lacerations, and therefore the incidence of infections directly attributable to the surgical procedure could not be determined. We have reviewed the available data on 20,713 patients who were delivered at the University of Alabama Hospitals between July 1983 and June 1988. These patients were delivered almost exclusively by the resident staff with attending supervision. All residents are given formal training in the techniques of performing and repairing episiotomy incisions and perineal lacerations. However, the decision to perform an episiotomy and the type of incision used were at the discretion of the physician

TABLE 2. Type of Episiotomy as Related to Parity

Incision	Primipara		Multipara	
	n	(%)	n	(%)
Median	4,822	(63)	4,371	(33)
Mediolateral	79	(1)	79	(<1)
None	2,774	(36)	8,588	(66)
Total	7,675		13,038	

performing the delivery. The resident physicians were neither asked to define their indications for an episiotomy nor were any indications recorded on the delivery records. Usually, episiotomies were performed either to shorten the second stage of labor or to protect the perineum from significant spontaneous lacerations. When spontaneous lacerations occurred, only those requiring repair were recorded.

There were 7,675 primiparas and 13,038 multiparas delivered during the reported time interval (Table 2). As expected, the majority (64%) of the primiparas vs. only 34% of the multiparas had an episiotomy. In both groups, the incidence of mediolateral episiotomy was at or below 1%, reflecting the general trend in obstetrics away from this type of incision.[6,7] As shown in Table 3, our data support the work of others[11,31] in that the incidence of third- and fourth-degree lacerations following a median episiotomy was higher in primiparas (20%) than in multiparas (9%) and that spontaneous lacerations involving the sphincter or rectum were very uncommon without an antecedent episiotomy incision (1% or less). Clearly, selection bias may account for some of the latter discrepancy because the patients believed to be at risk for a significant laceration were usually given an episiotomy. Therefore, the degree to which a median episiotomy predisposes to significant perineal trauma cannot be accurately determined. Nevertheless, the incidence of spontaneous third- and fourth-degree lacerations appears to be very uncommon if the perineum is left intact for the delivery.

Overall, infectious complications were rare, and only 10 infections in 20,713 patients (0.05%) were recorded. However, only those infections discovered prior to discharge were described on the delivery records and were available for analysis. The type of perineal trauma did not appear to have a significant bearing on infectious morbidity, since it was found to occur with vaginal sidewall lacerations, third- and fourth-degree lacerations, and also in cases where no significant extension of the episiotomy incision occurred. Slightly more infections were noted in the primiparas than in the multiparas (7 vs. 3, $P < .05$), and although the numbers are small, it is interesting to note that no infections were recorded in patients who did not have an episiotomy. There were no maternal deaths during this time period that could have been attributed to an episiotomy complication.

Recent studies have indicated that by selectively limiting the use of episiotomy, the overall incidence of perineal trauma is reduced.[11,31] It seems logical that an intact perineum is much less likely to become infected than one that was lacerated, regardless of the method. There are no data to support the concept that a cleanly made incision is less likely to become infected than a ragged tear. In fact, studies have shown that third- and fourth-degree lacerations rarely, if ever, occur without an antecedent midline episiotomy.[9] It is interesting to note that while mediolateral episiotomies are purported to prevent third- and fourth-degree tears, they still occur, albeit with low frequency, usually under 5% in reported series.[4] In our study, we found that 9 and 12% of mediolateral episiotomies in primiparous and multiparous patients resulted in either a third- or fourth-degree extension (Table 3). We are aware of no existing studies that compare the incidence of episiotomy infections with mediolateral as compared to median incisions. Whether higher-degree perineal lacerations are more likely to become infected than first- and second-degree tears has never been conclusively demonstrated; however,

TABLE 3. Degree of Laceration as Related to Type of Episiotomy and Parity

	Primipara						Multipara					
	No episiotomy		Median episiotomy		Mediolateral episiotomy		No episiotomy		Median episiotomy		Mediolateral episiotomy	
Type of laceration	n	(%)	n	(%)	n	(%)	n	(%)	n	(%)	n	(%)
None	2,073	(75)	2,134	(44)[a]	39	(49)	6,411	(75)	2,310	(43)[b]	37	(47)
2°	375	(14)	1,425	(30)	26	(33)	1,095	(13)	1,423	(33)	25	(32)
3° + 4°	52	(1)	968	(20)[a]	7	(9)	44	(<1)	409	(9)[b]	10	(12)
Other[c]	274	(10)	295	(6)[a]	7	(9)	1,038	(12)	229	(5)	7	(9)
Total	2,774		4,822		79		8,588		4,371		79	

[a]Total of seven infections (see text).
[b]Total of three infections (see text).
[c]Other, vaginal sidewall + periurethral + cervical lacerations.

surgical principles would predict that as tissue trauma increases and contaminated areas are entered, infectious complications would become more likely. Therefore, one should strive as much as possible to limit the extent of vaginal tears during delivery. Clearly, morbid outcomes such as rectovaginal fistulas and loss of sphincter function do not occur with lower-degree lacerations.

Episiotomy infections may be divided into four grades of severity as suggested by Shy and Eschenbach, who provide a detailed description and diagnostic criteria of the four types.[32] They point out that this classification scheme refers primarily to the depth of tissue involvement and represents a continuum of infection. Although primarily described in relationship to episiotomy incisions, this classification scheme is no doubt applicable to spontaneous lacerations as well. A condensed description of their work follows.

Simple episiotomy infections include infections limited to the skin and superficial fascia at the incision line. Skin necrosis, systemic symptoms, and bullae formation should not be present. Although this type of infection is rarely life threatening, it may be a cause of significant morbidity. If rapid resolution does not occur with broad-spectrum antimicrobial therapy, the suture line should be opened and debrided with attention to occult hematomas or abscesses. Ultimately the lacera-

tion may be closed and this will be discussed in the section on episiotomy dehiscence. *Superficial fascial infection* is an extension of the infection to the superficial fascia, but necrosis has not yet occurred. The overlying skin is generally edematous and may show rubor. Severe systemic manifestations should not be present. At times, the actual extent of the infection cannot be determined without surgical exploration. Broad-spectrum antibiotics may be tried initially with careful assessment of patient response. However, clinical worsening or failure to respond in 24 to 48 hours should prompt wound exploration.

Superficial fascial necrosis, otherwise known as necrotizing fasciitis, has also been described using many other terms, depending on the offending microbe. Numerous organisms have been cultured from the involved tissues, including gram-positive cocci (typically group A hemolytic streptococci), gram-negative aerobes, and various anaerobic strains. It is postulated that certain organisms may act synergistically to heighten the tissue destruction. In this instance infection has caused destruction of the superficial fascial layers (Colles' fascia on the perineum, Scarpa's fascia on the abdominal wall, and fascia lata on the medial thighs). Normally, these fascial layers prevent deeper invasion; however, at times the superficial fascia of the urogenital diaphragm and other deeper muscle tissues may become involved (myonecrosis).

The overlying skin may show marked edema and rubor early, but with advancing disease, the blood vessels supplying the skin may become occluded and the skin may evidence breakdown with bullae, ulceration, violaceous discoloration, or frank cutaneous necrosis. Crepitation may or may not be present, and negative radiologic demonstration of tissue gas is not of sufficient specificity to dismiss the diagnosis of such a devastating process.[33] While localized tenderness may also be an early feature, nerve ischemia and anesthesia may occur over time. Fisher and colleagues have outlined a descriptive classification for necrotizing fasciitis[34]: 1) extensive necrosis of the superficial fascia with peripheral undermining of normal skin, 2) moderate to severe systemic toxic reaction, 3) absence of muscle involvement, 4) absence of clostridia in wound and blood cultures, 5) absence of major vascular occlusion, and 6) extensive leukocyte infiltration, necrosis, or subcutaneous tissue and microvascular thrombosis on microscopic examination of debrided tissues.

Myonecrosis involves frank destruction of muscle tissue deep to the superficial fascia. Although classically described with clostridial infections, it may involve other organisms initially present in the superficial fascial necrosis.

The literature contains reports of 12 maternal deaths attributable to wound infections resulting from episiotomies and perineal lacerations; these are summarized in Table 4.[32,35-40] The first 11 cases involved necrotizing fasciitis or myonecrosis, while the last death resulted from a retroperitoneal abscess. These serious sequelae are fortunately rare; however, their rarity makes the recognition and treatment that much more difficult for the practicing obstetrician. The cause of death in severe perineal (episiotomy) infections appears to be a combination of massive extracellular fluid accumulation and bacterial sepsis leading to vascular collapse. Interestingly, while these patients may have extremely high white blood counts, they are often afebrile and may have a paucity of symptoms.

As in most pelvic infections, a variety of organisms including polymicrobial infestations may be involved. Often, it may be impossible to culture the offending microbes without surgical debridement, and attempts to culture the perineum and rectum would appear to be of little clinical benefit because of their inherent flora. In particular, obligate anaerobes may be very difficult to successfully culture and require special laboratory techniques and collection methods. The absence of a positive culture in a clear case of clinical infection may in fact be secondary to anaerobic bacteria, and, when suspected, antibiotic therapy should be directed at this possibility. Gram stains of deep tissues may be of use in determining the offending organism and provide immediate information.

Although the issue of underlying medical disease in cases of episiotomy infection has not been directly addressed, the surgical literature supports the concept that patients with impaired defenses, i.e., vascular disease, diabetes mellitus, and other chronic illness, are more susceptible to these types of serious infections. Since an obstetric population is for the most part younger and healthier than a surgical population, and since these infections are rarely seen in obstetrics, the exact contribution of maternal disease is unclear. In fact, the majority of case reports involve ostensibly normal gravidas.

We support the concept of aggressive surgical management in cases of higher-grade episiotomy infections. Reports where surgery was used late or not at all usually relate a poor outcome.[41] Surgery should be performed whenever significant skin changes, including edema, appear outside the local wound area. Failure to respond to antibiotic therapy or clinical worsening of the patient's condition, especially symptoms of systemic toxicity, should also prompt a wound exploration. Many adjunctive therapies have been suggested, including broad-spectrum antibiotics, aggressive fluid therapy, hemodynamic mon-

TABLE 4. Maternal Deaths Associated With Perineal Trauma

Report year	Age	Perineal trauma	Days to diagnosis	Final diagnosis	Initial treatment	Surgery	Pathogen recovered	Underlying medical disease
1986[35]	24	Med.,[a] 3° tear	4	Myonecrosis	Antibiotics and steroids	No[b]	Clostridia, E. coli, Klebsiella	None
1979[32]	21	Med.	6	Fascial necrosis	Local treatment and antibiotics	No	E. coli	None
1979[32]	22	Med.	9	Fascial necrosis	Local incision and antibiotics	No	E. coli, Bacteroides	None
1979[36]	23	Med.	4	Fascial necrosis	Antibiotics	No	Clostridia	None
1979[37]	30	Med., 4° tear	10	Presumed fascial necrosis	Antibiotics, steroids	No	None	None
1979[37]	19	Mediolateral episiotomy	3	Presumed myonecrosis	Antibiotics, hyperbaric O_2	No	E. coli, strep, clostridia	None
1979[38]	19	Procto-episiotomy	2	Presumed fascial necrosis	Antibiotics	Yes[c]	Not cultured	None
1979[38]	16	Med., 3° tear	2	Presumed fascial necrosis	Antibiotics and steroids	No	Not cultured[d]	None
1979[38]	24	Med.	3	Presumed fascial necrosis	Antibiotics and steroids	No	Strep, clostridia, staph	None
1977[39]	30	Med., 4° tear	5	Fascial necrosis	Antibiotics	No	Anaerobic strep, E. coli	None
1977[39]	23	Med., 3° tear	4	Fascial necrosis	Antibiotics and steroids	Yes	Staph, clostridia	None
1972[40]	23	Med., 3° tear[e]	5	Retroperitoneal abscess and hematoma	Antibiotics and heparin[f]	No	E. coli	None

[a]Med., median episiotomy.
[b]Died during preparation for surgery.
[c]Limited to exploration of ischiorectal fossa.
[d]Only lochia cultured.
[e]Suspected rectal involvement with suture or occult 4° tear.
[f]Had concurrent pulmonary embolism.

itoring, hyperbaric therapy, and MAST suit.[42] These techniques are based on sound surgical principles and extrapolations from reports of similar types of infections involving other areas of the body. No controlled studies of these ancillary measures in episiotomy infection are available.

When wound exploration is indicated, it is essential to carry the debridement to healthy tissue margins. Sutton et al. recommend electrocautery as an efficient means of removing obviously diseased tissue,[43] and when viable margins are questionable, the use of frozen sections have been suggested.[33] After adequate debridement has been performed, the resulting wound can be managed in a fashion similar to that of a full-thickness thermal injury. In this situation the use of temporary tissue grafts has been shown to hasten the healing process by reducing the bacterial contamination in preparation for permanent grafts. Several types of tissue have been used successfully for this purpose, including porcine xenografts, cadaveric homografts, and amnion.[44] Porcine xenografts have the advantages of availability and lower cost but must be changed every two days. Cadeveric tissue, while more expensive, may be left in place until the permanent grafts are established. Zarutskie and Silverberg reported the successful use of amnion in a patient with necrotizing fasciitis,[45] although the time required to begin permanent grafting may have been longer than is customary for other types of tissue.

Hematomas

There are few data available that address hematomas associated with episiotomy incisions or spontaneous lacerations. A 1938 series on mediolateral episiotomies by Huff reported a 0.23% incidence of hematomas (1 of 412).[46] We can find no other more contemporary report and postulate that it also is a rare complication. In fact, many hematomas are probably recognized very early, usually at the time of initial repair, and are managed by identification and suturing of the offending vessel.

Unrecognized hematomas, on the other hand, may become infected. The suture line, if it has not already spontaneously parted, should be opened, and the hematoma should be adequately drained. At times, abscess formation may have occurred. These too should be explored, carefully inspected, and permitted to drain. If an abscess or significant concurrent infection is identified, we recommend that antibiotic coverage for the commonly involved pathogens be started and that, after drainage, and wound be managed as a simple episiotomy infection. Clearly, small and nonexpanding vulvar and/or episiotomy hematomas can frequently be managed conservatively with observation, cold compresses, etc. However, there are no data of which we are aware that would give the lower limit of hematoma size that could be safely managed in a conservative fashion. It would seem prudent to evacuate any sizable and/or expanding vulvar or episiotomy hematomas that are clinically apparent remote from an occurrence at the time of vaginal delivery and initial episiotomy or perineal laceration repair.

Episiotomy Dehiscence

The techniques of episiotomy repair, including repair of the most frequent episiotomy complication, which is extension of the incision through the external sphincter ani muscle and rectal mucosa, have been well described.[1] The recommended approach is for a layered closure of all tissue planes beginning with the rectal mucosa, submucosa (rectovaginal septal fascia), the external sphincter ani muscle and fascia, the deep perineal tissue, and the vaginal mucosa and perineal skin. Fortunately, and most likely because of the abundant vascular supply of the perineal region, the vast majority of either median or mediolateral episiotomies heal with few or no long-term sequelae.

Superficial dehiscence. Uninfected simple dehiscence appears to occur rarely, and we are unable to find a reported incidence in the literature. It is conceivable that previous series on episiotomy infections included simple wound breakdowns that, in fact, may have been due to other causes such as mechanical trauma from early intercourse or sycabalous stool with subsequent bowel movement. Positive cultures of the wound should not be the sole criterion in determining if clinical infection is present; other signs of infection such as erythema, purulent drainage, and necrotic tissue should also be visible. The absence of severe pain, edema, and fever should further confirm that significant infection is not present. Management is secondary resuturing once the open wound is covered with healthy pink granulation tissue.

Complete dehiscence (third or fourth degree). Despite the reports in Table 1, little information exists on which to base the management of a dehiscence of a third- or fourth-degree episiotomy laceration repair in the early puerperium. Harris reported loss of external ani sphincter tone after a fourth-degree episiotomy extension but did not note the subsequent management of those women.[6] He did note that the one rectovaginal fistula in his series was repaired 4 months postpartum. Beynon alluded to early puerperal repair of some defects and stated that four cases of median episiotomy dehiscence were resutured before discharge from the hospital.[7] This puerperal resuturing approach has been adopted by other authors.[47,48] However, Beynon did not detail whether these complications involved the rectal mucosa and/or the external sphincter ani muscle.[7] Kaltreider and Dixon also referred to the early puerperal repair of some episiotomy dehiscences.[8] They reported that three of 15 episiotomy breakdowns were resutured on the 10th to 20th postpartum day with good results and that the remainder healed by secondary intention. These authors concluded that "episiotomy breakdowns may be treated by secondary repair in the hospital if infection has subsided," although none of their cases involved the external sphincter ani muscle or rectal mucosa. Jacobs and Adams reported one patient who developed incontinence of stool and required perineorrhaphy, but did not state when it was performed.[20] Sieber and Kroon repaired a single rectovaginal defect 6 weeks postpartum, even though it was discovered on the 6th postpartum day.[23]

Monberg and Hammen reported on 35 patients with a ruptured mediolateral episiotomy.[47] These 35 women were randomized to treatment with either clindamycin and resuturing (20 patients) or wound cleansing and spontaneous healing (15 patients). Patients who had the resuturing had a significantly shorter hospital stay, required fewer outpatient and home health care visits, and resumed coitus sooner. Clinical signs of infection were present in 20 of these 35 women at the time of diagnosis of episiotomy rupture; however, no mention was made whether the episiotomy involved the external sphincter ani muscle or the rectal mucosa. All remaining authors (Table 1) either provided too little detail as to how fourth-degree episiotomy repair dehiscences were

managed or reported no such complications. Cogan and Harris, however, stated that any infected rectal injury should not be repaired for at least 6 months and did not comment on the management of dehiscence without obvious infection.[49]

Thus, few data are available to detail the management of a dehiscence of a primary fourth-degree episiotomy repair. Some authors[50,51] have recommended deferring surgical repair for a minimum of 3 to 4 months, presumably to avoid formation of a rectovaginal fistula or further scarring of the dehiscence and to allow for complete vascularization and healing of the disrupted tissue. However, the evidence for these complications is sparse. We have surmised that the time-honored traditional approach to management of this complication of delaying repair for a minimum of 3 to 4 months was based on the fear of less than adequate local wound cleansing and continued fecal contamination. Additionally, Mattingly and Thompson express concern regarding the need to await revascularization of the tissue margins and the generation of healthy granulation tissue.[50] However, our experience with the biophysical response of these open wounds is similar to that described in Sabiston's *Textbook of Surgery*[52]: incised wounds allowed to remain open begin the healing process normally. An inflammatory exudate collects on the surface; marginal epithelial cells mobilize, divide, and migrate down the edges; injured venules bud, forming capillary networks; and fibroblasts invade the injured area. After 3 or 4 days, the wound surfaces can be closed with sutures or other mechanical devices and healing proceeds normally. Careful bacteriologic investigations demonstrate that heavily contaminated wounds left open can show a marked reduction in bacterial concentration during the first 3 to 6 days.

To avoid the definite disability associated with delayed repair, we have followed a protocol for early puerperal repair of these complications. Hauth et al. have reported eight women who had an early repair of an exter-

TABLE 5. Sequential Techniques for the Immediate Secondary Repair of a Fourth-Degree Episiotomy Dehiscence

Inspection and diagnosis
Initial debridement
Exclusion of infection
Exclusion of clotting abnormalities
Mechanical bowel preparation
Wound cleaning/debridement
Layered secondary wound closure
    Bowel rest
    Wound cleansing/drying
Extended pelvic rest

nal sphincter ani muscle and rectal mucosal dehiscence.[48] All eight presented within 10 days of delivery, six with complete dehiscence of the external sphincter ani muscle and rectal mucosa, one with an episiotomy abscess and complete dehiscence, and one with a large rectovaginal defect cephalad to an intact external sphincter ani muscle. None of these eight women had evidence of a coagulopathy; prothrombin and partial thromboplastin times, fibrinogen levels, platelet levels, as well as bleeding time, were all normal. No selection of patients occurred except the timing of the secondary closure in relation to the optimum local wound preparation.

Our treatment protocol is summarized in Table 5. Each patient underwent preoperative wound cleansing and debridement appropriate to the extent of superficial inflammation and necrosis. This ranged from 1 to 4 days in seven of the eight women and required 6 days in the one patient with an episiotomy abscess. Debridement consisted of removal of all visible suture material and initial superficial sharp resection of all devitalized tissue. Cleansing was accomplished with a povidone-iodine sitz bath three times daily and was continued until the wound was free of exudate and covered with healthy pink, well-vascularized granulation tissue. Well-vascularized wound edges and granulation tissue are pink and bleed superficially from newly formed venule buds when wiped with a gauze sponge. The one patient with the episiotomy abscess and surrounding soft tissue cellulitis was treated with cefoxitin during her preoperative wound preparation.

All eight women had a mechanical bowel preparation consisting of the administration of 6 liters of normal saline through a small nasogastric tube within 12 to 24 hours of admission to the hospital or discovery of the dehiscence. This was accomplished before wound preparation or surgical correction of the fourth-degree episiotomy dehiscence. The bowel flush solution was infused as rapidly (approximately 1 liter per hour) as tolerated, and senna extract or magnesium citrate was added to the first liter of normal saline solution. Potassium chloride (20 mEq) was added to the last liter to prevent hypokalemia and acidosis. Most recently, an oral bowel flush preparation, Golytely, was used, which obviates the need for a nasogastric tube and potassium or bicarbonate replacement.[53]

A similar surgical technique was used in all eight cases. The rectal mucosa was reapproximated with a running submucosal 0000 chromic surgical gut suture. This was reinforced with a layer of rectovaginal septal tissue that was approximated with a 000 chromic surgical gut running suture. No attempt was made to dissect free or specifically suture either the levator or puborectalis muscles. The external sphincter ani muscle was then approximated with four interrupted figure-of-eight suture of 00 chromic surgical gut or polyglactin suture material. Most recently we have sutured the external sphincter ani muscle with 00 polydioxanone (PDS-Ethicon), which retains a tensile strength of 50% at 4 weeks. The remainder of the wound was then repaired as described for a second-degree episiotomy in *Williams Obstetrics*.[1] All eight women were given a prophylactic broad-spectrum antibiotic at the time of the repair and for 7 days postoperatively. The bowel was rested for 10 days after the repair. This was accomplished initially by preventing any oral intake for 72 hours, and thereafter the

TABLE 6. Case Summaries of Eight Women With Dehiscence of a Fourth-Degree Episiotomy Laceration Repair

Presented postpartum day	Wound defect	Infection	Dyspareunia	Result
10	External sphincter ani intact, large rectovaginal defect	No	No	Healed
7	Dehiscence of external sphincter ani and rectal mucosa, vaginal mucosa intact	No	No	Healed
9	Dehiscence of external sphincter ani and rectal mucosa, vaginal mucosa intact	No	No	Healed
9	Complete dehiscence of external sphincter ani, rectal, and vaginal mucosa	No	No	Healed
10	Complete dehiscence of external sphincter ani, rectal, and vaginal mucosa	No	No	Healed
3	Complete dehiscence of external sphincter ani, rectal, and vaginal mucosa	Yes	No	Rectovaginal fistula (vaginal flatus)
2	Complete dehiscence of external sphincter ani, rectal, and vaginal mucosa	No	No	Healed
5	Complete dehiscence of external sphincter ani, rectal, and vaginal mucosa	No	No	Healed

eight women were given a commercial no-residue complete diet. This regimen was effective in preventing a bowel movement until the healing process was well under way and avoided the need for constipating agents and the subsequent passage of hard stool. During the bowel rest phase, local care of the repair consisted of povidone-iodine sitz baths followed by drying with a heating lamp or hair dryer. After 10 days of the above postoperative regimen, the eight women were begun on a regular diet and were provided stool softeners sufficient to prevent constipation with hard stool for at least 6 weeks. The women were discharged from the hospital after 10 days and upon resumption of bowel movements. Coitus was prohibited for 6 weeks.

Using the above prospective protocol, seven of the eight patients were successfully repaired with complete healing, normal ex-ternal sphincter ani muscle function, and no dyspareunia. The follow-up intervals in seven of eight women were 6 months or longer (Table 6). One patient complained of vaginal flatus but none of these eight women had any incontinence of stool on their follow-up visits. A small rectovaginal fistula causing vaginal flatus was found in one patient during an anoscopic examination 4 months postoperatively. The fistula coursed through the external sphincter ani muscle. This was repaired 6 months postpartum by an anal flap technique that consisted of covering the rectal end of the fistula tract with a mobilized 1 cm flap of anal mucosa and transrectal cauterization of the fistula tract. Anoscopic examination 3 weeks postoperatively was normal and this patient had no recurrent symptoms in 3 years of follow-up.

We have since expanded our observations with early repair of dehiscence of fourth-degree episiotomies from eight to 22 cases.[54] Significant complications were limited to the development of a small rectovaginal fistula in two (9.1%) of the 22 women with early repair of a fourth-degree dehiscence. This complication rate is similar to that reported with delayed repairs, which have a reported failure rate of approximately 10%.[51] Both pinpoint fistulae in our series were corrected by creation of a small rectal flap. While 18% of these women had occasional incontinence for stool or flatus at 6 months post repair, all were fully continent by 9 months.

Our results indicate that dehiscence of a fourth-degree episiotomy laceration repair and large rectovaginal defects can be successfully accomplished in the puerperium. The repairs were safe, effective, and avoided the prolonged period of disability and stool incontinence inherent to a delayed secondary repair. We must emphasize, however, that preoperative bowel and wound preparation is of paramount importance. Under no circumstances should the wound be secondarily closed unless the wound margins are covered with healthy pink, well-vascularized granulation tissue. In the absence of healthy tissue margins, the risk of subsequent rectovaginal fistula formation could be a serious complication of an early closure. In a review of 32 women who had a delayed repair of complete perineal lacerations, Given and Browning also emphasized the importance of a careful mechanical and antimicrobial bowel preparation.[51] In their series, all six patients who had a Warren flap method of repair had function completely restored. Of the 20 women who had a layered repair and adequate follow-up, 16 had function completely restored, two had improved function, and two failures occurred (10%). Overall function was improved in 92% and completely restored in 85%. It is likely that some of these failures with a delayed closure and the need for paradoxical sphincterotomies, as suggested by Miller and Brown in 1937[55] and as recommended by Given and Browning,[51] relate to the marked wound and tissue contracture

that occurs with open wounds if secondary closure is not accomplished. If delayed closure is not performed or if tissues have been lost, a remarkable change in the physical dimensions of the wound occurs with time. After a delay of 2 or 3 days, open wound margins move toward each other, making the surface defect smaller. The propensity of open wounds to contract is well known. In areas where mobile skin is important, contraction produces serious functional abnormalities and deformities, such as in the perineum and rectovaginal septum.

Remaining questions relate to the initial presence of infection as a contraindication to immediate as compared to delayed secondary repair of a fourth-degree episiotomy dehiscence. To date we have successfully repaired two women whose fourth-degree episiotomy dehiscence was complicated by an episiotomy abscess and surrounding cellulitis. Within 4 and 7 days, abscess drainage, wound debridement, local wound care, and antimicrobial therapy resulted in a healthy wound with normal granulation tissue and no surrounding cellulitis. The dehiscence was successfully closed secondarily on the 8th and 13th postpartum days in these two patients.

Is the described mechanical bowel preparation, local wound care, and postoperative bowel rest essential for a successful secondary closure? Given and Browning reported 14 successful repairs in patients who had an adequate bowel preparation, and two failures occurred in the 10 women with an inadequate bowel preparation.[51] We also used a mechanical bowel preparation and prolonged bowel rest in our first series of eight women who had a secondary closure in the immediate puerperium. Cogan and Harris[49] and Mattingly and Thompson[50] argue against an early secondary closure of a fourth-degree episiotomy dehiscence because an unacceptably high failure or rectovaginal fistula rate has previously resulted. However, these adverse results occurred prior to the use of the outlined perioperative techniques. Therefore, in consideration of prior adverse results, we favor use of the described protocol until an unselected series of successful early secondary closures of fourth-degree episiotomy dehiscence is reported without the use of bowel preparation, etc.

Lastly, we can find little data on which to base recommendations regarding subsequent routes of delivery. Following secondary closure in the immediate puerperium we have recommended a trial of labor if the patient's bowel function and perineal anatomy are normal and in the absence of extensive and palpable rectovaginal septum scar formation. However, following delayed repair of old complete perineal lacerations, Given and Browning reported that one of these women developed a 1.5 cm rectovaginal fistula following a vaginal delivery.[51] Those authors recommended that the safest course would be a cesarean delivery.

SUMMARY

This chapter has described some general aspects about the use of the episiotomy in obstetrics, with an emphasis on infections and the management of other serious complications. Our review was constrained by the paucity of recent well-designed research studies in this area, and it is apparent that numerous important questions about episiotomies remain without conclusive answers. The older literature appears to be based to a large extent on anecdotal opinions and not scientific fact. To some extent, our current obstetric practices appear to be a carryover from this era, and we would encourage the infusion of new data into the literature. Of particular interest would be controlled studies of the incidence of infections associated with episiotomies and spontaneous lacerations, significant risk factors for complications, pertinent microbiologic data, and optimum management strategies and repair techniques. Other valuable goals would be attempts to better determine the incidence of long-term genital complications from vaginal birth with respect to the type of perineal trauma at delivery and to better define the indications for and benefits of an intentional incision of the perineum.

REFERENCES

1. Pritchard JA, MacDonald PC, Gant NF: "Williams Obstetrics," 17th edition. Norwalk, CT: Appleton-Century-Crofts, 1985, chapter 17.
2. Hofmeyr GJ, Sonnendecker EWW: Elective episiotomy in perspective. S Afr Med J 71:357–359, 1987.
3. Harrison RF, Brennan M, North PM, Reed JV, Wickham EA: Is routine episiotomy necessary? Br Med J 288:1971–1975, 1984.
4. Thacker SB, Banta HD: Benefits and risks of episiotomy: An interpretative review of the English language literature, 1860–1980. Obstet Gynecol Surv 38:322–338, 1983.
5. Smith SH: The median episiotomy. Its technique and a review of 1500 cases. West J Surg 59:102–109, 1949.
6. Harris RE: An evaluation of the median episiotomy. Am J Obstet Gynecol 106:660–665, 1970.
7. Beynon CL: Midline episiotomy as a routine procedure. J Obstet Gynaecol Br Commonw 81:126–130, 1974.
8. Kaltreider DF, Dixon DM: A study of 710 complete lacerations following central episiotomy. South Med J 41:814–820, 1948.
9. Gass MS, Dunn C, Stys SJ: Effect of episiotomy on the frequency of vaginal outlet lacerations. J Reprod Med 31:240–244, 1986.
10. Legino LJ, Woods MP, Rayburn WF, McGoogan LS: Third- and fourth-degree perineal tears. 50 years' experience at a university hospital. J Reprod Med 33:423–426, 1988.
11. Thorp JM Jr, Bowes WA Jr, Brame RG, Cefalo R: Selected use of midline episiotomy: Effect on perineal trauma. Obstet Gynecol 70:260–262, 1987.
12. Ingraham HA, Gardner MM, Heus EG: A report on 159 degree lacerations. Am J Obstet Gynecol 57:730–735, 1949.
13. D'Errico E, Mckeogh RP: Complete perineotomy. Am J Obstet Gynecol 62:1333–1337, 1951.
14. McNulty JV: Third degree laceration at delivery. Etiological considerations and a technique for repair. Calif Med 77:326–329, 1952.
15. Hofmeister FJ: Reconstructive perineal repair of rectovaginal fistulas and injuries occurring at partuition. Am J Surg 84:566–573, 1952.
16. Dodek SM: Anal and rectal injuries during delivery. Am J Proctol 5:42–46, 1954.
17. Cunningham CB, Pilington JW: Complete perineotomy. Am J Obstet Gynecol 70:1225–1231, 1955.

18. Fulshear RW, Fearl CL: The third degree laceration in modern obstetrics. Am J Obstet Gynecol 69:786–793, 1955.

19. Fleming AR: Complete perineotomy. Obstet Gynecol 16:172–174, 1960.

20. Jacobs WM, Adams BD: Midline episiotomy and extension through the rectal sphincter. Surg Gynecol Obstet 111:245–246, 1960.

21. Brantley JT, Burwell JC: A study of fourth degree perineal lacerations and their sequelae. Am J Obstet Gynecol 80:711–714, 1960.

22. Barter RH, Parks J, Tyndal C: Median episiotomies and complete perineal lacerations. Am J Obstet Gynecol 80:654–662, 1960.

23. Sieber EH, Kroon JD: Morbidity in the third-degree laceration. Obstet Gynecol 19:677–680, 1962.

24. Wendt WP, Wolfgram R: Episirectomy. Obstet Gynecol 18:626–630, 1961.

25. Pilkington JW, Cunningham C, Johnson R: Median episiotomy and complete perineotomy. South Med J 56:284–286, 1963.

26. Norris F: Episioproctotomy. Surg Clin North Am 42:947–954, 1962.

27. Taylor W: Continuing use of episirectomy. Nebr Med J 43:329–330, 1963.

28. O'Leary JL, O'Leary JA: The complete episiotomy. Analysis of 1224 complete lacerations, spincterotomies, and episioproctotomies. Obstet Gynecol 25:235–240, 1964.

29. Walker JL: Complete perineal incision for delivery. South Med J 67:265–268, 1974.

30. Coats PM, Chan KK, Wilkins M, et al.: A comparison between midline and mediolateral episiotomies. Br J Obstet Gynaecol 87:408–412, 1980.

31. Sleep J, Grant A, Garcia J, Elbourne D, Spencer J, Chalmers I: West Berkshire perineal management trial. Br Med J 289:587–590, 1984.

32. Shy KK, Eschenbach DA: Fatal perineal cellulitis from an episiotomy site. Obstet Gynecol 54:292–298, 1979.

33. Stamenkovic I, Lew PD: Early recognition of potentially fatal necrotizing fasciitis. N Engl J Med 310:1689–1693, 1984.

34. Fisher JR, Conway MJ, Takeshita RT, et al: Necrotizing fasciitis. Importance of roentgenographic studies for soft-tissue gas. JAMA 241:803–806, 1979.

35. Soper DE: Clostridial myonecrosis arising from an episiotomy. Obstet Gynecol 68:26S–28S, 1986.

36. Scott WC: Discussion of reference 40. N Engl J Med xxx:177, 1979.

37. Hibbard LT: Discussion of reference 40. N Engl J Med xxx:178, 1979.

38. Ewing TL, Smale LE, Elliott FA: Maternal deaths associated with postpartum vulvar edema. Am J Obstet Gynecol 134:173–179, 1979.

39. Golde S, Ledger WJ: Necrotizing fasciitis in postpartum patients: A report of four cases. Obstet Gynecol 50:670–673, 1977.

40. Jewett JF: Committee on Maternal Welfare: Fatal perineal sepsis. N Engl J Med 286:1213–1214, 1972.

41. Stone HH, Martin JD: Synergistic necrotizing cellulitis. Ann Surg 175:702–711, 1972.

42. Pearse CS, Magrina JF, Finley BE: Use of MAST suit in obstetrics and gynecology. Obstet Gynecol Surv 39:416–422, 1984.

43. Sutton GP, Smirz LR, Clark DH, Bennett JE: Group B streptococcal necrotizing fasciitis arising from an episiotomy. Obstet Gynecol 66:733–736, 1985.

44. Salisbury RE, Carnes R, McCarthy LR: Comparison of the bacterial clearing effects of different biological dressings on granulating wounds following thermal injury. Plast Reconstr Surg 66:596–598, 1980.

45. Zarutskie P, Silverberg F: Amniotic membranes as a temporary wound dressing in necrotizing fasciitis. Obstet Gynecol 64:284–287, 1984.

46. Huff GD: Mediolateral episiotomy. Calif West Med 48:177–179, 1938.

47. Monberg J, Hammen S: Ruptured episiotomia resutured primarily. Acta Obstet Gynecol Scand 66:163–164, 1987.

48. Hauth JC, Gilstrap LC, Ward SC, Hankins GDV: Early repair of an external sphincter ani muscle and rectal mucosal dehiscence. Obstet Gynecol 67:806–809, 1986.

49. Cogan JE, Harris JW: Rectal complications after perineorrhaphy and episiotomy. Arch Surg 93:634–637, 1966.

50. Mattingly RF, Thompson JD: "Te Linde's Operative Gynecology," 6th edition. Philadelphia: J.B. Lippincott, 1985.

51. Given FTJr, Browning G: Repair of old complete perineal lacerations. Am J Obstet Gynecol 159:779–784, 1988.

52. Sabiston DC: "Davis-Christopher Textbook of Surgery," 12th edition. Philadelphia: W.B. Saunders, 1981.

53. Beck DE, Harford FJ, DiPalma JA: Comparison of cleansing methods in preparation for colonic surgery. Dis Colon Rectum 28:491–495, 1985.

54. Hankins GDV, Hauth JC, Gilstrap LC, Hammond TL, Yeomans ER, Snyder RR: Early surgical repair of episiotomy dehiscence. (in press).

55. Miller NF, Brown W: The surgical treatment of complete perineal tears in the female. Am J Obstet Gynecol 34:196–209, 1937.

9

Soft Tissue Infection

Sebastian Faro, M.D., Ph.D.

Postoperative wound infections are among the most frequently occurring nosocomial infections, second to postoperative endometritis, and may result in significant morbidity and, rarely, mortality. The incidence of wound infection varies according to the preceding events. In clean operations, 1–5% of patients will develop a postoperative wound infection, whereas in clean-contaminated procedures, the incidence is 3 to 10%. In contaminated procedures, the incidence ranges between 15 and 20%, and in dirty cases, the incidence may be as high as 30 to 40%.[1] The areas in which wound infections can occur are the episiotomy site, the infraumbilical incision following minilaparotomy for bilateral tubal ligations, and the abdominal incision following cesarean section. The perineum is extremely resistant to infection and can withstand a considerable amount of bacterial contamination. However, the tissues of the abdominal wall are less resistant to infection, and therefore the frequency of wound infection following cesarean section is much higher. The consequences of a wound infection are an increase in the length of hospital stay, the frequency of outpatient visits, increased hospital costs, and a greater loss of personal income, not to mention the patient'

mental anguish and anger. Wound infections are also a common cause of litigation.

CLASSIFICATION

Wounds are classified as clean, clean-contaminated, contaminated, or dirty, depending upon areas of the body entered or events preceding the creation of a wound (Table 1). The classification of the wound is important, because the particular type of wound or circumstances concerning the wound have a bearing on the relative risk of infection. A clean wound, made by sharp incision with sterile instruments, is nontraumatic. The wound is not infected nor is it inflamed. These wounds are elective, closed primarily, and drains are not used. Clean-contaminated wounds are elective wounds that enter an area contaminated with bacteria, e.g., the genitourinary tract. Contaminated wounds are usually recent traumatic wounds, but also include elective wounds where there has been a major break in sterile technique and incisions made in an area of acute, nonpurulent inflammation. A dirty wound involves an area of infection or perforated viscera.

Infections in Pregnancy, pages 75–90
© 1990 Alan R. Liss, Inc.

TABLE 1. Classification of Wounds

Clean
  Nontraumatic
  No inflammation
  Sterile technique maintained

Clean-contaminated
  Bacterial contaminated areas entered
  Urinary tract
  Respiratory tract
  Gastrointestinal tract
  Minor break in sterile technique

Contaminated
  Significant spillage from gastrointestinal tract
  Traumatic wound, recent major break in sterile
    technique
  Entrance of urinary tract in presence of infected
    urine

Dirty wound
  Presence of pus or infection
  Incision of noninfected tissue to achieve drainage
    of abscess
  Perforated viscus
  Traumatic wound with necrotic tissue, foreign
    bodies, fecal contamination

TABLE 2. Risk Factors for Wound Infection

Endogenous
  Age
  Malnutrition
  Obesity
  Presence of remote infection
  Chronic disease, e.g., diabetes

Exogenous and environmental
  Improper handwashing
  Improper preparation of operative site
  Preoperative hospitalization
  Duration of operation

PREVENTION

Factors that contribute to an increase in the incidence of wound infections can be divided into three categories: exogenous, environmental, and endogenous (Table 2). A major exogenous factor that contributes to an increased risk in wound infection is the transportation of bacteria on the hands of medical personnel coming in contact with the patient. The most important preventive measure in reducing the risk of infection is hand washing prior to examining or tending to the patient. Physicians, nurses, phlebotomists, respiratory technicians, or anyone who comes into physical contact with a patient should wash their hands immediately after concluding their examination or procedure. When making ward rounds, hands should be washed when entering the ward and after each time contact has been made with a patient. The preoperative scrub significantly reduces the bacterial count on the hands; however, with prolonged operative procedures, the bacterial count increases in direct relationship to the time required to complete the operative procedure.[2] Several studies have shown that during operative procedures, 30% of the gloves worn by surgeons are perforated at sometime during the procedure.[3] A preoperative scrub of 6 minutes reduces the bacterial count of the skin by approximately one-half.[2] Dineen, in 1969, reported no difference in bacterial counts of surgeons' hands at the conclusion of operative procedures, regardless of whether the preoperative scrub lasted 5 or 10 minutes.[4] The antiseptic agent used to wash the hands is also important. Povidone-iodine has an immediate effect of killing bacteria, but has no prolonged effect. After the hands are dried, there is no inhibitory or killing effect of the povidone-iodine while the surgeons' hands are gloved, thus allowing the bacteria present to reproduce. During the operation, especially procedures lasting longer than 2 hours, the hands become moist, the temperature becomes elevated, and conditions are conducive for bacterial growth.[5] Thus, antiseptics have been developed that have a lasting killing effect. Studies have shown that a hexachlorophene scrub leaves a residue on the skin and has the advantage over povidone-iodine of having a prolonged bactericidal effect. The disadvantages of hexachlorophene are that its action is slow, it is absorbed slowly through the skin, and thus may exhibit toxicity to the individual user. It is for the latter reason that hexachlorophene has been replaced by chlorohexidine, which combines the antiseptic action of povidone-iodine and hexachlorophene but does not have the toxicity of the latter.

A preoperative shower with chlorohexidine has been shown to be as effective as a hexachlorophene shower in reducing the incidence of wound infections.[6] Comparative studies have shown that preoperative showers with an antiseptic vs. soap and water reduce the incidence of wound infection by 5%. In one double-blinded control study, patients who showered with 4% chlorohexidine had lower mean colony counts of bacteria at the surgical incision site prior to the final scrub than patients who showered with povidone-iodine or medicated bar soap. Bacteria were recovered from 4% of the patients who were scrubbed with chlorohexidine, 9% of the patients who were scrubbed with povidone-iodine, and 15% of those who showered with medicated soap and were scrubbed with povidone-iodine.[7] Local skin preparation and the timing of and mechanism of removal of hair prior to the operation have a major effect on the infection rate. Patients who are shaved more than 2 hours prior to surgery had an infection rate of 2.3%, whereas patients who had their hair clipped had an infection rate of 1.7%. Patients who did not undergo hair removal had an infection rate of 0.9%.[8] Mechanical removal of hair just prior to the operative procedure does not allow for enough time to elapse for the bacteria to colonize and reproduce in the minute lacerations of the skin.[8,9]

The operative site and adjacent areas should be thoroughly cleansed with a germicide (antiseptic), taking care not to cause breaks in the skin. Germicides (agents that kill microorganisms) are divided into two categories: antiseptics (agents applied to living tissue) and disinfectants (agents used to sterilize inanimate objects). Disinfectants should not be used on living tissue because these agents denature protein and are toxic to living tissue. Therefore, instruments that are sterilized in a disinfectant should be thoroughly rinsed in sterile water prior to being used. Antiseptics such as chlorohexidine are well suited for cleansing the operative site because they are active against gram-positive and gram-negative bacteria. In addition, their action is prolonged because a residue remains on the skin. Preoperative scrubbing of the patient should be performed by trained personnel, using meticulous aseptic technique.

Another contributing factor that can influence the nosocomial infection rate is the duration of preoperative hospitalization. There is a direct correlation between the incidence of infection and the length of time the patient is hospitalized preoperatively. A 1-day preoperative hospitalization is associated with a wound infection rate of approximately 1%. Patients who are hospitalized for 7 days prior to their operation have a 2% risk of developing a wound infection, and if the hospitalization exceeded 14 days, the expected rate of infection is 3–4%.[10]

The duration of the operation also contributes to the risk of infection. Each hour required to complete the operation may result in a doubling of the risk of infection. The reasons for this significant increasing risk of infection are not understood, but several possibilities exist. The bacterial inoculum size, commonly found in wound infections, increases with time. Many of these organisms have short reproductive times, especially the gram-positive aerobes and gram-negative facultative anaerobes. The rapid metabolic and reproductive rates cause a change in the environment within the wound, producing an ever-increasing anaerobic environment, which factors the growth of obligate anaerobes. Because there is a great likelihood that bacteria colonizing the wound originate from the lower genital tract, the anaerobes are likely to be present. Women who have labor with ruptured membranes and are delivered by cesarean section, especially for cephalopelvic disproportion, are at significant risk for developing a polymicrobial mixed aerobic and anaerobic wound infection. Where the presenting part is elevated out of the pelvis, vaginal fluid containing many bacteria is brought up through the abdominal incision with delivery of the fetus. In addition, prolonged exposure of the tissue to the atmosphere causes tissue drying, which results in cellular damage and breakdown, and thus the leakage of serum-containing nutrients into the wound. The tissue is also traumatized by the surgical instruments, i.e., retractors, clamping of tissue-containing vessels, placing of suture to achieve hemostasis and to obliterate dead space, again resulting in cellular breakdown.

Improper use of electrocoagulation can contribute to a great deal of tissue necrosis, which may not be readily apparent, and thus lead to the collection serum that serves as an excellent culture material. The common errors made when using electrocoagulation are coagulating large areas of tissue surrounding a bleeding vessel, grasping large amounts of tissue surrounding a bleeding vessel for coagulation, and grasping tissue with sharp instruments instead of atraumatic instruments. Another common error made when using electrocoagulation is "the dabbing technique," in which the flat blade of the electrocautery is used and the operator dabs it over a large area to reduce oozing of blood. This results in the destruction of large surfaces of tissue and also causes deeper tissue damage (Figs. 1, 2). Impairment of deeper capillaries results in tissue hypoxia, which contributes to infection rates.

Incisions made with the use of electrosurgery are three times more likely to become infected than those made with a scalpel.[11] Cruse and Foord, in a prospective study, found that incisions made with electrosurgery became infected twice as often as those made by traditional means.[6] Thus, electrocoagulation should not be used for the purpose of cutting through skin, subcutaneous tissue, fascia, muscle, or peritoneum. Instead, pinpoint electrocoagulation should be used for achieving hemostasis, and the voltage should be set at the lowest value needed to cause thrombosis of a vessel. Large vessels should

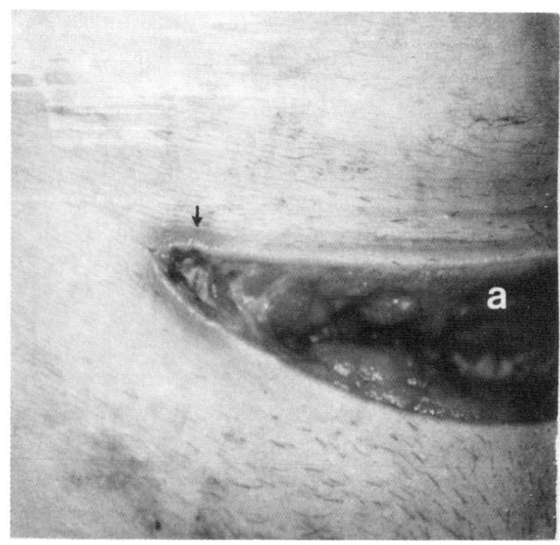

Fig. 1.   Arrow indicates necrotic tissue secondary to electrocauterization to achieve hemostasis. a, open abdominal wound.

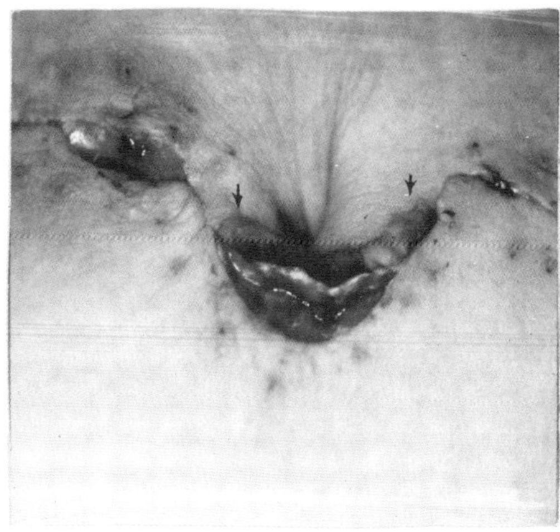

Fig. 2.   Arrows indicate area of burn secondary to electrocautery. Wound edges separated spontaneously because of necrosis.

be ligated and not coagulated, as coagulation results in the destruction of a large amount of tissue. Heated instruments used to make incisions, such as the heated scalpel, have been shown to interfere with the wound's inherent resistance to infection and healing.[12] Thus, the use of electrocautery or coagulation in the patient undergoing cesarean section should be limited to cauterization of small vessels, using pinpoint electrocoagulation, and employing minimum power.

In tissue that tends to weep, or if dead space is present, the use of drains should be considered when the wound is closed. Drains should not exit through the wound and closed suction drains should be employed.[6,13] Studies have demonstrated that higher infection rates are associated with Penrose drains exiting through the incision (7–8%), as compared to a Penrose exiting through a separate incision well away from the original incision (2%). A lower infection rate is associated with a closed suction drainage system (1%), exiting through a stab wound away from the operative incision. The advantage of a closed drainage system over a Penrose drain is that the latter acts as a wick providing a two-directional flow—fluid exits out of the drain but bacteria from the skin can migrate up the drain—thereby colonizing and infecting the deeper tissues of the wound. The closed drainage system allows for the removal of stagnant fluid and blood, allowing for the replacement of fresh fluid containing opsonins, which are necessary to prepare the bacteria for phagocytosis by the host's WBCs. Fluid can also be removed for Gram staining and culture in patients who are suspected of being infected.

The presence of dead space in an incision has always been considered to be a potential site for a wound infection. The tendency for almost all surgeons is to close the dead space by approximating opposing tissue with suture; however, closing the dead space may contribute to the risk of infection.[14,15] Closing or obliterating dead space by suturing results in tissue ischemia and necrosis (Fig. 3). The presence of suture in the tissue that may have become contaminated by bacteria during the operative procedure may encourage infection, since the inoculum required is much lower in the presence of suture. If it is necessary to place suture in the subcutaneous tissue to approximate the cut surfaces and to facilitate obliteration of the dead space, this can be accomplished by placing a few inter-

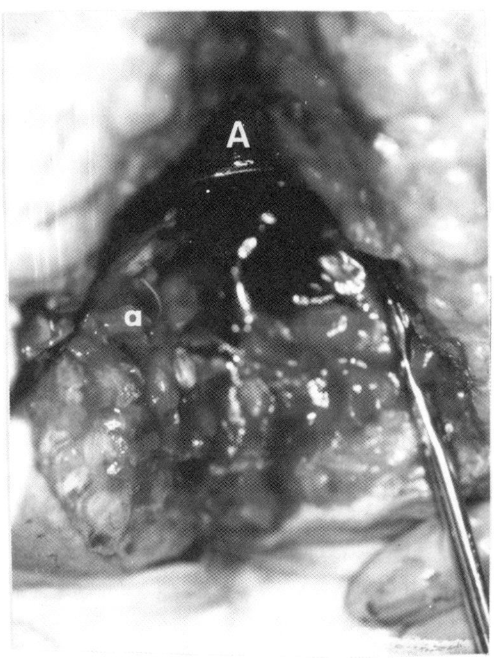

Fig. 3. Vertical abdominal incision with hematoma (A), which prevented wound healing. Note presence of subcutaneous suture (a), the probable cause of bleeding in the wound. Subcutaneous drains larger than 2 inches may have helped prevent this complication.

rupted sutures that are loosely tied. Care should be taken not to cause tissue necrosis or tearing of the tissue (Fig. 4). It serves no beneficial purpose to close the subcutaneous tissue with running sutures in multiple layers. The dead space should be obliterated by approximating the tissue edges by using a dressing that applies gentle pressure to oppose the tissue edges and collapse the potential space that may be present.

The patient herself may have inherent significant risk factors. Nutritional status of the patient is important. Patients who are malnourished are definitely at increased risk for the development of postoperative infection. Altered nutritional status, such as diabetes and obesity, is associated with increased frequency of postoperative infection. The incidence of wound infection for these groups of

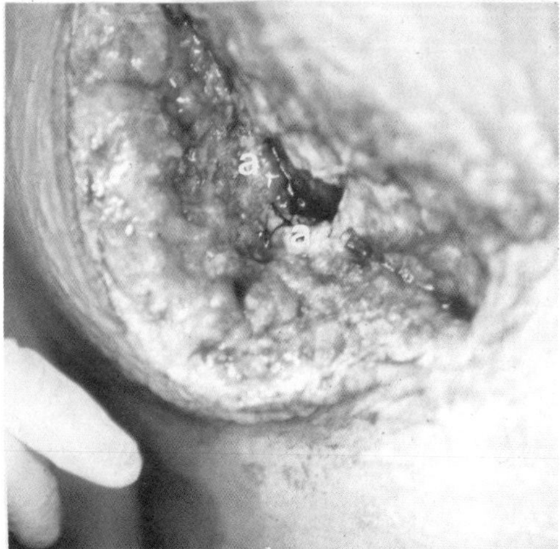

Fig. 4. Fascial dehiscence. The suture (a) was placed close to the fascial edge and was placed under too much tension, which resulted in tearing of the fascia.

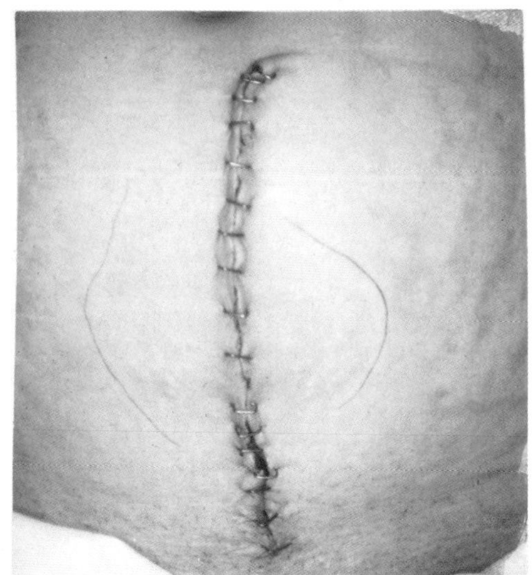

Fig. 5. Lines drawn on abdomen mark the borders of cellulitis. This area is erythematous and indicates early wound infection.

patients was found to be 16% for malnourished patients, 8% for diabetic patients, and 7% for obese patients.[16] Perhaps the most important endogenous host factor is local tissue resistance factors. Halsted stressed that the most important factors in reducing the risk of postoperative infection were strict adherence to the principles of surgical technique.[44] The surgeon must be meticulous in his or her surgical technique, achieving complete hemostasis while maintaining an adequate blood supply. In addition, the physician should debride devitalized tissue, obliterate dead spaces, utilize fine suture, and should not place the layers of the wound under tension. Obeying the principles of good surgical technique will not interfere with the host's inherent resistance to infection. Elegant studies performed by Elek and Conen demonstrated that if silk or monofilament suture were placed in the skin that only 100 colonies of *Staphylococcus aureus* were necessary to establish an infection. If the suture were omitted, then more than a million colonies of bacteria were necessary to establish an infection.[17] Other investigators have

shown that the inoculum size required to induce infection could be reduced if tissue were incorporated into the ligation. The bacterial count or inoculum size is critical in establishing an infection. Experimental studies revealed that for a wound to become infected, a million bacteria or greater per gram of tissue are required.[18,19] The specific type of aerobe or facultative anaerobic bacteria is not important; it is the inoculum size that is critical, which can be influenced by the presence of a foreign body.

If a wound contains pus or exudate, it is best to aspirate this fluid and place it in an anaerobic container and process for aerobic as well as anaerobic bacteria (Figs. 5, 6). If the wound requires significant debridement, excision of tissue measuring $2 \times 1 \times 0.5$ cm should be performed. The specimen, like all specimens, should be placed in an anaerobic transport vial. This specimen can be processed for quantitative bacteriology.[20,21] All specimens should be Gram stained because this will allow the appropriate choice of antibiotic; for example, if the Gram stain reveals the presence of mainly gram-positive

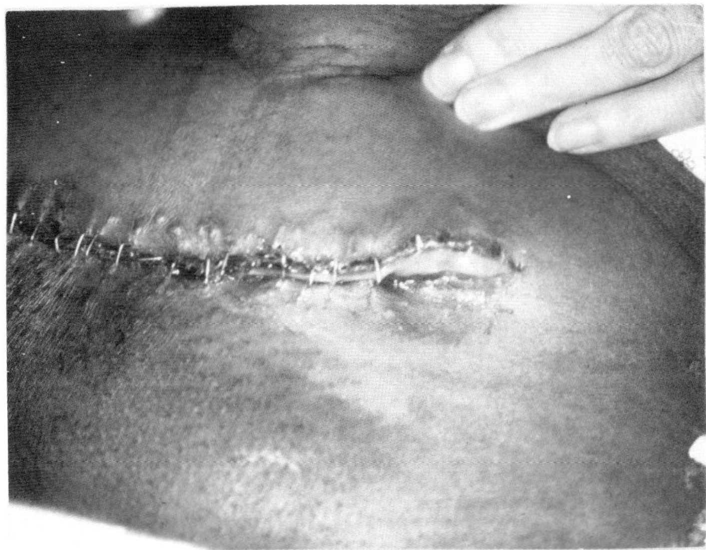

Fig. 6. Spontaneous separation of the wound edges with purulent fluid draining from left side of the wound.

cocci, then a broad-spectrum penicillin such as ticarcillin/clavulanic acid or ampicillin/sulbactam should be used. However, if only gram-negative rods are present, perhaps a broad-spectrum cephalosporin should be used (cefotaxime, cefotetan, cefoxitin, or ceftizoxime).

The bacteriologic makeup of a wound infection varies from patient to patient, because of the circumstances preceding the development of a wound infection. The most common bacteria isolated from abdominal wound infections tend to reflect organisms normally found to inhabit the skin and lower genital tract. In addition, there tends to be a selection for resistant bacteria in those patients who received antibiotic prophylaxis. In one report, the most common bacteria isolated from infected wounds were *Staphylococcus aureus, Streptococcus faecalis,* and *Escherichia coli,* which is not too dissimilar from those organisms isolated from patients delivered by cesarean section. However, it is not uncommon to isolate anaerobes from such wounds.

The principal host's defensive mechanism, located in the wound to combat infection, is the neutrophil. Bacteria must be opsoninized in order to be phagocytosized. Opsonins are antibodies found in serum that originate from antigenic stimulation by different but antigenically related bacteria. Specific antibody of the IgG and IgM class are potent opsonins. These antibodies or opsonins attach to bacteria and facilitate attachment of the bacterium to the phagocyte. Phagocytosis and opsoninization are enhanced by complement, which further enhances the adherence of the bacteria to the phagocyte membrane. This system becomes impaired in the wound with the presence of dead space that has not been drained. Thus with all the factors mentioned in the above discussion, the effect of the wound on the neutrophil becomes of paramount importance on whether or not infection occurs. Neutrophils must reach the site of contamination to be effective, and unimpeded neutrophils can usually accommodate an inoculum of up to one million bacteria. However, certain factors may work against the neutrophil. For example, when a wound is made, the cut vessels usually form thrombosis back to the nearest perfused capillary loop impeding neutrophil migration. In uncoagulated tissue, this distance creates a dead space (an area of unperfused tissue) of approximately 50 to 100 μm. The absence of blood perfusing the tissue results in an area of hypoxia. The oxygen concentration of the tissue is important to neutrophil function, which requires an oxygen concentration of greater than 15 mm Hg. The oxygen concentration of wound space is approximately 5–10 mm Hg with a gradual increase toward the skin and earliest perfusing capillaries.[22,23] Phagocytosis of bacteria requires a number of metabolic actions that result in approximately a 20-fold increase in oxygen requirements.[22] Meticulous handling of tissue and prudent use of pinpoint electrocoagulation will not result in significant tissue hypoxia, and therefore will not create a hostile environment for the neutrophil.

EPISIOTOMY INFECTION

The two most common types of wound infection in the postpartum patient are episiotomy and abdominal wound infections. The perineum, regardless of whether the episiotomy is made mediolateral or in the midline, is typically resistant to infection. The perineum has adapted to overcome a large inoculum, because the episiotomy is often exposed to feces and thus is subjected to a large inoculum. This area seems to contradict the principles outlined above regarding inoculum size and suture as factors contributing to infection. The reason that infection sometimes, although rarely, occurs in the episiotomy is because of poor hemostasis, strangulation of tissue, overuse of suture, and failure to recognize a defect in the rectal mucosa. If a fourth-degree episiotomy has occurred, it may contribute to infection if the rectal serosa is not properly closed, allowing for fecal material to contaminate the rectovaginal space created by the episiotomy.

Episiotomy infection occurs in approximately 0.5 to 3% of patients delivered vaginally.[24] The factors contributing to the development of infection in the episiotomy site are not known, but would appear to be similar to those of any clean or clean-contaminated wound. The perineum apparently possesses an inherent resistance because this area does not readily become infected even after exposure to a large inoculum and the presence of suture. Signs of an infected episiotomy are erythema, edema, weeping of purulent exudate along the suture line, and pain associated with marked swelling. If the incision has not spontaneously broken down, and if the area has abscessed, it is best to open the episiotomy to allow for drainage. Necrotic tissue should be debrided until healthy tissue is found. The wound edges should not be reapproximated for closure at this time as this is likely to result in recurrent abscess formation. The patient should cleanse the episiotomy site by taking sitz baths or using a gentle spray of antiseptic followed by cleansing with water. The wound can be allowed to granulate and close by secondary intention, or closed when the entire wound is covered with a layer of granulation tissue. If the patient had a third- or fourth-degree episiotomy and, subsequently, a dehiscence occurs that requires reestablishing a third- or fourth-degree situation, it would be best to repair this when all signs of infection and inflammation has resolved. Episiotomy infections and dehiscence are discussed in further detail in chapter 8.

ABDOMINAL WOUND INFECTION

The incidence of abdominal wound infection following cesarean section varies from institution to institution and population to population; however, the general range of infection is 3 to 16%, with an average of 7%. Overall, the wound infection rate in patients who received antibiotic prophylaxis is approximately 3 to 4%, with a range of 2 to 8%.[25,26] The factors that place patients at risk for the development of a wound infection are age, obesity, diabetes, liver disease, malnutrition, steroid therapy, and immuno-suppression (Table 2).[26] Additional factors are poor hemostasis, the presence of a he-matoma, necrotic tissue, anoxic tissue, for-eign bodies, and anemia.[27]

Wound infection not involving group A beta-hemolytic streptococci occurs usually between the 5th and 7th days. However, most wound infections do make their appear-ance known early, although the changes in the wound are very subtle. The earliest signs may become apparent 48 to 72 hours after surgery. The initial signs are an advancing margin of erythema, the skin may develop a sheen or resemble that of an orange skin, and induration may be present. All too often, the erythema that is initially seen is not carefully examined. The wound may initially be weep-ing and the drainage is usually serous, but it often contains blood and becomes darker each day or the fluid is cloudy and becomes purulent. The patient often exhibits a low-grade fever, with a range of 99 to <100.4°F, and the pulse rate is usually not significantly elevated. A wound that develops an abscess with a large area of cellulitis is usually accom-panied with high temperatures, >101°F. The patient usually has a characteristic diurnal variation, but unlike the normal variation, the fever does not reach baseline (98.6°F). Again, the pulse rate does not parallel the fever pattern, as is seen in patients with sys-temic infection, unless there is a large area of cellulitis.

In contrast to the slow development of a wound infection seen with gram-positive and/or gram-negative infections, two types of rapidly developing infection are those due to beat-hemolytic streptococci and necrotizing cellulitis or fasciitis. Infections due to group A beta-hemolytic streptococci and some-times group B hemolytic streptococci appear within 24 hours of surgery. The patient usu-ally develops high spiking temperatures and tachycardia. The infection spreads rapidly, causing a marked cellulitis.

The evaluation should begin by examining the surface of the skin in the overlying area adjacent to the incision. The edge of the area of erythema should be marked and the time recorded, the wound should be reexamined in 1 to 2 hours, and note made of whether or not the margin of erythema has advanced be-yond the previous margin. The wound should be palpated and the examiner should deter-mine if there is crepitance or pain, or if there is absence of pain in the presence of indura-tion or swelling and erythema. The presence of crepitance or the absence of pain in the face of swelling and erythema may indicate the presence of necrotic tissue, even though the overlying skin has not become discol-ored. If there is spontaneous drainage, the area should be cleansed with a topical anti-septic and then wiped with sterile gauze. A sterile needle can be inserted directly through the site of drainage, and since this is usually along the incision line, it will not cause the patient pain. The area should be aspirated by gentle retraction on the plunger. If no fluid returns, aspiration should be con-tinued for a few seconds before withdrawing the needle, allowing for the evacuation of gas that may be present if anaerobic bacteria are present. Any fluid that is aspirated should be placed in an anaerobic transport vial. The aspirate should be Gram stained and pro-cessed for the isolation of aerobic and anaer-obic bacteria as well as *Mycoplasma*.[28] If no fluid is draining spontaneously, the abdomen and surrounding incision can be examined with the aid of ultrasonography. If a collec-tion of fluid is detected supra- or subfascial, this can be aspirated under direct vision with the aid of ultrasonography.

The use of ultrasonography is beneficial in that it can lead the physician to avoid aspi-ration if no fluid pocket is detected. This technique also can be used to determine if there is a fascial dehiscence and if bowel has protruded through the defect, thus avoiding the creation of an evisceration by opening the skin on the wound. In turn, the patient can be taken to the operating suite and the wound opened under sterile conditions.

If the fascia is intact, the wound can be

opened in a treatment room; precautions should be taken to maintain sterile conditions. The wound should be opened widely to allow for complete exploration of the infected areas and drainage of all fluid. The wound should be probed for defects and loculations of pus. Necrotic tissue should be debrided back to the presence of healthy tissue. The correct amount of debridement can be determined by noting the occurrence of bright red bleeding and the patient's development of pain. Debridement of necrotic tissue does not elicit pain from the patient. The wound should be copiously irrigated with sterile normal saline or another surgical irrigant. An acceptable protocol is to irrigate with saline or hydrogen peroxide and then pack the wound with cotton gauze that has been moistened with 0.25% acetic acid. The gauze should not be soaking wet, but should be wrung tightly to remove all excess acetic acid. The gauze should then be fluffed and placed into the wound, but not tightly packed into the wound. The gauze should come in direct contact with the entire surface of the wound. The dressing and packing should be changed at least three times a day. When the packing dries, it will stick to the tissue and all necrotic tissue will cling to the gauze and be removed when the packing is removed. The 0.25% acetic acid is not toxic to newly generated tissue and does not provide a good medium for bacterial growth. The wound should be managed in this fashion until there is a layer of granulation tissue covering the entire wound. It is at this point that closure of the wound can be undertaken. The closure can be accomplished by suturing the wound or by bringing the skin edges together from the base, being careful not to leave any dead space, and steri strips can be used to approximate the skin edges. It is important that a layer of granulation tissue be completely formed and that no dead space is left because this will serve as a focus for the secretion of serum and allow for the formation of a seroma.

Otherwise, the process will repeat itself, and a wound infection is likely to be reestablished.

ABDOMINAL WOUND CELLULITIS

In contrast to the formation of a wound abscess, infections caused by group A beta-hemolytic streptococci usually cause a cellulitis. This type of infection is not characterized by the accumulation of pus. A wound that is characterized by cellulitis does not need to be opened and drained, as there is no fluid collection to drain. The mainstay of treatment is antibiotics. Although these infections tend to be monobacterial, it is best to institute therapy with a broad-spectrum agent such as ticarcillin/clavulanic acid, ampicillin/sulbactam, cefoxitin, cefotetan, ceftizoxime, etc. These agents will provide activity against gram-positive cocci and also gram-negative bacteria. It is important to remember that not only are the organisms that inhabit the skin likely to contaminate the wound, but also those bacteria that are brought up from the lower genital tract and washed across the tissues of the abdominal wall at time of cesarean section.

NECROTIZING INFECTION

The most serious type of wound infections that are associated with a significant mortality are necrotizing cellulitis and necrotizing fasciitis. Gangrenous infection rarely occurs today, but when it does, the mortality rates range between 20 and 50%, even with the availability of broad-spectrum antibiotics.[29–31] The high mortality associated with necrotizing infections and septic shock can be reduced significantly if the infection is recognized early.

Necrotizing infections start out slowly, but once initiated, become rapidly fulminating and are associated with increasing morbidity and mortality with progression of the infection. The degree of infection is dependent upon the layers of tissue involved. Infection involving the skin and subcutaneous tissue is referred to as "necrotizing cellulitis," but if the fascia is involved, the term "necrotizing fasciitis" is used. Necrotizing infections can occur following any type of incision, e.g., abdominal wall incision, episiotomy, vulva biopsy, and Bartholin's gland abscess.[32,33] Basically, these infections can be divided into two broad microbiological groups— those involving *Clostridium* and nonclostridial infections. The latter group are often referred to as "nonclostridial anaerobic cellulitis" or "synergistic necrotizing cellulitis." Other terms are gram-negative anaerobic cutaneous gangrene, necrotizing cutaneous myositis, and synergistic nonclostridial anaerobic myonecrosis. Synergistic necrotizing cellulitis is a variant of necrotizing fasciitis.

Clostridium perfringes, the most commonly involved species involved in clostridial soft tissue infections, are introduced in the soft tissues of the abdominal wall, perineum, and vulva by contamination at the time of the operative procedure. The infection may be limited to the subcutaneous tissue and only superficially involve the fascia; it is referred to as "clostridial anaerobic cellulitis." However, the infection may involve the deeper tissues, fascia, and muscle, and this is referred to as "clostridial myonecrosis."

Clostridial anaerobic cellulitis usually becomes evident 3 or more days after the surgical procedure. It may have a slow onset, but subsequently spreads rapidly.[35] Typically, the signs and symptoms of infection are not pronounced; on the contrary, they are usually mild. However, there is usually a watery, dark, frequently foul-smelling discharge exiting from the wound. There is also usually frank crepitance that may extend widely, indicating the evolution of extensive tissue gas formation. Aspiration of the exudate will reveal the presence of blunt-ended gram-positive bacilli and numerous polymorphonuclear leukocytes. An x-ray of the soft tissue will show a collection of gas in the tissue. The presence of crepitance or gas is not pathognomonic of clostridial infection and

TABLE 3. Differential Diagnosis of Crepitance in Soft Tissues

Common
  Clostridial cellulitis
  Nonclostridial anaerobic cellulitis
  Infected vascular gangrene

Noninfectious causes
  Injuries involving compressed air
  Loosely sutured wounds
  Irrigation of wounds with hydrogen peroxide
  Intravenous catheter placement

Less common
  Clostridial myonecrosis
  Necrotizing fasciitis
  Synergistic necrotizing cellulitis

Uncommon
  Streptococcal myositis

may be the result of other infections or noninfectious etiologies (Table 3).

Clostridium perfringes is found in up to 80% of the cases of myonecrosis, frequently referred to as gas gangrene.[36] Other species isolated from cases of myonecrosis are *C. novyi, C. septicum,* and *C. sordelli.* It may be difficult to distinguish initially between myonecrosis and necrotizing fasciitis or cellulitis. Usually *Clostridium* is absent in the latter infections, but a synergy exists between multiple bacteria such as *Staphylococcus aureus, Staphylococcus epidermidis, Streptococcus* sp., *Streptococcus agalactiae, Pseudomonas, Escherichia coli, Citrobacter,* and *Enterobacter,* as well as several opportunistic bacteria.

Clostridial myonecrosis occurs following muscle injury and contamination with spores of *C. perfringes* or other histotoxic clostridial species. Predisposing conditions include compound fractures, penetrating wounds, surgical wounds involving the bowel or biliary tract, arterial nonsufficiency in an extremity, and tissue devitalization or trauma associated with surgery, abortion, or delivery (vaginal or cesarean section). It is important to remember that *C. perfringes* is found as part of the normal vaginal flora in approximately 8% of the population.[34,35]

Clostridium perfringes produces a variety of

exotoxins that cause necrosis of normal tissue, especially muscle, thereby allowing vast areas to be invaded by bacteria. The exotoxin may cause renal tubular necrosis and anuria hemolysis with hemoglobinemia and hemoglobulinuria and progressive jaundice. The exotoxin is also neurotoxic and may cause delirium and coma. The exotoxin becomes fixed to the tissues and cannot be neutralized with polyvalent antitoxin.

The exotoxins facilitate spread of the bacteria by causing necrosis and anoxia. The organism produces a characteristic lesion that consists of a central dead zone, a dying zone, and a normal zone.[35,37] The central zone consists of necrotic tissue, blood clot, and bacteria. The dying zone contains hemodynamically compromised muscle that demonstrates an inflammatory response and bacteria. The normal zone contains viable muscle, but there is a marked inflammatory response.

Progressive accumulation of gas and fluid creates pressure in the tissue spores, which can cause necrosis of muscle. In addition, this pressure is exerted on the lymphatics and vessels, which results in anoxia. The muscles initially appear hemorrhagic and friable, and they exude a brownish red, watery, foul-smelling fluid.

The incubation period from time of injury to development of clostridial myonecrosis is 2 to 3 days, but symptoms may occur within 6 hours of injury. The earliest symptom is pain, which increases rapidly and is out of proportion to the surgical procedure form. Shortly after the onset of pain, the patient appears ill, pale, and diaphoretic. The pulse is rapid, hypotension develops, and shock and renal failure follow. Fever is present, but usually is not over 101°F (38.3°C). The patient may become hypothermic, which is usually associated with shock.

Early in the course of infection, there is edema and localized tenderness. Drainage is usually serosanguinous, dirty, and contains numerous bacteria but few polymorphonuclear leukocytes. The wound has a foul odor and gas bubbles may be present in the discharge. Crepitance may or may not be present or may be obscured by the presence of edema. The skin adjacent to the wound appears normal in color at first, but if swollen, it rapidly changes to a yellow or bronze discoloration. This is an extremely aggressive and fulminate infection and changes occur over 2 to 4 hours.

Treatment for clostridial cellulitis or myonecrosis involves the immediate institution of antibiotics, 20–40 million units of penicillin daily. Alternate drugs are tetracycline and chloramphenicol. If a nonclostridial infection is suspected, the addition of an aminoglycoside as well as clindamycin is indicated. Prompt surgical debridement is imperative, and in many instances the patient will have to undergo several surgical debridements. Hyperbaric oxygenation is indicated and has proved to be beneficial.[38] Hyperoxygenation is bacteriostatic to the organism, and toxins are eliminated by tissue metabolism and the advancement of infection is halted.[39,40] Patients with gas gangrene of the anterior abdominal wall have a higher mortality and will benefit from hyperbaric oxygenation. Adverse effects of hyperbaric oxygenation are middle ear syndrome during compression, oxygen intoxication, and the bends (caisson disease), which occurs during decompression. Hyperbaric oxygenation prior to surgery facilitates differentiation between viable and necrotic tissue, thus allowing a more precise debridement without sacrificing healthy tissue.

Necrotizing fasciitis differs from clostridial cellulitis and myonecrosis in that it is a polymicrobial mixed aerobic and anaerobic infection.[32] Bacteria frequently involved in this infection include *Staphylococcus*, *Streptococcus*, *Escherichia coli*, *Proteus*, *Klebsiella*, *Pseudomonas*, *Enterococcus*, *Peptostreptococcus*, and *Bacteroides*. The infection can occur following a major surgical incision or what may be considered a minor invasion of the skin or surface epithelium, such as paracervical and pudendal blocks.[33,41–43]

The disease is extremely serious and is fulminate with the patient being acutely ill and toxic. The changes that occur in the cutaneous tissues occur hourly. Initially, the wound is extremely painful, but with necrosis comes anesthesia. Areas of cellulitis are accompanied by the formation of blisters, which are filled with hemorrhagic and serous fluid. The skin surrounding the blisters forms a halo of necrotic, black tissue. Adjacent areas become edematous and ecchymotic. The pathognomonic sign of necrotizing fasciitis is a dusky discoloration of the skin and purple ecchymotic areas. These skin lesions become gangrenous, which is a late sign.

The subcutaneous and fascial necrosis is associated with formation of "dishwater" exudate or drainage from the wound. The muscle is usually not involved, unless it becomes secondarily involved in the infection process. Thrombosis of the vessels within the necrosis fascia and subcutaneous tissue leads to gangrene of the skin.

The cornerstone of treatment is early diagnosis, institution of broad-spectrum antibiotics, and surgical debridement. The finding of dusky discoloration of skin in the wound or adjacent area, with or without ecchymosis, should be the clue to the presence of this severe infection. The next step, and this should not be overlooked, is to obtain cultures from the affected area and venous blood. Specimens from the wound should include an aspirate obtained under anaerobic conditions, and if tissue is debrided, a specimen should be sent to the laboratory. All specimens should be transported in anaerobic vials and processed for aerobic and anaerobic bacteria. A Gram stain should be performed to determine whether the infection is unimicrobial or polymicrobial, gram-positive or gram-negative.

Because this is an extremely fulminate infection and frequently polymicrobial, it is best to use combination antibiotics. Penicillin or ampicillin should be used to provide coverage for beta-hemolytic streptococci. An aminoglycoside should be included to provide coverage of gram-negative facultative anaerobes. In addition, the aminoglycoside will act synergisticly with ampicillin against *S. faecalis.* Clindamycin or metronidazole will round out the therapeutic regimen to provide coverage against anaerobes, particularly *Bacteroides* sp.

The foundation of the therapeutic regimen is immediate and extensive surgical debridement of all necrotic and infected tissue. There is no reason to delay examining the patient under general anesthesia. These patients' wounds should not be examined in their rooms or a treatment room. Delay in appropriate management results in increased morbidity. All layers of involved tissue should be excised, and the debridement should be continued until the different layers of tissue cannot be easily separated, e.g., subcutaneous tissue from fascia.

Following debridement, the wound should be packed with loose gauze packs moistened with a topical agent, e.g., Dakin's solution, hydrogen peroxide, zinc peroxide, or neomycin and polymyxin. It is of paramount importance to change the dressings every 8 hours, which allows for passive and active debridement. When the dressings are removed, they should have dried considerably, and necrotic tissue clinging to the gauze will be removed. The wound should be inspected for debridement of necrotic tissue.

Postoperative management of these patients is critical because they can easily develop septic shock. Therefore, it is imperative that their fluid and electrolyte status be monitored continuously. If debridement is extensive, there is a tendency for sequestering large amounts of fluid, which may result in electrolyte imbalance. A bacterium such as group B beta-streptococcus can cause hemolysis of red blood cells. The anemia that results is worsened by the surgical debridement.

Calcium depletion may occur secondary to sequestration in areas of tissue necrosis. Replacement can be accomplished by the administration of calcium gluconate or calcium chloride.

Another variant of necrotizing wound infections is synergistic bacterial gangrene, which is a more insidious type of infection. The onset of this infection is slower than necrotizing fasciitis. This infection is due to the synergistic activity of aerobic and anaerobic bacteria, usually involving two or more distinct species that have markedly different oxygen requirements. The most frequent bacterial isolates are microaerophilic, nonhemolytic *Streptococcus* and *Staphylococcus aureus* along with facultative gram-negative anaerobes and obligate anaerobes. The basic microbiological difference between synergistic bacterial gangrene and necrotizing fasciitis is that the former usually contains hemolytic *Staphylococcus* plus nonhemolytic, microaerophilic streptococcus and the latter does not, but the latter usually has group A beta-hemolytic streptococcus. Both may contain facultative gram-negative anaerobes and obligate anaerobes.

Synergistic bacterial gangrene may not appear to be different from uncomplicated wound infection at the onset. The infection is slow to progress, however it differs from other infections in that it fails to heal and the margins of the lesion become gangrenous. There is ischemia in the wound and the margins appear purple. The wound is painful. Usually, these patients do not manifest systemic signs until late in the course of the infection.

Treatment consists of broad-spectrum antibiotics and surgical debridement. Again, as in the preceding discussions, the debridement must be extensive in order to prevent recurrent infection. The excision must be taken beyond the zone of erythema. The wound should be packed as described earlier.

All wound infections should be approached as being serious infections. The surface skin overlying the deeper tissues does not reflect the potentially serious underlying infection that may be present. All too frequently this misleads the physician into improperly assessing the wound, and therefore embarking on an inappropriate course of management. This unfortunate delay results in more drastic measures being taken and a prolonged hospital course, not to mention the possible increased risk of mortality. Therefore, all wound abnormalities suspected of having an origin in infection should be approached aggressively.

Steps that can be taken are to characterize the appearance of the wound as to presence of erythema and to mark the edges to determine if progression occurs and over what period of time. This will give some estimate of how aggressive the bacterial infection is. It is also important to determine if there is induration, pain, and drainage. Ultrasound and/or x-ray of the soft tissue should be obtained to determine if there is a collection of fluid and/or gas. Any fluid that is present should be aspirated, Gram stained, and transported in anaerobic vials for isolation of aerobes, anaerobes, and *Mycoplasma*. The wound should be probed to determine if the fascia is intact, unless ultrasonography reveals the presence of bowel above fascia. If the fascia is not intact, the patient should be taken to the operating room for exploration and debridement.

Antibiotic therapy should provide coverage against three main groups of bacteria—the gram-positive aerobes, facultative gram-negative anaerobes, and obligate anaerobes—if the wound infection is either gangrenous or necrotizing or both. An uncomplicated wound abscess that has not caused necrosis of the subcutaneous tissue or fascia can be treated by incision and drainage followed by packing. However, if the abscess is associated with a large area of cellulitis, then antibiotics are indicated. Beta-lactam antibiotics such as ticarcillin/clavulanic acid or ampicillin/sulbactam should be considered in these patients.

Proper management of the infected wound requires thorough examination early in the course of infection followed by multiple daily examinations until the wound is healed.

REFERENCES

1. Ortona L, Federico G, Fantoni M, et al.: A study on the incidence of postoperative infections and surgical sepsis in a university hospital. Infect Control 8(8):320–324, 1987.
2. Price PB: The bacteriology of normal skin: A new quantitative test applied to a study of the bacterial flora and the disinfectant action of mechanical cleansing. J Infect Dis 63:301–318, 1938.
3. Taylor FW: An experimental evaluation of operative wound irrigation. Surg Gynecol Obstet 113:465–470, 1961.
4. Dineen P: An evaluation of the duration of the surgical scrub. Surg Gynecol Obstet 129:1181–1184, 1969.
5. Lowbury EJL, Lilly HA, Bull JP: Methods for disinfection of hands and operation sites. Br Med J 5408:531–536, 1964.
6. Cruse PJE, Foord R: A five-year prospective study of 23,649 surgical wounds. Arch Surg 107:206–210, 1973.
7. Garibaldi RA, Skolnick D, Lerer T, et al.: The impact of preoperative skin disinfection on preventing intraoperative wound contamination. Infect Control 9(3)109–113, 1988.
8. Seropian R, Reynold BM: Wound infections after preoperative depilatory versus razor preparation. Am J Surg 121:251–254, 1971.
9. Altemeier WA, Burke JF, Pruitt BA Jr, Sandusky WR (eds): Preoperative preparation of the patient. In: "Manual on Control of Infection in Surgical Patients." Philadelphia: Lippincott, 1984, p 74.
10. Cruse PJE: Wound infections: epidemiology and clinical characteristics. In Howard RJ, Simmons RL (eds): "Surgical Infectious Disease." Norwalk, CT: Appleton and Lange, 1988, p 319.
11. Madden JE, Edlick RF, Custer JR, et al.: Studies in the management of the contaminated wound. IV. Resistance to infection of surgical wounds made by knife, electrosurgery, and laser. Am J Surg 119:222–224, 1970.
12. Keenan KM, Rodeheaver GT, Kenney JG, Edleck RF: Surgical cautery revisited. Am J Surg 147:818–821, 1984.
13. Alexander JW, Korelitz J, Alexander NS: Prevention of wound infections—A case for closed suction drainage to remove wound fluids deficient in opsonic proteins. Am J Surg 132:59–63, 1976.
14. Ferguson DJ: Clinical application of experimental relations between technique and wound infection. Surgery 63:377–381, 1988.
15. deHoll D, Rodeheaver G, Edgerton MT, Edlick RF: Potentiation of infection by suture closure of dead space. Am J Surg 127:716–720, 1974.
16. Levenson SM, Seifter E: Dysnutrition, wound healing and resistance to infection. Clin Plast Surg 4:375–388, 1977.
17. Elek SD, Conen PE: The virulence of *Staphylococcus pyogenes* for man: A study of the problems of wound infection. Br J Exp Pathol 38:573–577, 1957.
18. Howe CW, Marston AT: A study of sources of postoperative staphylococcal infection. Surg Gynecol Obstet 115:266–275, 1962.
19. Roettinger W, Edgerton MT, Kurtz LD, et al.: Role of inoculation site as a determinant of infection in soft tissue wounds. Am J Surg 126:354–358, 1973.
20. Robson MC, Lea CE, Dalton JB, Heggers JP: Quantitative bacteriology and delayed wound closure. Surg Forum 19:501–502, 1968.
21. Edlich RF, Rodeheaver GT, Spengler M, et al.: Practical bacteriology monitoring of the burn victim. Clin Plast Surg 4:561–569, 1977.
22. Klebunoff S: Oxygen metabolism and the toxic properties of phagocytosis. Ann Intern Med 93:480–485, 1986.
23. Hohn DC, MacKay RD, Holiday B, Hunt TK: The effect of O_2 tensions on the microbicidal function of leukocytes in wounds and in-vitro. Surg Forum 27:18–20, 1976.
24. Thacker SB, Banta HD: Benefits and risks of episiotomy: An interpretative review of the language literature, 1860–1980. Obstet Gynecol Surv 38:322–338, 1983.
25. Mead PB: Prophylactic antibiotics and antibiotic resistance. Semin Perinatol 1:101–106, 1977.
26. Polk HC, Miles AA: Enhancement of bacterial infection by ferric iron kinetics, mechanisms and surgical significance. Surgery 70:71–77, 1971.
27. Stage AH, Silberman R, Greene CM: Wound infection following cesarean section. Surg Gynecol Obstet 145:882–884, 1977.
28. Phillips LE, Faro S, Martens MG, et al.: The microbiology of postpartum endometritis in high risk patients delivered by cesarean section. Curr Ther Res 42(6): 1157–1165, 1987.
29. Golde S, Ledger WJ: Necrotizing fasciitis in postpartum patients: A report of four cases. Obstet Gynecol 50:670–673, 1977.
30. Dellinger EP: Severe necrotizing soft tissue infections. JAMA 246:1717–1721, 1981.
31. Casali RE, Tucker WE, Petrino RA, et al.: Postoperative necrotizing fasciitis of the abdominal wall. Am J Surg 140:787–790, 1980.
32. Pruyn SC: Acute necrotizing fasciitis of the endopelvic fascia. Obstet Gynecol 52:25–29, 1978.
33. Roberts DB, Hester LL: Progressive synergistic bacterial gangrene arising from abscesses of the vulva and Bartholin's gland duct. Am J Obstet Gynecol 114:285–291, 1972.
34. O'Neill RT, Schwartz RH: Clostridial organisms in septic abortions. Obstet Gynecol 35:458–461, 1970.
35. Altemeier WA, Furste WL: Gas gangrene: Collec-

tive review. Surg Gynecol Obstet 84:507–523, 1947.

36. Altemeier WA, Fullen WE: Prevention and treatment of gas gangrene. JAMA 217:806–811, 1971.

37. McNally JB, Price WB, Wood MD: Gas gangrene of the anterior abdominal wall. Am J Surg 116: 779–783, 1968.

38. McAllister TA, Stark JM, Worman JN, Ross RM: Inhibitory effects of hypertonic oxygen on bacteria or fungi. Lancet 2:1040–1042, 1963.

39. Brummelkanp WH, Boerema I, Hogendijk J: Treatment of clostridial infections with hyperbaric oxygen drenching: A report on 26 cases. Lancet 1:235–238, 1963.

40. Brummelkanp WH, Hogendijk J, Boerema I: Treatment of anaerobic infections (clostridial myositis) by drenching the tissues with oxygen under high atmospheric pressure. Surgery 49:299–302, 1961.

41. Hubbard LT, McVann RM, Snyder EM: Subgluteal and retopsoal infections in obstetric practice. Obstet Gynecol 39:137–142, 1972.

42. Crosthwait RW Jr, Crosthwait RW, Jordan GL: Necrotizing fasciitis. J Trauma 4:149–157, 1964.

43. Rea WJ, Wyrick WJ Jr: Necrotizing fasciitis. Ann Surg 172:957–964, 1970.

44. Halsted WS: "An Account of the Introduction of Gloves." Menaska, Wisconsin: George Banta Publishing, 1939.

10

Pregnancy and Septic Shock

Gary D.V. Hankins, M.D., Russell R. Snyder, M.D., and Wesley Lee, M.D.

The classic triad of infection, hemorrhage, and hypertension has accounted for most of the maternal mortality in the United States during the last 25 years. Infections, whether unique to the pregnancy state, as in chorioamnionitis, or merely temporally associated, as in acute appendicitis, remain commonplace. One-half percent to 1% of all pregnant women are estimated to develop chorioamnionitis,[1] 1 to 4% of women delivering vaginally develop postpartum endomyoparametritis,[2] and 15 to 85% of women undergoing cesarean section develop postpartum endomyoparametritis.[3-5] Additional sources of infection, all capable of producing septic shock, are listed in Table 1.[1-19]

The goal of therapy with each of these infections is either primary prevention or early identification and aggressive treatment with eradication of the septic focus. If the infection continues unabated, septic shock will occur, accompanied by a mortality variously reported as from 11 to 80%.[20-22] The mortality with septic shock in the obstetric patient should be less than that quoted above, however, because the pregnant woman is usually healthy before the acute infectious event, has no underlying malnutrition or irreversible disease such as a malignancy, and

is not on immunosuppressive therapy nor has she received radiotherapy. In addition, the pregnant woman will usually have an identifiable and readily treatable source of infection.[23,24] Even so, septic shock can be lethal for both the woman and her fetus, as demonstrated by the recent series by Lee and associates, who reported a 20% maternal mortality rate.[25]

MICROBIOLOGY

Traditionally the term "septic shock" has been associated with the gram-negative Enterobacteriaceae group and liberation of endotoxin. It is estimated that these endotoxin-forming organisms account for 95% of septic shock.[18,26,27] As demonstrated in Table 2, however, a host of gram-positive organisms can also cause bacteremia in pregnant women and account for 5% of the septic shock seen during pregnancy or in the puerperium.[14,15,28-31] Among these gram-positive organisms are group B streptococcus, a not uncommon uropathogen and a signifi-

The opinions expressed in this chapter are those of the authors and not necessarily those of the United States Air Force or the Department of Defense.

Infections in Pregnancy, pages 91–114
Published 1990 by Alan R. Liss, Inc.

TABLE 1. Conditions Associated With Septic Shock in Pregnancy or the Postpartum Period

Obstetric
  Postpartum endomyoparametritis
  Chorioamnionitis
  Septic abortion
  Septic pelvic thrombophlebitis
Nonobstetric
  Acute appendicitis
  Acute biliary disease
  Pyelonephritis
  Bartholin's gland abscess
  Toxic shock syndrome
  Mastitis/breast abscess
Procedures
  Amniocentesis
  Infected cerclage
  Necrotizing fasciitis, postoperative
  Chorionic villus sampling

TABLE 2. Principal Pathogens Responsible for Bacteremia in Obstetric Patients

Gram negative
  Escherichia coli
  Klebsiella-Enterobacter
  Proteus mirabilis
  Bacteroides sp.
  Serratia
  Fusobacterium nucleatum or *necrophorum*
  Pseudomonas
Gram positive
  Group A streptococci
  Group B streptococci
  Group D streptococci (*Enterococcus*)
  Streptococcus pneumoniae
  Staphylococcus aureus
  Clostridia sp.
  Listeria monocytogenes
  Peptostreptococcus
  Peptococcus

cant contributor to neonatal morbidity and mortality, several anaerobes, and the exotoxin-producing *Staphylococcus*. The mechanism of gram-positive shock differs from that of the gram-negative organisms with their classic endotoxin effects. For example, *Clostridia* sp. produces alpha exotoxin, which is a phospholipase C capable of damaging lipid membranes. Phospholipase C will principally affect erythrocytes, platelets, leukocytes, vascular endothelium, and the plasma membrane of muscle cells. The end result is fulminant intravascular hemolysis and myonecrosis, reflecting cell death of erythrocytes and myocytes. Similarly, *Staphylococcus aureus* produces enterotoxin B and F, the latter also known as exotoxin C. These exotoxins can then effect a host of organ system derangements, which in fact are required for the case definition of the toxic shock syndrome (Table 3).[32]

PATHOPHYSIOLOGY OF SEPTIC SHOCK—ENDOTOXIN

In all gram-negative bacteria, whether cocci or rods, the outer cell wall is composed of endotoxin lipopolysaccharides (LPS). The basic chemical structure of LPS is similar from organism to organism and is composed of three moities: 1) lipid A, linked via ketodeoxyoctonoic acid, 2) a common polysaccharide core structure, and 3) O-specific sugars on the outermost portion of the lipopolysaccharide molecule, usually present in repeating multiple layer sequences. The innermost lipid portion, lipid A, which is identical from organism to organism, possesses all of the biological activities associated with endotoxin.

Release of endotoxin from the bacterial cell wall, whether as a consequence of the normal life cycle of reproduction and death of the bacteria or of the antibiotic-induced death of the bacteria, will simultaneously activate a number of host defense mechanisms. Gram-negative bacteria and/or endotoxin have been shown to bind and activate Hageman factor (factor XII) in the blood, which, in turn, can activate four distinct but interrelated plasma pathways: 1) the coagulation pathway, 2) the fibrinolytic pathway, 3) the complement pathway, and 4) the kinin pathway.

COAGULATION/FIBRINOLYSIS

Activated factor XII, through activation of factor XI and the intrinsic coagulation path-

TABLE 3. CDC Case Definition for Toxic Shock Syndrome

Fever	T ≥ 38.9°C
Rash	macular erythroderma
Desquamation	especially palms and soles at 7–14 days
Systolic BP	<90 mm Hg
Multisystem involvement	at least 3
GI	vomiting, diarrhea
Muscular	severe myalgias, CPK > twice normal
Mucus membrane	oral, conjunctival, vaginal
Renal	BUN or Cr > twice normal pyuria, > 5 WBC without infection
Hepatic	bilirubin, SGOT, SGPT > twice normal
Hematologic	platelets <100,000/mm^3
CNS	disorientation or alteration in consciousness without focal neurologic signs when fever and hypotension are absent
If ordered, negative test for:	
Cultures	blood, urine, CSF
Serologies	Rocky Mountain spotted fever, leptosperosis, measles

way, will result in the eventual conversion of fibrinogen to fibrin. Hageman factor also activates factor VII and again leads to the conversion of fibrinogen to fibrin via the extrinsic coagulation pathway. Simultaneously, factor XII will activate the fibrinolytic pathway with conversion of plasminogen to plasmin. Each of these pathways carry significant potential for tissue injury when uncontrolled activation takes place. Disseminated intravascular coagulation (DIC) is a frequent problem in bacteremic patients and is often part of the septic shock syndrome. DIC results when extensive turnover of blood factors results in intravascular thrombosis. The clotting process will consume both platelets and clotting factors, resulting in their depletion in the blood with a resultant thrombocytopenia and hypofibrinogenemia. Concomitantly, the accelerated activity of the fibrinolytic pathway will result in an accumulation of fibrin split products. If unchecked, the disseminated intravascular coagulation can disrupt the microcirculation and ultimately produce tissue ischemia, necrosis, widespread hemolysis, shock, and death.

COMPLEMENT

Activated Hageman factor also leads to activation of the complement system through the intermediary of plasmin. While the complement system is critical during infection for its capacity to mediate the inflammatory response, to render bacteria susceptible to phagocytosis, and to directly lyse organisms, this system is also responsible for much of the injury that the host itself ultimately sustains. The complement system is a cascade in which inactive proteins circulating in the blood become biologically active and promote inflammation through a complex sequence of events. The system consists of 18 plasma proteins, 15 of which promote the inflammatory responses and three to serve as natural inhibitors to control and deactivate the process. Complement can be activated through either the classical pathway, so called because it was discovered first, or the alternative pathway (Fig. 1).

Although the system appears to be exceedingly complex, an understanding of the nomenclature greatly simplifies this system. The 11 protein components of the classical pathway are designated with a capital letter "C," and are assigned a number in the order of their discovery. Each of these components, C1 through C9, represents an individual plasma protein. C1 has three subcomponents, called C1q, C1r, and C1s. During activation, the individual components interact in a sequential manner. Unfortunately the first four components of complement do not interact in the sequence in which they were discovered. The actual order of activation and interaction is C1, 4, 2, 3, 5, 6, 7, 8, 9. The alternative pathway (properdin) follows the same activation pattern, beginning at C3. Different proteins initiate the activation sequence, however, and the alternative

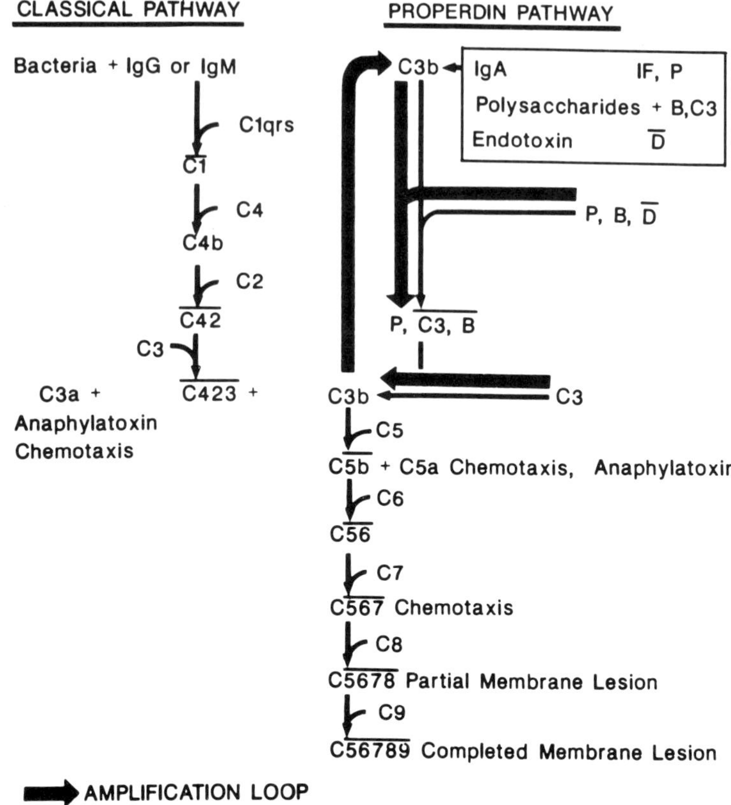

Fig. 1. Complement cascade demonstrating classical and alternate pathways, as well as the amplification loop.

pathway does not include classical pathway components C1, 4, or 2. During activation of either pathway the individual complement proteins are enzymatically cleaved. An activated component is indicated by a bar placed above it. The cleavage also yields a small fragment that remains in solution, designated by the letter "a," and a large fragment that remains bound to the complex formed by the previous complement component, designated by the letter "b." The one exception to this rule is C2, in which the larger fragment is designated C2a and the smaller C2b. The classical activating system is initiated when an antigen–antibody complex is formed. In the septic patient this complex would involve the bacteria or endotoxin and its specific antibody. This complex is capable of binding to C1qrs by interaction of the crystalline fragment portion of the antibody molecule with the C1q component. Once bound, activated C1 in turn activates the next two components to bind, C4 followed by C2. This results in a complex, $C\overline{42}$, which is the unique portion of the classical pathway. By splitting off a small fragment of C3a, the $C\overline{42}$, complex activates C3. The C3a fragment is an anaphylatoxin, while the larger active fragment, C3b, may either remain in solution or join the assembling complex to form $C\overline{423}$. $C\overline{423}$ then activates C5 to release C5a, a second anaphylatoxin and potent chemotactic factor. The formation and binding of C5b on the bacterial membrane begins the so-called membrane-attack sequence. The binding of C6,

7, 8, and 9 eventuates in bacterial lysis and death.

The alternative pathway, also referred to as the properdin pathway, can be initiated by endotoxin, polysaccharide antigens, or aggregated IgA. Properdin is one of three plasma proteins that interact to form an enzyme capable of activating C3. Properdin is a gamma-globulin with a molecular weight of 220,000. Factor B is a beta-globulin with a molecular weight of 100,000, and factor D is an alpha-globulin with a molecular weight of 25,000. Although the mechanism of their activation is unknown, these initiating factors bind C3b to their surfaces. C3b then forms a complex with properdin and factor B, while activated factor $\overline{D}$ activates factor B. This complex, P,C$\overline{3}$,$\overline{B}$, is the functional equivalent of the classical pathway's $\overline{C42}$ complex, i.e., it cleaves and activates C3 and C5. It is significant that factor B can bind with C3b, as in the presence of activated $\overline{D}$, C3b generated by either pathway can create a complex capable of cleaving C3 into still more C3b. This sequence is responsible for an amplification loop through which both the classical and alternative pathways enjoy an autocatalytic boost that bypasses the initial stages of each to accelerate the activation of C3. It is $\overline{C3}$ and the effector sequence that follows that have real impact, whether beneficial or harmful, with respect to the host defense mechanisms. The classical and alternative pathways are illustrated in Figure 1, and the various functional activities of the components and/or fragments of complement are detailed in Table 4.

Several control mechanisms act as brakes to prevent the complement activation sequence, once initiated, from running away with itself. There is an inactivator of $\overline{C1}$ that modulates the subsequent cleavage of C4 and C2. Once formed, $\overline{C2}$ is unstable and loses activity relatively quickly, thus limiting the effective biologic life of $\overline{C42}$ and $\overline{C423}$. In addition, there is a serum carboxypeptidase that acts upon both C3a and C5a, destroying their biological activity. Finally,

TABLE 4. Components or Fragments of Complement and Their Biological Activities

Component/fragment	Activity
C4b, $\overline{C423}$	Virus neutralization
C3a, C5a	Anaphylatoxin
C3a, C5a, $\overline{C567}$	Chemotaxis of PMNs, monocytes, eosinophils
C3b	Opsonization—PMNs, macrophages
$\overline{C56}$	Endotoxin inactivation
$\overline{C5678}$	Lysis—virus-infected cells
$\overline{C56789}$	Bacteriolysis

an inactivator of C3b destroys the function of this key complement fragment.

The production of C3b on the surface of the gram-negative organism is of particular importance for host defense mechanisms against serum-resistant bacteria. Leukocytes, which have migrated to the site of infection through the chemotactic and anaphylatoxic action of split products of C3 and C5, recognize C3b on the bacterial surface by means of the C3b receptor on the phagocytic cell membrane. This results in phagocytosis and subsequent death of the bacterium within the leukocytes. Thus the complement system not only prepares the bacterium for phagocytosis by coating it with C3b, but it also produces substances that attract phagocytic cells to the bacterium itself. Secondary effects of the activation of the complement cascade include the release of inflammatory mediators by leukocytes attracted to the area of injury, which in turn can result in damage to the vascular endothelium with resultant exposure of collagen, aggregation of platelets, release of platelet factor III, and intensification of the coagulation cascade. Additionally, components C3a and C5a cause degranulation of mast cells and release of histamine. Histamine in turn disrupts the vascular endothelium and results in increased capillary permeability with extravasation of fluid into the interstitial spaces and a resultant fall in plasma volume.

KININ PATHWAY

Activated Hageman factor also triggers the kinin-forming system, which generates kallikrein and in turn bradykinin. Bradykinin contributes to tissue damage through its effects on the margination of leukocytes, smooth muscle stimulation, vasodilatation, and increased vascular permeability. These changes, similar to those of histamine, result in leakage of fluid into the interstitial space, further contributing to intravascular hypovolemia. Further, bradykinin evokes a profound fall in systemic vascular resistance secondary to its vasodilitary effects, clinically seen as hypotension in the early phases of "warm" septic shock.

INTERLEUKIN-1

The complexity and multiplicity of the pathophysiologic processes of septic shock is demonstrated by the vast number of factors/substances hypothesized to play roles in this process (Table 5). Of most significance among these additional mediators are interleukin-1, the prostaglandins, and myocardial depressant factor. It is uncertain whether interleukin-1 is a single compound or group of similar compounds. Interleukin-1 has previously been called endogenous pyrogen, because of its role in the mediation of fever; leukocyte endogenous mediator, because of its ability to promote neutrophilia; and lymphocyte-activating factor, because of its ability to facilitate the proliferation of lymphocytes in suboptimal concentrations of various plant lectins. In addition to stimulating bone marrow production of neutrophils, it also appears to activate neutrophils to release lactoferrin, which binds serum iron that is subsequently taken up by the reticuloendothelial cells of the liver, resulting in hypoferremia. Interleukin-1 reduces zinc levels and promotes a host of acute-phase proteins. Production of immunoglobulins, enhancement of killer-cell lymphocyte activity, and stimulation of fibroblasts to elaborate collagen and

TABLE 5. Humoral Factors That Potentially Mediate Sequential Organ Failure in Sepsis

Interleukin-1
Eicosanoids
Opioids/neuropeptides
Glucagon
Insulin
Corticosteroids
Growth hormone
Thyroxin
Myocardial depressant factor
False neurotransmitters
Activated complement
Kinin
Histamine
Serotonin
Free-oxygen radicals
Hydrogen peroxide
Superoxide radicals
Hydroxyl radicals
Lysosomal enzymes
Proteases
Collagenase
Elastases
Myeloperoxidase
Fibronectin

promote fibrosis also seem to be mediated by interleukin-1. Additionally, the bulk of current evidence suggests that interleukin-1 mediates many of the catabolic processes that result in protein and caloric malnutrition and render the host more vulnerable to multiple organ system failure.[33]

PROSTAGLANDINS

The prostaglandins also appear to play a prominent role in the pathophysiology of septic shock. Of these compounds, prostacyclin (PGI_2) and thromboxane (TBX) are of most importance. Prostacyclin is a potent vasodilator synthesized principally within the vascular endothelium. Although the parent compound is unstable, prostacyclin's metabolite (6-keto-PGF_1-a) can be measured and has been reported to be elevated commensurate with the level of sepsis.[34,35] The stable metabolite of PGI_2 was 4 pg/ml in uninfected control patients, 30 pg/ml in septic patients who ultimately survived, and 229 pg/ml in patients who died of sepsis. Prostacyclin likely exerts its most significant effect within the lung. In the uninjured lung the pulmonary vasculature autoregulates to match the degree of perfusion to the ventilation present; this regulation of flow is the so-called hypoxic reflex. This regulation of the amount of blood flow to the hypoventilated alveolus allows the amount of shunting, and hence hypoxemia, to be minimized. In animal models, the hypoxic pulmonary vasoconstriction response is inhibited by the administration of endotoxin and thereby con-tributes even further to the intrapulmonary shunt.[36] This is generally a delayed response to injury manifest 6 to 24 hours after the initial insult and detected clinically by falling arterial PO_2 values.[36,37] Prostacyclin may also play a role similar to that of the histamine, serotonin, and bradykinins with respect to being a general vasodilator during the early "warm" phases of septic shock.

TBX's effects are essentially the reverse of those of prostacyclin, being a potent vascular and bronchiolar smooth muscle constrictor. Most TBX is of platelet origin. Direct vessel damage by either endotoxin, the complement system, or other mediators of the inflammatory process will expose collagen and cause platelet aggregation with release of a number of factors that include TBX. The vasoconstriction that accompanies the release of TBX contributes to further formation of microemboli, thrombin clots, and perpetuation of tissue ischemia. In experimental models, TBX mediates the early pulmonary hypertension and increased airway resistance, effects that can be negated by cyclooxygenase inhibitors.[37] The vascular constriction, decreased blood flow, and sludging play an important permissive role in polymorphonuclear leukocyte aggregation. Aggregation is also enhanced by the hydroxyl fatty acid arachidonate products that are potent granulocyte chemotaxins.[38] Other products of the prostaglandin cascade and lipoxygenase enzymes are the leukotrienes, one of which has been identified as a slow reactive substance of anaphylaxis (SRS-A). Both activated granulocytes and platelets can produce the cyclooxygenase products of arachidonate and thereby contribute to the increased vascular permeability.

MYOCARDIAL DEPRESSANT FACTOR

An additional humoral factor proposed to play a role in septic shock, especially in the terminal phases, is myocardial depressant factor (MDF).[39,40] Several studies in both laboratory animals and humans have identified this factor, which is apparently released from the ischemic pancreas during evolution of the shock state. Although MDF has only partially been characterized, it is thought to be a peptide or glycopeptide with a molecular weight of 500 to 1,000.[41] During shock in experimental animals, MDF accumulates in plasma in direct proportion to the severity of splanchnic ischemia.[39] MDF acts principally as a direct depressant of myocardial contactility and does not alter heart rate, rhythm, or coronary blood flow. It does, however, enhance vasoconstriction of the splanchnic blood bed, thereby accelerating its own production. It also depresses the phagocytotic activity of the reticuloendothelial system, resulting in impaired clearance of lysosomal enzymes and MDF from within the circulation.

In brief summary, the occurrence of gram-negative bacteremia or endotoxemia will simultaneously trigger a number of important events, including 1) activation of the coagulation system, 2) activation of the fibrinolytic system, 3) activation of the complement system, and 4) stimulation of interleukin-1 (Fig. 2). Secondary to these primary events, a number of the body's host defense mechanisms—leukocytes, macrophages, and platelets—will be called into play. By-products of these elements will then trigger a series of further events to include the elucidation of vasoactive substances varying from the histamine, bradykinin, and serotonin compounds, to the prostaglandins, to MDF. The end re-

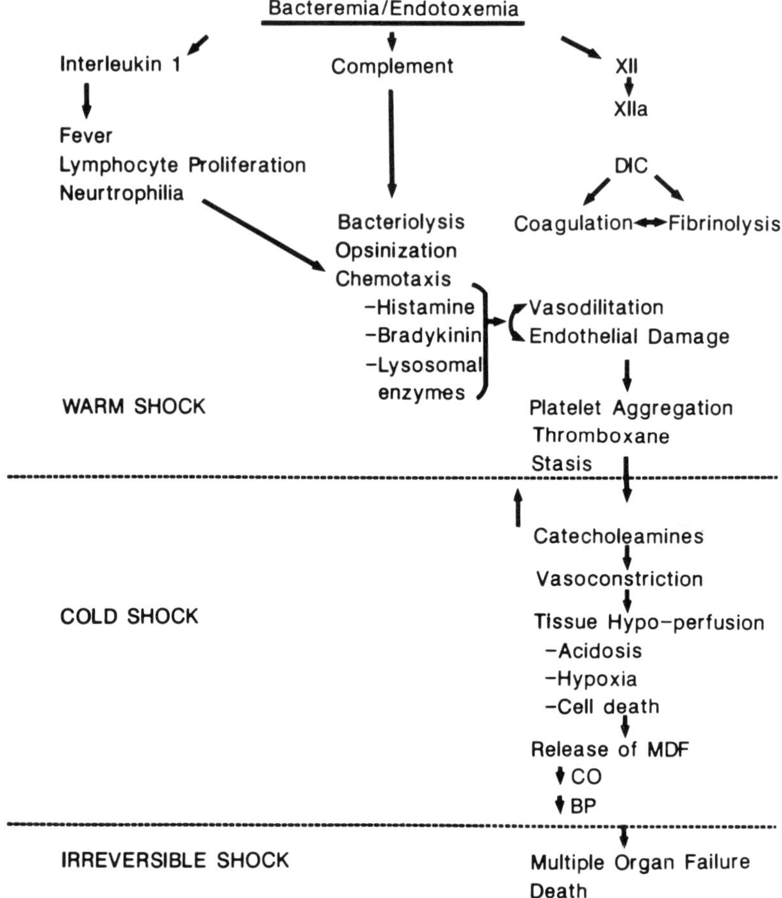

Fig. 2. Schematic representation of the pathophysiology of gram-negative endotoxic shock.

sult of all these pathways is increased endothelial cell damage throughout the body with disruption of the microcirculation and resultant tissue hypoperfusion, acidosis, hypoxia, and ultimately cell death. If the principal process, i.e., bacteremia/endotoxemia, is not eradicated then the process will proceed to multiple organ system failure and a maternal and/or fetal death.

PREGNANCY AND SEPTIC SHOCK

Since 1935, when Apitz first observed during his studies on endotoxin that one rabbit died after application of less endotoxin than that received by the rest of the group,[42] and he further noted that this animal was pregnant, the question of increased sensitivity to endotoxin as a result of the pregnancy state has been raised. Subsequently an assortment of information collected from both animal models and clinical observations in humans supports the hypothesis that pregnancy may potentiate the effects of endotoxin and that milligram per milligram, the effects of endotoxin are much greater in the pregnant woman than in her nonpregnant counterpart. McKay reviewed the accumulated data concerning the generalized Schwartzman reaction in pregnant and nonpregnant rabbits and concluded that pregnant animals at term required less endotoxin for the development of shock and organ necrosis, the latter resulting from disseminated intravascular coagulation, than did their nonpregnant controls.[43] Using the gravid ewe as a model, Beck-Jansen and associates noted that the pregnant animals died after exposure to lesser amounts of endotoxin than did nonpregnant controls.[44] Beller and coworkers also used a large animal model, the minipig, and produced similar results.[45] Using *Escherichia coli* B6 polysaccharide in a dosage of 0.2 mg/kg body weight as a continuous infusion, they noted that the nonpregnant animals' mean survival was 16 hours, as compared to only 3½ hours in near-term pregnant animals. These investigators found no significant difference in the coagulation/fibrinolytic/DIC picture, but noted that the pregnant animals had a much more pronounced metabolic acidosis than did their nonpregnant counterparts. Pregnant animals died of cardiovascular collapse, never mounting a compensatory tachycardia as might be expected, considering the profound drop in cardiac output and mean arterial pressure with a concomitantly high systemic vascular resistance. In fact, these animals appeared to progress very rapidly into the cold shock phase followed by irreversible shock. Also notable was that all pregnant animals were oliguric by 3 hours into the study, whereas none of the nonpregnant animals were oliguric at that point in time. Another potentially important observation by these investigators was the development of uterine ischemia, perhaps etiologic in the premature labor that frequently characterizes these critically ill women. Morishima and associates also demonstrated a predilection for premature labor in the setting of endotoxic shock.[46] In the pregnant baboon (*Papio* sp.) they used *E. coli* endotoxin in a dosage of 5 mg/kg, equivalent to one-fifth of the lethal dose. Following administration of this supposed sublethal dose of endotoxin, all animals labored, the average Montevideo units during the control phase of the study being 35 mm Hg compared to 255 mm Hg at the conclusion of the study. Because this study lacked a control group it can be argued that the acute experimental preparation, not the administration of the endotoxin, precipitated the labor. Notwithstanding, acute increases in both maternal and fetal temperatures, a pronounced fall in maternal mean arterial pressure, and a compensatory increase in heart rate occurred. Although the fetal blood pressure remained stable until near the point of maternal death, all four fetuses developed severe late decelerations, most pronounced with the increasing uterine activity. By 120 minutes into the experiment, the maternal pH had fallen from 7.44 to 7.32, and the fetal pH had fallen from 7.34 to 6.93 with a corresponding drop in the PaO_2 from 29 mm Hg to 7 mm Hg. Again, with the administration of what was calculated to be only 20% of a lethal dose of endotoxin, all fetuses died and three of four maternal preps died. Cunningham and colleagues reported a large series of pregnant women who developed a significant lung injury in association with pyelonephritis.[7,12] In addition to pulmonary injury, these women manifest multiple organ system derangements to include hypothalamic thermoregulatory instability, abnormalities of liver function, derangements of renal function, and thrombocytopenia and anemia. Such associated dysfunction is decidedly unusual in the nonpregnant patient with pyelonephritis, and a significant lung injury is yet to be reported in the nonpregnant woman with otherwise uncomplicated pyelonephritis. This assortment of data indicates that the pregnant woman is indeed more sensitive to the effects of endotoxin and at greater risk of sustaining injury to one or many different organ systems. Nonetheless, these women are usually young and otherwise healthy, and if survivability is to occur in the setting of endotoxic shock, then it should be excellent in the pregnant woman.[47]

CLINICAL PRESENTATION

Patients admitted with septic shock will show a varied clinical picture depending

TABLE 6. Clinical Description of Septic Shock and Effects on Multiple Organ Systems

	Stage I	Stage II	Stage III	Stage IV
General appearance	No obvious signs	"Ill," labile	Obviously unstable	Terminal, moribund
Cardiovascular system	↑ Volume requirements	Hyperdynamic, volume dependent	Shock, decreased CO, edema	Inotropes required, volume "overload"
Respiratory function	Mild respiratory alkalosis	Tachypnea, hypocapnia, hypoxia	Severe hypoxia	Hypercapnia, barotrauma
Renal function	Limited responsiveness	Fixed output, minimal azotemia	Azotemia	Oliguria
Metabolism	↑ Insulin requirements	Severe catabolism	Metabolic acidosis, hyperglycemia	Severe acidosis, increased oxygen consumption
Hepatic function		Chemical jaundice	Clinical jaundice	Encephalopathy
Hematology		↓ Platelets ⇕ WBC	↓ Platelets ↓ Fibrinogen ↑ FSP ↑ PT, PTT	Immature cells, continued coagulopathy
Central nervous system	Confusion	Variable	Some response to noxious stimuli	Coma

upon the severity and duration of the process when they first present. The earliest phase of septic shock is termed "warm shock." Ideally the process will be interdicted and reversed at that point in time. Failure to so do will result in progression of the disease into cold shock and ultimately into irreversible shock characterized by multiple organ failure and death (Fig. 2). If the process is allowed to progress to the stage of multiple organ failure, as occurs in 30 to 50% of operations performed for intraabdominal sepsis,[33] then the associated mortality varies from 30 to 100% depending upon the number of organs involved. Knaus and associates have reported that with a single organ system failure lasting more than 1 day the mortality rate approached 40%, with two organ system failures for longer than 1 day the mortality increased to 60%, and with three or more organ system failures persisting for more than three days the mortality was 98%.[47] Survival of the patient is dependent upon prompt recognition and reversal of the septic process.

In describing the clinical appearance of the patient, the classic description of the stages of respiratory failure developed in the late 1960s can be applied to critical organ systems and stages assigned (Table 6). Clinical stages I and II correspond to the warm shock phase (Fig. 2). During the first stage the patient often shows no obvious signs of impending septic shock. At most the clinical examination may reveal mild confusion or alteration of mental status and a tachypnea with resultant mild respiratory alkalosis. With continued showering of bacteria or endotoxin the patient can move quite rapidly into stage II. During this stage release of histamines, serotonins, and bradykinins will produce peripheral vasodilitation and the patient will appear warm and flushed. Unless obviously volume depleted, the cardiovascular system will be hyperdynamic. From a respiratory standpoint the patient will continue to manifest tachypnea and may for the first time have concomitant hypoxemia. At this stage the patient will commonly manifest thrombocytopenia and the white blood cell count can range from abnormally low to a frank leukocytosis. Urine output will generally be adequate, particularly if volume replacement has been instituted. Renal function tests may show a mild increase in both the BUN and creatinine levels. If the disease goes unchecked or the patient fails to present

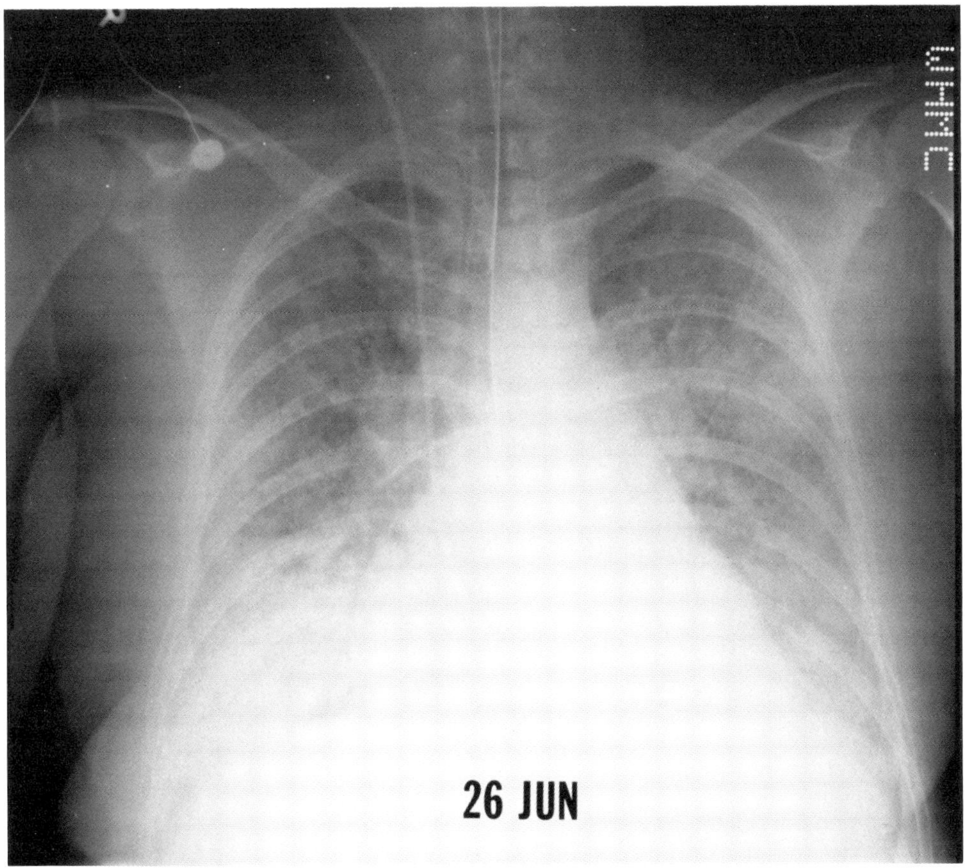

Fig. 3. Chest radiograph of a woman with septic shock and the adult respiratory distress syndrome (ARDS). Note fine ground-glass appearance of all lung fields.

for treatment, the patient will enter into stage III. General appearance will show an obviously unstable patient with marked alteration of consciousness due to hypoperfusion of the central nervous system. This stage will correspond to "cold shock," characterized by a very high systemic vascular resistance with shunting of blood flow from the skin and gut and preferential flow to the heart, brain, and kidneys. Despite autoregulatory attempts at maintaining perfusion of vital organs, there will be a rapid deterioration in renal function manifest by a rising serum creatinine level and a decreased creatinine clearance. Pulmonary gas exchange will be significantly altered and the arterial oxygen content will be markedly depressed. On chest radiograph the lungs will show diffuse involvement with a fine ground-glass appearance throughout all lung fields (Fig. 3). During this phase both the coagulation system and the fibrinolytic system will be activated, resulting in thrombocytopenia, hypofibrinogemia, and elevations in fibrin split products. Simultaneous impairment of liver function and consumption of coagulation factors will result in elevations of both the PT and PTT. The patient will retain some responsiveness to noxious stimuli. Stage IV is the final clinical stage of septic shock. The patient is in a coma and is terminal or moribund. A failing myocardium will result in worsening pulmonary edema and worsening of the adult respiratory distress syndrome (ARDS) on the basis of back pressure. Concomitantly the myocardium will be unable to generate enough forward flow to adequately maintain a systemic blood pressure in the absence of significant inotropic and/or vasopressor support. The degree of ARDS will be such that neither ventilation, manifest by an increasing PCO_2, nor oxygenation, manifest by a continued decline in the PO_2, can be supported, and chest radiographs may show a complete whiteout of all lung fields. The patient will have marked oliguria, a continued rise in creatinine level, and a fall in creatinine clearance, and may at this point be dialysis dependent. The combination of renal and lung failure will result in a severe mixed metabolic and respiratory acidosis. While the overall oxygen demands in this setting may be greatly increased, these demands cannot be met because of dual failure of the cardiovascular system manifest both by pump failure and by vessel failure with a tremendous increase in extravasation of fluids into the interstitium, impeding diffusion of gases into and out of the cells. The liver's ability to either synthesize or metabolize will be greatly impeded, as will the function of its reticuloendothelial cells. The hematologic system will remain in shambles and immature forms will be seen in the peripheral circulation.

SOURCE EVALUATION

Microbiologic studies are of paramount importance in establishing the diagnosis of septic shock and a determination of the origin of the infection. Depending upon the clinical setting, certain cultures may be of greater significance than others. Notwithstanding, a urine specimen should be obtained by catheterization and examined by the clinician in addition to being analyzed for culture and sensitivity. As a minimum, blood cultures, both aerobic and anaerobic, should be obtained upon admission and repeated when the patient experiences rigors or a temperature elevation. If antibiotic therapy has been instituted prior to obtaining subsequent cultures, the specimens should be collected in culture bottles containing antibiotic binding resins and the laboratory notified of the antibiotics that the patient was receiving at the time the cultures were obtained. Some authors recommend that blood cultures be obtained in triplicate from the same puncture site in order to discriminate contaminants from pathogens. Using this technique, the growth of an organism such as *Staphylococcus aureus* in the first culture bottle, but not from the subsequent bottles, would be considered a contaminant and not a pathogen. While the majority of obstetric and gynecology patients' sputum cultures will be of little benefit, sputum cultures may prove invaluable in the patient admitted to the intensive care unit who has required intubation and ventilatory support. The likelihood of an infectious pneumonia is much higher in this subgroup of patients than in other obstetric and gynecology patients. If a wound exists, whether traumatic or surgical, it should be closely examined and cultures obtained. In instances where debridement is necessary, aerobic, anaerobic, and fungal cultures should be obtained and tissue submitted for histologic examination and staining to identify any infectious etiology. In the woman who is still pregnant and presents with sepsis, it is prudent to obtain a specimen of amniotic fluid for examination and culture unless another obvious source of the infection exists. Similarly, cervical, vaginal, and endometrial cultures should be considered depending upon the individual clinical circumstances. If an unusual organism is under consideration, such as *Listeria monocytogenes*, then the laboratory should be alerted so that the cultures are not discarded prematurely or the organism incorrectly dismissed as a diphtheroid contaminant. In selection of specific cultures to be obtained and the weight given to the culture results one cannot overemphasize the importance of the clinical examination and assessment.

Routine chest radiographs, including a posterior anterior and lateral view, and a flat plate and upright abdominal film are standard in the evaluation of patients with presumed bacteremia, especially if the patient has progressed to septic shock. Additional radiologic studies that may be of assistance include ultrasound examination of the biliary tree, pancreas, and pelvis. CT scans can be used to study virtually any area of the body, as can magnetic resonance imaging studies.[48] An area of infection that is often overlooked in the critically ill patient is a sinusitis. This condition often is not the process that precipitated the admission to the intensive care unit but is a by-product of therapies to include endotracheal tubes and nasogastric tubes. Failure to diagnose and appropriately treat such infections can lead to continuous bacterial seeding and a progressive worsening of multisystem failure.

Although a subject of debate, multiple organ failure is considered by many, including the authors, to be an indication for abdominal exploration in the absence of another defined etiology for the infection.[19,33,49,50] Finally, a phenomenon of "nonbacteremic clinical sepsis," characterized by patients who manifest all the usual characteristic findings of sepsis including fever, leukocytosis, and remote organ dysfunction, appears to exist. In these patients multiple repeated blood cultures are negative, yet the clinical course and outcome is essentially equal to that of patients with demonstrable bacteremia. It is hypothesized that the gastrointestinal system serves as the reservoir for their continued low-grade sepsis. A change in intestinal flora, coupled with impairment of the normal barrier function of the GI tract, allows the bowel to serve as a reservoir of pathogens that can enter the portal and systemic circulations and fuel the ongoing septic process. Evidence to support this hypothesis includes oral-pharyngeal colonization with gram-negative organisms, which commonly occurs during critical illness. Following oral-pharyngeal colonization, these organisms seed to the stomach and proximal small bowel. It has been well demonstrated that among these organisms are the gram-negative Enterobacteriaceae and *Enterococcus.* Their overgrowth within the bowel, in conjunction with impaired intestinal function and compromise of normal barriers by hypoperfusion, tissue hypoxia, and acidosis, invariably leads to increased permeability of the gut wall to these organisms. The two largest reticuloendothelial organs in the body, the liver and the lungs, are connected in series and if functioning normally can clear bacteria from the blood draining the GI tract. However, with septic shock both the liver and lungs are also hypoperfused and have sustained significant injury such that they are unable to effectively clear bacteria seeding from the gut. Clinically, the patient manifests an ileus with distention of the bowel and perhaps accumulation of ascitic fluid. Here again an argument can be made for exploration of the patient with multiple organ failure and no identifiable source for the sepsis to exclude intraabdominal abscess or infarcted bowel. Even if negative, the celiotomy will allow any infected ascitic fluid to be drained, the abdomen to be thoroughly irrigated, and mechanical decompression of the intestines to be carried out.

PATIENT MANAGEMENT

The patient with septic shock or with impending septic shock is critically ill and requires management in an intensive care setting. For the purposes of treatment and discussion we will divide management into four areas: 1) stabilization, involving principally the cardiovascular and respiratory systems, 2) institution of broad-spectrum antibiotic coverage after appropriate diagnostic cultures have been obtained, 3) erradication of the septic focus, and 4) avoidance of further organ system deterioration and/or appropriate management of those complications. While discussed separately in this chapter, in clinical practice many or all of these therapies will be instituted either simultaneously or in close temporal relationship to one another.

VOLUME RESUSCITATION AND INITIAL STABILIZATION

The stability of the cardiovascular system can be quickly assessed by the patient's blood pressure, pulse rate, quality of the pulse, and skin color, turgor, and moisture. The adequacy of the circulation can be assessed by the patient's mental status and urine output. In the pregnant woman the fetus also serves as an excellent indicator of the adequacy of the circulatory system by an assessment of the fetal heart rate from a standpoint of both the absolute rate as well as any periodic deceleration patterns.

The patient with bacteremia, especially if in septic shock, will be intravascularly depleted because of the increased permeability of the vascular tree and extravasation of water, albumin, and other plasma proteins, and even red blood cells, into the interstitial spaces. Accordingly, it is reasonable to give such patients an initial volume infusion of 2 liters of a crystalloid solution, especially if they have tachycardia and/or hypotension. Failure of this initial volume infusion to stabilize the patient will necessitate the use of invasive hemodynamic monitoring in order to optimize the patient's outcome.[25,51] In the patient manifesting severe hypotension with refractoriness to the initial volume infusion, or in whom vascular access is difficult secondary to intravascular depletion, the military antishock trousers (MAST) or antishock garments have been successfully employed.[52–54] These devices work by mobilizing blood and fluids that have pooled in the lower extremities and lower abdomen and returning them to the central circulation, thereby preventing further myocardial and cerebral ischemia secondary to continued hypotension. It is estimated that 750 to 1,000 ml of autologous blood is returned to the central circulation by this very simple

maneuver without compromising the arterial supply to the lower abdomen or legs. An additional benefit accrued from the use of these devices is the prevention of the crystalloid and other resuscitative fluids from pooling in the extremities. Such devices are only a temporizing measure, however, and the devices should be slowly deflated and removed once the central circulation has been stabilized. Both congestive heart failure and cerebral edema are contraindications for the use of antishock garments.

If invasive hemodynamic monitoring is necessary, we prefer the pulmonary artery catheter over the central venous pressure (CVP) catheter.[51,55] The pulmonary artery catheter will allow monitoring of the filling pressures of both the right and left ventricles, measurements of the pulmonary artery pressure and of cardiac output, calculations of the pulmonary and systemic vascular resistances, and measurement of mixed venous blood gases. In contrast, a CVP catheter will allow the measurement of only the right ventricular filling pressure, which may not accurately reflect left ventricular function. Moreover, the morbidity of both the pulmonary artery catheter and the CVP line is related principally to the acquisition of venous access, i.e., they are virtually identical. The risk-to-benefit ratio of the pulmonary artery catheter in the obstetric and gynecology patient was addressed by Clark and associates, who reported that among 90 patients requiring a pulmonary artery catheter during an 18-month period, none had any significant clinical morbidity associated with the procedure itself.[51]

Once invasive monitoring has been established, a number of algorithms exist to guide further management. Lee and associates have recommended a sequential hemodynamic approach for stabilizing obstetrical septic shock with volume repletion, inotropic therapy, and peripheral vasoconstrictors, as outlined in Figure 4.[25] Rackow and Wheel recommend the administration of 5 to 20 ml/kg body weight of crystalloid solution administered

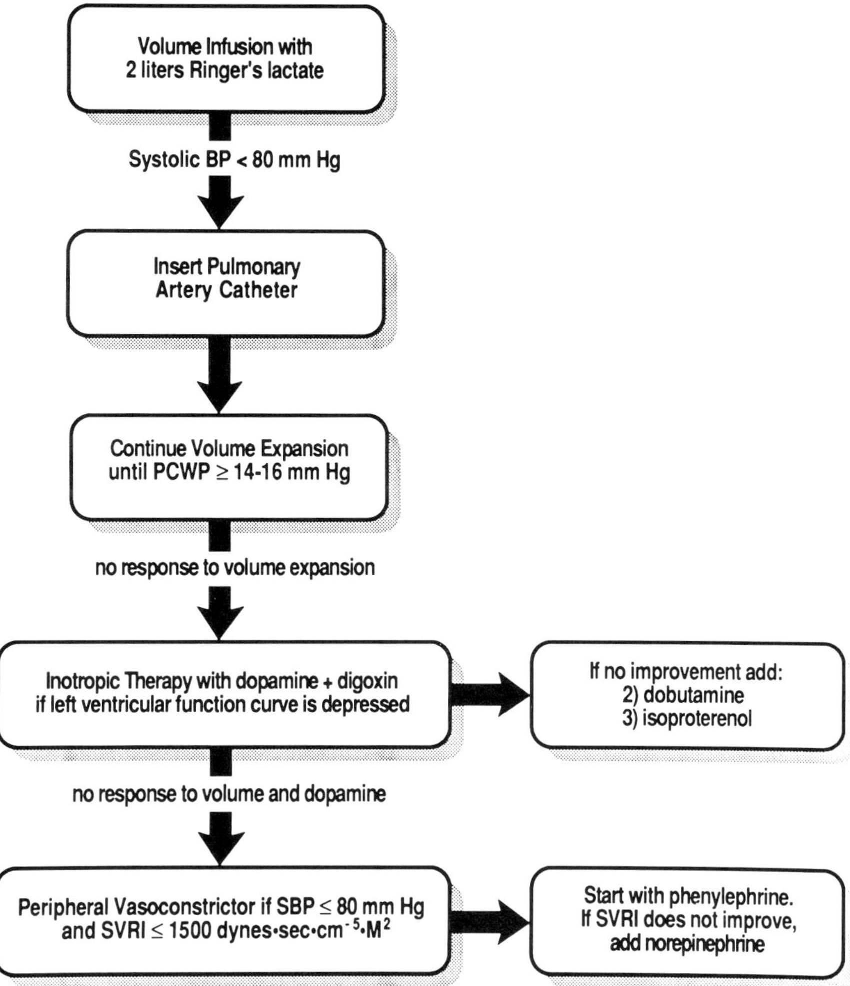

Fig. 4. Hemodynamic algorithm for obstetrical septic shock. (From Lee et al.,[25] with permission of the publisher.)

over 10 minutes while monitoring the patient's pulmonary capillary wedge pressure.[50] If the pulmonary capillary wedge pressure increases by 7 mm Hg or greater, the infusion is cut back to a maintenance dose, whereas if the increase of the wedge pressure is less than 3 mm Hg, the fluid challenge is repeated.[50] These investigators refer to this as the 7-3 rule. Failure to have achieved stabilization of the patient's blood pressure by volume expansion alone is an indication for inotropic support. The commonly used sympathomimetic

and pressor drugs used for the treatment of obstetrical septic shock are listed in Table 7. It is important to emphasize that the patient's volume status should be repleted prior to initiation of these potent medications. Further, in the setting of obstetric hemorrhage or other causes for blood loss, the use of packed red blood cells or blood component therapy may be the indicated and preferred means of volume resuscitation.

Failure of volume resuscitation to correct the patient's blood pressure implies that the

TABLE 7. Sympathomimetic, Vasopressor, and Vasodilator Drugs Useful for Therapy of Obstetrical Septic Shock

Agent	Dosage range	Therapeutic goals
Inotropic		
Dopamine	2–10 μg/kg/min	Cardiac index ≥ 3 liters/min/M^2,SBP ≥ 80 mm Hg
Dobutamine	2–10 μg/kg/min	
Isoproterenol	0.01–0.30 μg/kg/min	
Vasopressors		
Phenylephrine	0.1–0.7 μg/kg/min	SVRI ≥ 1,500 dynes · sec · cm^{-5} · M^2
Norepinephrine	0.05–1 μg/kg/min	
Vasodilators		
Nitroprusside	0.4–5 μg/kg/min	SVRI ≤ 2,400 dynes · sec · cm^{-5} · M^2
Phentolamine	0.5–20 μg/kg/min	
Chlorpromazine	5–10 mg IV q 30 min	

problem is either with the heart itself, and resultant inadequate cardiac output, or else a problem of too little or too much systemic vascular resistance. During the warm phase of shock the cardiac output will usually be normal or high and the systemic vascular resistance will be low, accounting for the low systemic blood pressure. Indeed, among the 10 obstetric patients with septic shock reported by Lee and associates, the hemodynamic profile upon institution of invasive monitoring showed only a mild increase in heart rate, a low systemic vascular resistance, and a slightly elevated cardiac index (Table 8).[25] When compared to values after reversal of the process and immediately prior to discontinuation of the pulmonary artery catheter, the only significant changes effected by treatment were an absolute increase in the mean arterial pressure of 19 mm Hg, an increase in the left ventricular stroke work index of 15 g·M·M^2 and an increase in systemic vascular resistance of 787 dynes·sec·cm^{-5}·M^2. The cardiac output had declined by almost a liter per minute in these women. Importantly, two of the women reported by Lee and associates had mildly depressed ventricular function upon initial presentation, while three had markedly depressed ventricular function (Fig. 5).[25] Additionally, no woman in their series with a left ventricular stroke work index less than 20 g·M·M^2 survived.

TABLE 8. Presenting Invasive Hemodynamic Parameters From Eight Surviving Obstetrical Septic Shock Patients Compared to Period Immediately Prior to Discontinuation of Pulmonary Artery Catheter

Parameter	Mean initial value	Mean final value
Mean arterial pressure[a] (mm Hg)	66 ± 5	85 ± 9
Heart rate (beats/min)	114 ± 28	91 ± 18
Stroke volume index (ml/beat/M^2)	40 ± 14	43 ± 8
Cardiac index (liters/min/M^2)	4.58 ± 1.91	3.86 ± 0.89
Pulmonary capillary wedge pressure (mm Hg)	10 ± 6	11 ± 4
Central venous pressure (mm Hg)	6 ± 5	8 ± 4
Systemic vascular resistance index[a] (dyne · sec · cm^{-5} · M^2)	885 ± 253	1,672 ± 413
Left ventricular stroke work index[a] (g · M · M^2)	30 ± 10	45 ± 11

From Lee et al.,[25] with permission of the publisher.
[a]Indicates statistically significant difference at $P < .05$, paired Student's t-test.

Table 9 presents the invasive hemodynamic parameters from eight surviving and two nonsurviving obstetrical septic shock patients reported by Lee and associates. This table demonstrates quite dramatically that

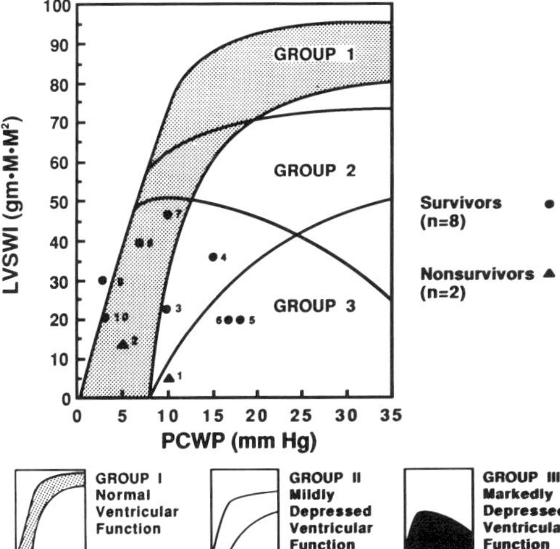

Fig. 5. Presenting left ventricular function of 10 pregnant women with septic hypotension. LVSWI, left ventricular stroke work index; PCWP, pulmonary capillary wedge pressure. (From Lee et al.,[25] with permission of the publisher.)

TABLE 9. Presenting Invasive Hemodynamic Parameters From Eight Surviving and Two Nonsurviving Obstetrical Septic Shock Patients

Parameter	Survivor	Nonsurvivor
Mean arterial pressure (mm Hg)	66 ± 5	50 ± 5
Heart rate (beats/min)	114 ± 28	137 ± 67
Stroke volume index (ml/beat/M²)	40 ± 14	18 ± 8
Cardiac index (liters/min/M²)	4.58 ± 1.91	2.66 ± 2.24
Systemic vascular resistance index (dyne · sec · cm⁻⁵ · M²)	885 ± 253	1,871 ± 1,554
Left ventricular stroke work index (g · M · M²)	30 ± 10	11 ± 6

From Lee et al.[25]

the woman presenting in late or cold septic shock generally will be a nonsurvivor.

INOTROPIC AGENTS

Dopamine serves as a first-line drug for treating septic hypotension when inotropic therapy is indicated. A precursor of norephineprine, dopamine has dopaminergic, beta- and alpha-receptor-stimulating actions depending upon the dosage at which it is administered. At dosages of 0.5 to 5 µg/kg/min the effects will be principally dopaminergic, leading to vasodilatation and improved perfusion of the renal and mesenteric vascular beds. These effects can be of great value in protecting the kidneys and maintaining urine output. Additionally, the improved blood flow to the mesenteric vascular beds and pancreas may prevent elucidation of myocardial depressant factor, which could result in a further decline in cardiac function. In dosages of 5 to 15 µg/kg/min, the principal effects will be on the beta-1 receptors of the heart. Stimulation of the beta-1 myocardial receptors will result in improved myocardial contractility, stroke volume, and cardiac output. In dosages exceeding 15 µg/kg/min, the principal effects will be on the alpha-adrenergic system and result in generalized vasoconstriction. In this regard dopamine can be used as a vasopressor in much the same fashion as phenylephrine, metaraminol, or norephinephrine. Generally, however, if these very potent vasopressor agents are required, then we would maintain the dopamine infusion in the dopaminergic range and add a pressor agent if an increase in systemic vascular resistance was required in order to maintain sufficient blood pressure to perfuse vital organs, i.e., brain, heart, kidneys, and uteroplacental circulations. Myocardial performance during the administration of inotropic agents can be assessed by construction of ventricular function curves, by using absolute criteria that will satisfy most patients' needs, such as a cardiac index above 3 liters per minute per M², or by assessment of the adequacy of the cardiac output by clinical parameters such as maintaining normal acid-base status, maintaining a normal urine output, and maintaining normal mental status.

Rao and Cavanagh have reported very favorable results of dopamine in a septic shock model. Using nonpregnant female baboons given lipopolysaccharide of *E. coli* suspended in normal saline, these investigators were able to show significant ameliorating effects of a simultaneous dopamine infusion. In their studies they saw a significant increase in both systolic and diastolic blood pressure as well as mean arterial pressure in those animals receiving the dopamine. Endotoxins' effects were obviated principally by an increase in cardiac output, which occurred on the basis of an increase in stroke volume. They further noted a decrease in renal vascular resistance and an increase in renal blood flow with a concomitant increase in urine output of those animals receiving dopamine relative to the control animals receiving only the *E. coli* endotoxin.[56]

The inability to obtain appropriate inotropic support with dopamine may necessitate the use of either dobutamine or isoproterenol. Dobutamine is a much purer inotropic agent than is dopamine and will have less effects on heart rate. Isoproterenol is considered a third-line drug as it is a potent beta-1 and beta-2 agent and is associated with increased arrhythmias relative to the other agents listed.

VASOPRESSORS

Vasopressor drugs such as those listed in Table 7 may also be required in the treatment of obstetrical septic shock. With respect to these agents it is important to emphasize the continued use of clinical parameters such as adequate urinary output, ability of the patient to maintain a normal acid-base status, and, if still pregnant, the ability to maintain a normal fetal heart-rate tracing. In the absence of an abnormality of the above we would not add these potent alpha agents merely on the basis of continued maternal hypotension resulting from a profound decrease in her systemic vascular resistance. It has been our experience that although the addition of the agents can normalize the blood pressure, they do so at the expense of end-organ perfusion as shown by a decline in

urine output or worsening of the acid-base status.

VASODILATORS

A final class of drugs that may be required in the management of the patient with obstetrical septic shock are the vasodilators. In patients presenting with myocardial failure and a very high systemic vascular resistance, such as the nonsurvivors represented in Table 9, the combined use of an inotropic agent and a vasodilator may prove to be life saving. In this instance the systemic vascular resistance may simply be so great that it is playing a major role in the myocardial failure, a role such that correction of myocardial contractility alone cannot overcome the failure. In this setting combination therapy is likely to be the only successful pharmacologic therapy that can be employed, if indeed any therapy will be successful.

ANTIBIOTICS

Once specimens for bacteriologic cultures are obtained, and simultaneous with hemodynamic stabilization, antibiotic therapy should be instituted. In obstetric and gynecologic patients, excluding gynecologic oncology patients, the major organisms responsible for bacteremia and soft tissue pelvic infections are the aerobic gram-negative rods, group B streptococcus, anerobic *Streptococcus*, and *Bacteroide* sp.[6,7,20,57,58] If the infection is pyelonephritis, then the overwhelming majority of organisms will be from the Enterobacteriaceae group.[7,12] Accordingly it is appropriate to begin broad-spectrum antibiotic coverage that will target and cover the most frequently encountered organisms pending identification and sensitivities of a specific organism. Several acceptable regimens are listed in Table 10.

Each drug listed has known side effects for which the clinician must be alert. The patient with septic shock will usually have some degree of renal compromise and will be sus-

TABLE 10. Antibiotic Regimens Recommended for the Obstetric Patient in Septic Shock

Duff and Gibbs[20]	Penicillin
	    5 million U q 6 h
		Tobramycin 3–5 mg/kg/d
		    or
			Clindamycin 600 mg q 6 h

Gonik[21]		Gentamicin	
Lee et al.[25]	Ampicillin 2 g q 6 h	Gentamicin 2 mg/kg load then 1.5 mg/kg q 8 h	Clindamycin 900 mg q 8 h
Hawkins[19]	Penicillin or Cephalosporin	Gentamicin	Metronidazole

Knuppel et al.[22]	Penicillin
	    10 million U q 4 h or
	    Ampicillin 2 g q 4 h or
	    Oxacillin 2 g q 4 h
		Tobramycin
		    1.5 mg/kg q 8 h
			Clindamycin 600 mg q 6 h
			Chloramphenicol 1 g q 6 h
			Metronidazole 1 g load
			    then 500 mg q 6 h

ceptible to nephrotoxicity from aminoglycosides. The risk of nephrotoxicity is minimized when peak serum levels are maintained in the range of 6 to 10 μg/ml and trough levels are maintained at less than 2 μg/ml. If unable to obtain serum drug levels, then the dosage of aminoglycosides can be adjusted by either decreasing the amount of drug or spacing out the interval between dosages. One simple means to accomplish this is an adjustment of the dosing interval calculated as the serum creatinine value (mg/dl) multiplied by 8, which yields the dosing interval in hours. Other potential toxicities of the aminoglycosides include their ability to potentiate the neuromuscular blockade effects of both succinylcholine and magnesium sulfate.

The high dosages of penicillin recommended to treat septic shock will be accompanied by significant administration of potassium. The regimen recommended by Knuppel and associates, 60 million units of potassium penicillin G per day, would yield a 90 mEq load of potassium.[22] If the patient is in renal failure or impending renal failure, then she will have difficulty handling such a potassium load and a sodium salt, such as ampicillin, may be preferred. Finally, pseudomembranous colitis, resulting from an overgrowth of *Clostridium difficile*, has been reported with a number of the antibiotics routinely recommended for the patient in septic shock, including ampicillin, penicillin, cephalosporins, and clindamycin. The

diagnosis is suspected on the basis of diarrhea and can be confirmed by obtaining *C. difficile* titers and by proctosigmoidoscopy with demonstration of characteristic greyish white plaques on the colonic mucosa. The occurrence of pseudomembranous enterocolitis will require discontinuation of the presumed offending drug and treatment with vancomycin, 500 mg orally every 6 hours until the diarrhea resolves. Relapses have been reported, and if they occur, administration of binding resins, specific antitoxin, and additional antibiotics active against *C. difficile*, including metronidazole, miconazole, and bacitracin, may be required.

SURGICAL TREATMENT

Unless the source of the infection is identified and eradicated, and the intermittent or continuous showering of bacteria and endotoxin is disrupted, the patient will die. Majority opinion today is that failure to identify a source of infection in the face of continued clinical deterioration of the patient warrants surgical exploration. Accordingly, once initial hemodynamic stabilization has been achieved and antibiotic therapy has been instituted, one should proceed with draining any sources of obvious infection. If the patient is presenting with a septic abortion, or is septic following instrumentation of the uterus to perform an abortion, then a dilatation and curettage is indicated. Failure to achieve significant improvement in the clinical status within a period of 48 hours implies that a septic focus persists, either in the form of myometrial microabscesses or septic pelvic thrombophlebitis, which can extend to involve both ovarian and hypogastric vessels. Differentiation of these two entities is of great clinical importance as the therapy for the former is hysterectomy, whereas for the latter it would be full heparinization. A number of authors have reported success in diagnosing septic pelvic thrombophlebitis using combinations of venography, computed axial tomography, and magnetic resonance imaging studies.[22,48] The imaging studies may provide additional information as to the presence of discrete collections of fluids in abscess cavities or of the more ill-defined inflammatory phlegmon.

If the septic shock is on the basis of chorioamnionitis, the pregnancy is at a gestation consistent with fetal viability, and the fetus is still living, then the optimal approach at evacuating the uterus is less clear. Here again the initial steps would consist of stabilization of the cardiovascular systems and broad-spectrum antibiotic coverage. While some authors recommend that cesarean section be performed if vaginal delivery cannot be effected within 12 hours,[22] it is notable that 13 of 14 maternal deaths occurring from chorioamnionitis in the series reported by Gogoi occurred in women delivered by cesarean section.[59] With respect to outcome for the fetus, neither Gibbs and coworkers[60] nor Hauth[13] were able to demonstrate a critical interval from diagnosis of chorioamnionitis to delivery with regard to serious neonatal morbidity or mortality. Accordingly, while we strongly agree that expeditious delivery is indicated, we feel that there is no absolute time limit that should be placed on a vaginal delivery so long as one is successful in stabilizing the mother. In such settings we feel that electronic fetal monitoring with a scalp electrode and an intrauterine pressure catheter are mandatory and, given sufficient maternal stability to be proceeding toward vaginal delivery, we

would also perform a cesarean section for evidence of significant fetal distress.

With respect to other surgical conditions associated with septic shock in pregnancy or in the postpartum period as outlined in Table 1, the gallbladder bed should be drained in the patient with acute biliary disease, as should the area of appendiceal abscess. An infected Bartholin's gland with abscess would be marsupialized, packed open, and followed with frequent repackings and wound care. Failure of the patient with pyelonephritis to respond to appropriate therapy within 72 hours necessitates evaluation for obstruction to drainage or perinephric abscess and, if present, surgical drainage. Finally, deterioration in the patient's status after any initial surgery will necessitate a thorough review for an alternate source of infection and a redirection of therapy toward any new source identified. The absence of an identifiable source is considered to be reason for surgical reexploration.

During any surgical procedure involving infected tissue and/or abscesses, one should anticipate showering of bacteria and endotoxin with manipulation of the infected tissues. Concurrent with this bacteremia/endotoxemia, the patient's clinical status may undergo significant deterioration. Surgical technique may minimize these effects by assiduous attention to handling tissue gently and to ligation of vascular pedicles draining infected areas as soon as it can safely be achieved. Abscess cavities should be evacuated carefully and efforts made to avoid intraperitoneal spill of contents. If intraperitoneal spillage does occur, copious irrigation, using 10 to 20 liters of normal saline, should be carried out. When intraperitoneal spillage of abscess cavity content occurs, an ileus is virtually certain to ensue and a nasogastric tube should be used for bowel rest to avoid distention and potential bacterial seeding from the bowel.

ANTIENDOTOXIN ANTIBODIES

McCabe and associates reported that mortality in gram-negative bacteremia is signifi-

cantly reduced in patients who develop antibodies directed against certain common
antigens shared by the Enterobacteriaceae.[61]
In a group of 175 patients with bacteremia due
to gram-negative bacilli, they noted that both
shock and death were only one-third as frequent in patients with high titers of antibody
directed against an antigen present in the cell
wall of rough mutant strains of bacteria. From
a pathophysiologic standpoint this observation would support the use of passive immunization of patients presenting with septicemia.[62] In treatment of septic shock, the
administration of antibiotics will result in
death of bacteria; however, with their death
will come the release of lipopolysaccharide
(endotoxin), which is the mediator of the
majority of the patient's morbidity and mortality. Further, antibiotics do not clear endotoxin from the woman's circulation.

Lipopolysaccharide is present in the gut in
large amounts and may enter the circulation
and cause toxic reactions when the gut is
damaged by almost any mechanism, including radiotherapy. Normally small amounts of
LPS leaving the gut will be cleared by the
reticuloendothelial system, i.e., the liver,
lungs, and spleen. With significant damage
of the intestines, massive amounts of LPS
may overwhelm the capacity of the reticuloendothelial system to clear it. Such massive
damage may accompany hypoperfusion of the
mesenteric bed during septic shock. Anti-
LPS antibodies, both IgG and IgM, are involved in LPS detoxification through the
complement cascade. Using the ischemic
bowel injury model, analogous to the nonbacteremic clinical sepsis described by
Meakins and colleagues,[49] Gaffin reported a
survival in control animals of 12.5% compared to a survival of 87.5% in animals who
received anti-LPS antibody.[62]

Anti-LPS antibody can be prepared
through the identification of human plasma,
which is rich in this IgG antibody for specific
organisms, including *E. coli, Pseudomonas,
Klebsiella, Salmonella,* and *Proteus.* Such
plasma, once identified to have greater than

40 µg/ml of anti-LPS IgG, can be freeze-
dried and stored until needed to treat a patient with septic shock. Lachman and associates used such a preparation and achieved
excellent results in a well-controlled study.[27]
Entry criteria included a temperature of
38.5°C, an obvious source of sepsis, and a
systolic blood pressure less than 80 mm Hg
after volume resuscitation to a central venous
pressure greater than 6 mm Hg. These investigators treated all patients in both groups
with appropriate antibiotics and surgery was
performed as indicated. One group received
anti-LPS human plasma, 2 units rapidly upon
presentation followed by 1 unit every 4
hours, whereas the other group received
plasma that was not rich in anti-LPS. The
mortality rate in the control group was 9 of
19 (47%) vs. 1 of 14 (7%) in the treated
group. These investigators noted an increase
in the mean arterial pressure from 45 mm Hg
to 69 mm Hg within 75 minutes of treatment, whereas controls who received identical volumes of fluids and plasma had no such
blood pressure response. Clearly this is an
exciting area of treatment that gives hope for
improved survival in the future.

OTHER ORGAN SYSTEM SUPPORT

Multisystem effects of endotoxin have been
emphasized throughout this review to include
those on the hypothalamus, liver, kidneys,
coagulation system, myocardium, and gastrointestinal tract, and to especially include
the small bowel and pancreas. A daily assessment of each of these organ systems, both
clinically and from a laboratory standpoint, is
in order and correction of any abnormalities
should be undertaken. A final organ system
deserving of special attention is the pulmonary system. It has now been 25 years since
Ashbaugh and associates described the adult
respiratory distress syndrome and emphasized
that this was primarily a lung injury as opposed
to heart failure.[63] Notwithstanding, this area
of medicine has received little attention in the
obstetric literature and there are no reported

frequencies of the condition per se in pregnancy. Sepsis is among the most frequent sources of pulmonary injury, and if sustained, and if it progresses into the adult respiratory distress syndrome, the mortality will be 90%. Because most pregnant women are young and in excellent health before their acute injury, their survival should exceed that of the general population. Accordingly, we advocate aggressive management of the suspected lung injury including early intubation and the institution of invasive hemodynamic monitoring. This approach ensures the most thorough assessment of the extent of the initial lung injury and allows rapid assessment of therapeutic maneuvers and their subsequent adjustment. Our goal is to reverse the initial insult early while avoiding further iatrogenic injury. Excellent reviews of this topic are available that deal specifically with pregnancy.[24,64] Recent detailed reviews of ARDS and patient management are also available.[24,64]

PREMATURE LABOR AND SEPTIC SHOCK

Frequently the critically ill woman, especially if acutely hypoxic, enters into spontaneous labor. With acute respiratory failure on the basis of a permeability lung lesion, we feel the use of beta-sympathomimetic tocolytic agents is contraindicated. The tendency to retain water and to develop mild elevations of the pulmonary capillary wedge pressure with these tocolytics worsens the permeability lung injury.[65–67] We accordingly allow the labor to progress and deliver the infant in the intensive care unit. Similarly, in critically ill women, we proceed with vaginal delivery irrespective of the type or number of prior cesarean deliveries and reserve operative delivery for obstetric indications.

REFERENCES

1. Gibbs RS, Castillo MS, Rodgers PJ: Management of acute chorioamnionitis. Am J Obstet Gynecol 136:709–713, 1980.
2. Gibbs RS, Rodgers PJ, Castaneda YS, Ramzy I: Endometritis following vaginal delivery. Obstet Gynecol 56:555–558, 1980.
3. Depalma RT, Leveno KJ, Cunningham FG, et al.: Identification and management of women at high risk for pelvic infection following cesarean section. Obstet Gynecol 55:185–192, 1980.
4. Duff P, Smith PN, Keiser JF: Antibiotic prophylaxis in low risk cesarean section. J Reprod Med 27:133–138, 1982.
5. Cunningham FG, Hauth JC, Strong JD, Kappus SS: Infectious morbidity following cesarean section. Obstet Gynecol 52:656–661, 1978.
6. Gilstrap LC, Cunningham FG: The bacterial pathogenesis of infection following cesarean section. Obstet Gynecol 53:545–549, 1979.
7. Cunningham FG, Lucas MJ, Hankins GDV: Pulmonary injury complicating antepartum pyelonephritis. Am J Obstet Gynecol 156:797–807, 1987.
8. Muggah HF, D'Alton ME, Hunter AGW: Chorionic villus sampling followed by genetic amniocentesis and septic shock. Lancet i:867–868, 1987.
9. Orzel JA, Cohen DL, McDonald ED, Gandy G: Clostridium perfringens sepsis involving mother and neonate with survival of both. Pediatr Infec Dis 2:457–459, 1983.
10. Carson GD, Smith P: Escherichia coli endotoxic shock complicating Bartholin's gland abscess. Can Med Assoc 122:1397–1398, 1980.
11. Chow AW, Wittmann BK, Bartlett KH, Scheifele DW: Variant postpartum toxic shock syndrome with probable intrapartum transmission to the neonate. Am J Obstet Gynecol 148:1074–1079, 1984.
12. Cunningham FG, Leveno KJ, Hankins GDV, Whalley PJ: Respiratory insufficiency associated with pyelonephritis during pregnancy. Obstet Gynecol 63:121–125, 1984.
13. Hauth JC, Gilstrap LC, Hankins GDV, Connor KD: Term maternal and neonatal complications of acute chorioamnionitis. Obstet Gynecol 66:59–62, 1985.
14. Barela AI, Kleinman GE, Golditch IM, Menke DJ, Hogge WA, Golbus MS: Septic shock with renal failure after chorionic villus sampling. Am J Obstet Gynecol 154:1100–1102, 1986.
15. Katoh H, Ogihara T, Iyori S: Postpartum toxic shock syndrome: A report of a case. Jpn J Med 27:71–73, 1988.
16. Bowen LW, Sand PK, Ostergard DR: Toxic shock syndrome following carbon dioxide laser treatment of genital tract condyloma acuminatum. Am J Obstet Gynecol 154:145–146, 1986.
17. Tweardy DJ: Relapsing toxic shock syndrome in the puerperium. JAMA 253:3249–3250, 1985.
18. Beller FK, Schmidt EH, Holzgreve W, Hauss J: Septicemia during pregnancy: A study in different

species of experimental animals. Am J Obstet Gynecol 151:967–975, 1985.

19. Hawkins DF: Management and treatment of obstetric bacteraemic shock. J Clin Pathol 33:895–896, 1980.

20. Duff P, Gibbs RS: Maternal sepsis. In Berkowitz R (ed): "Critical Care of the Obstetric Patient." New York: Churchill Livingstone, 1988, pp 189–217.

21. Gonik B: Septic shock in obstetrics. Clin Perinatol 13:741–754, 1986.

22. Knuppel RA, Rao PS, Cavanagh D: Septic shock in obstetrics. Clin Obstet Gynecol 27:3–10, 1984.

23. Bryan CS, Reynolds K, Moore EE: Bacteremia in obstetrics and gynecology. Obstet Gynecol 64:155–158, 1984.

24. Hankins GDV: Acute pulmonary injury and respiratory failure during pregnancy. In Clark S, Phelan J (eds): "Critical Care Obstetrics." Oradell, New Jersey: Medical Economics, 1987, pp 290–314.

25. Lee W, Clark SL, Cotton DB, Gonik B, Phelan J, Faro S, Giebel R: Septic shock during pregnancy. Am J Obstet Gynecol 159:410–416, 1988.

26. Henry S, DeMaria A, McCabe WR: Bacteremia due to fusobacterium species. Am J Med 75:225–231, 1983.

27. Lachman E, Pitsoe SB, Gaffin SL: Anti-lipopolysaccharide immunotherapy in management of septic shock of obstetric and gynaecological origin. Lancet i:981–983, 1984.

28. Boucher M, Yonekura ML, Wallace RJ, et al.: Adult respiratory distress syndrome: A rare manifestation of listeria-monocytogenes infection in pregnancy. Am J Obstet Gynecol 149:686–688, 1984.

29. Fleming AD, Ehrlich DW, Miller NA, Monif GRG: Successful treatment of maternal septicemia due to Listeria monocytogenes at 26 weeks gestation. Obstet Gynecol 66:52S–53S, 1985.

30. Zervoudakis IA, Cedergvist LL: Effect of Listeria monocytogenes septiciemia during pregnancy on the offspring. Am J Obstet Gynecol 129:465–467, 1977.

31. Katz VL, Weinstein L: Antepartum treatment of Listeria monocytogenes septicemia. South Med J 75:1353–1354, 1982.

32. FDA Drug Bulletin: Toxic shock syndrome update. 10:17–19, 1980.

33. Carrico CJ, Meakins JL, Marshall JC, Fry D, Maier RV: Multiple-organ-failure syndrome. Arch Surg 121:196–208, 1986.

34. Reines HD, Halushka PV, Cook JA, et al.: Plasma thromboxane levels are elevated in patients dying with septic shock. Lancet 2:174–175, 1982.

35. Halushka PV, Reines HD, Barrow SE, et al.: Elevated plasma 6-keto-prostaglandin F-1-alpha in patients in septic shock. Crit Care Med 13:451–453, 1985.

36. Weir EJ, Mlezoch J, Reeves JT, et al.: Endotox-

emia and prevention of hypoxic pulmonary vasoconstriction. J Lab Clin Med 88:975–983, 1976.

37. Brigham KL: Mechanisms of lung injury. Clin Chest Med 3:9, 1982.

38. Ford-Hutchinson A, Bray M, Doig M, et al.: Leukotriene-B, a potent chemokinetic and aggregation substance released from polymorphonuclear leukocytes. Nature 286:264–265, 1980.

39. Lefer AM: Role of a myocardial depressant factor in shock states. Mod Concepts Cardiovasc Dis 42:59–64, 1973.

40. Raffa J, Trunkey DD: Myocardial depression in sepsis. J Trauma 18:617–622, 1978.

41. Goldfarb RD, Weber P: The chemical nature of a pancreatic cardiodepressant factor. Circ Shock 4:95–100, 1977.

42. Apitz K: A study on the generalized Schwartzman phenomenon. J Immunol 29:255–266, 1935.

43. McKay DG: "Disseminated Intravascular Coagulation, an Intermediary Mechanism of Disease." New York: Harper & Row, 1965.

44. Beck-Jansen P, Brinkmann CR, Johnson CH, Assali NS: Circulatory shock in pregnant sheep: I. Effects of endotoxin on uteroplacental and fetal umbilical circulation. Am J Obstet Gynecol 112:1084–1094, 1972.

45. Beller FK, Schmidt EH, Holzgreve W, Hauss J: Septicemia during pregnancy: A study in different species of experimental animals. Am J Obstet Gynecol 151:967–975, 1985.

46. Morishima HO, Niemann WH, James LS: Effects of endotoxin on the pregnant baboon and fetus. Am J Obstet Gynecol 131:899–902, 1978.

47. Knaus WA, Draper EA, Wagner DP, Zimmerman JE: Prognosis in acute organ-system failure. Ann Surg 202:685–693, 1985.

48. Brown CEL, Lowe TW, Cunningham FG, Weinreb JC: Puerperal pelvic thrombophlebitis: Impact on diagnosis and treatment using x-ray computed tomography and magnetic resonance imaging. Obstet Gynecol 68:789–794, 1986.

49. Meakins JL, Wicklund B, Forse RA, et al.: The surgical intensive care unit: Current concepts in infection. Surg Clin North Am 60:117–132, 1980.

50. Rackow EC, Weil MH: Recent trends in diagnosis and management of septic shock. Curr Surg 40:181–185, 1983.

51. Clark SL, Horenstein JM, Phelan JP, Montag TW, Paul RH: Experience with the pulmonary artery catheter in obstetrics and gynecology. Am J Obstet Gynecol 152:374–378, 1985.

52. McSwain NE: Pneumatic trousers and the management of shock. J Trauma 17:719–724, 1977.

53. Paris PM: Antishock garments. N Engl J Med 305:960, 1981.

54. Waeckerle JF: Antishock garments. Crit Care 2:15, 1980.

55. ACOG Technical Bulletin #121: Hemodynamic monitoring in obstetrics and gynecology. October 1988.

56. Rao PS, Cavanagh D: Endotoxic shock in the primate: Some effects of dopamine administration. Am J Obstet Gynecol 144:61–66, 1982.

57. Faro S: Group B beta-hemolytic streptococci and puerperal infection. Am J Obstet Gynecol 139:686–689, 1981.

58. Gibbs RS, Jones PM, Wilder CJ: Antibiotic therapy of endometritis following cesarean section. Obstet Gynecol 52:31–37, 1978.

59. Gogoi MP: Maternal mortality from cesarean section in infected cases. Br J Obstet Gynaecol 78:373–376, 1971.

60. Gibbs RS, Castillo MS, Rodgers PJ: Management of acute chorioamnionitis. Am J Obstet Gynecol 136:709–713, 1980.

61. McCabe WR, Kreger BE, Johns M: Type specific and cross-reactive antibodies in gram-negative bacteremia. N Engl J Med 287:261–267, 1972.

62. Gaffin SL: Gram-negative bacteraemia: New therapeutic possibilities with anti-endotoxin antibodies. Hamatol Bluttransfus 29:107–111, 1985.

63. Ashbaugh DG, Bigelow DB, Petty TL, et al.: Acute respiratory distress in adults. Lancet ii:319–323, 1967.

64. Rafferty TD, Niederman MS: Ventilator therapy and care of the patient with ARDS. In Berkowitz R (ed): "Critical Care of the Obstetric Patient." New York: Churchill Livingstone, 1988, pp 21–46.

65. Hauth JC, Hankins GDV, Kuehl TJ: Ritodrine hydrochloride infusion in pregnant baboons. I. Biophysical effects. Am J Obstet Gynecol 146:916–924, 1983.

66. Hankins GDV, Hauth JC, Kuehl TJ, Brans YW, Cunningham FG: Ritodrine hydrochloride infusion in pregnant baboons: II. Sodium and water compartment alterations. Am J Obstet Gynecol 147:254–259, 1983.

67. Hankins GDV, Hauth JC: A comparison of the relative toxicities of B-sympathomimetic tocolytic agents. Am J Perinatol 2:338–346, 1985.

11

Syphilis During Pregnancy

George D. Wendel, Jr., M.D., and Larry C. Gilstrap, III, M.D.

Untreated syphilis during pregnancy may result in significant perinatal morbidity and mortality. It has been observed that untreated primary or secondary syphilis in pregnant women may result in symptomatic congenital syphilis in 40 to 50% of cases.[1] Congenital syphilis should be a preventable disease if early maternal infection is properly diagnosed and treated with penicillin. The practicing clinician, who rarely encounters syphilis infections, must still be aware of the many presentations of this maternal/fetal infection. The main emphasis of this chapter will be on the treatment, prevention, and fetal effects of syphilis occurring during pregnancy.

INCIDENCE AND EPIDEMIOLOGY

The exact incidence of syphilis in pregnant women is unknown. However, at Parkland Memorial Hospital in Dallas, approximately 2% of pregnant patients have a positive serologic test for syphilis and the approximate rate of probable and/or definite congenital syphilis[2] has been 1.2 per 1,000 livebirths.[3]

According to the statistics from the Centers for Disease Control (CDC), there was a 25% increase in primary and secondary syphilis in the United States in 1987 compared to the previous year.[4] The 1987 incidence of 14.6 cases per 100,000 persons was the highest rate in the last 27 years, equaled only in 1950 and 1982.[4] Even more disconcerting, during 1987 primary and secondary syphilis increased 43, 24, and 22% for black, Hispanic, and white women, respectively. Not unexpectedly, this increase in syphilis in women has resulted in a concomitant increase in congenital syphilis (Fig. 1).[4-6] From 1978 to 1987, there was a fourfold increase in the number of cases of congenital syphilis in infants under 1 year of age reported in the United States.[4,5]

What is the major reason for the recent increase in antepartum early (primary, secondary, and latent syphilis of less than 1 year's duration) syphilis and congenital syphilis? The greatest increases in early syphilis are occurring in urban, heterosexual, minority group adults, often in areas plagued with "crack" abuse and HIV infection.[4,7] One study has suggested a relationship between increases in primary and secondary syphilis in Connecticut and Philadelphia to illicit drug use and prostitution.[8] As pointed out in recent reviews, a primary factor in pregnancy

Infections in Pregnancy, pages 115–124

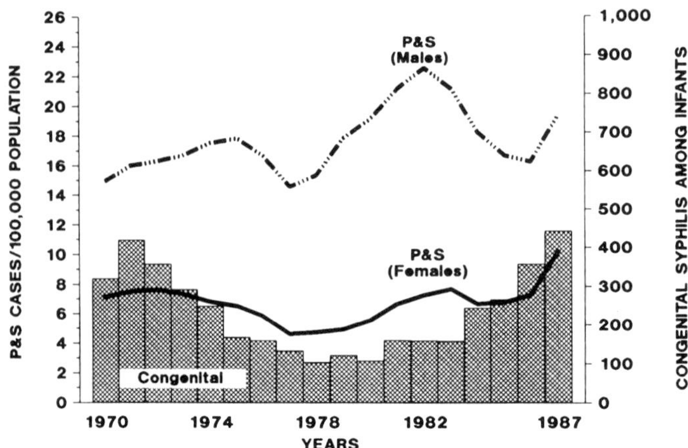

Fig. 1.   Syphilis (primary and secondary) by sex and congenital syphilis under 1 year of age in the United States, 1970–1987. (From Centers for Disease Control.[6])

appears to be inadequate prenatal care, mostly in the indigent patient.[3,4,9] It is not known whether underutilization of available services, inaccessibility of care in urban areas, or other impediments to antepartum care is the main determinant of the observed lack of prenatal care in this population. Nearly one-half of the women delivering an infant with congenital syphilis have had no prenatal care.[5] Unfortunately, congenital syphilis still occurs in infants born to mothers with prenatal care. The reason for this is basically twofold: either the patients enroll late for prenatal care and are treated late in pregnancy or there is failure in making the diagnosis of syphilis in the mother.[9,10] Thus, the most successful strategy in preventing congenital syphilis would be to 1) encourage early enrollment for accessible prenatal care and 2) ensure that proper serologic screening for syphilis is accomplished at the first prenatal visit and in the third trimester of pregnancy.

DIAGNOSIS

Pregnancy probably does not affect the course of syphilis, so the diagnosis in the pregnant patient is made essentially in the same manner as in the nonpregnant patient.

In women with primary syphilis, the diagnosis usually can be confirmed by identification of the causative organism, *Treponema pallidum*, in dark-field examination of material taken directly from a lesion. However, the majority of pregnant women who are at risk for giving birth to a baby with congenital syphilis do not have obvious lesions at time of presentation for prenatal care. Thus, the diagnosis of antepartum syphilis is most often made by serologic screening.[3] Additionally, cervical chancres may be difficult to diagnose unless a speculum examination is performed. Signs of secondary syphilis such as condylomata lata, mucous patches, adenopathy, alopecia, and skin rashes often are present for weeks prior to complaints from patients. Unfortunately, most of these syphilitic skin lesions or findings are painless, and thus patients do not seek immediate attention by a health-care provider. By the time some gravidas at Parkland Memorial Hospital present with symptoms of primary or secondary syphilis, the signs have been present for 2 to 4 weeks.

The most commonly used screening tests for detection of syphilis during pregnancy include the rapid plasmin reagin (RPR) test and the venereal disease research laboratory (VDRL) test.[11] These tests will be positive in the majority of pregnant women with a lesion of primary syphilis and in virtually all with secondary syphilis.[11,12] Both of these tests detect nontreponemal antibody, and positive tests are reported as reactive with a titer. The titer is highest in patients with active disease, i.e., secondary (generally the highest titer) and primary (somewhat lower) syphilis.[11] Patients with latent infection (reactive serology without lesions) generally have the lowest titers.

Specific antitreponemal antibody tests, the microhemagglutination assay for antibodies to *T. pallidum* (MHA-TP) and the fluorescent treponemal antibody-absorption (FTA-ABS) test, are used to confirm positive nontreponemal antibody tests.[11] These tests also identify patients with false-positive RPR or VDRL tests. The latter patients generally have "weakly reactive" or low titer nontreponemal antibody tests, but negative specific antitreponemal tests. Reported etiologies of false-positive tests include a recent febrile illness, intravenous drug abuse, autoimmune disease, and, arguably, pregnancy.[11–13] There are infrequent false-positive treponemal tests.[11,12] Antitreponemal antibody tests remain positive for life in adults and should not be used to diagnose current clinical infection.

The serial evaluation of the quantitative titer of nontreponemal tests over time may be used to evaluate the efficacy of therapy. This is particularly important in monitoring response to therapy in patients with latent disease, who have no lesions to monitor. Titers tend to fall faster with primary, secondary, and early latent (less than 1 year's duration) disease, in that order. Generally, the titers will decrease fourfold (two dilutions) by 3 months posttherapy with primary and secondary syphilis.[14] Most patients with primary and secondary disease revert to negative nontreponemal testing by 1 year of follow-up,[15] while others, mostly with latent syphilis, will remain "serofast" with persistent low-titer antibody.[15]

In diagnosing latent syphilis (reactive serologic test without clinical lesions) in a pregnant woman, one must try to confirm the duration of infection and rule out prior treatment resulting in a serofast positive nontreponemal test. It is best to be conservative, overtreating probable serofast-titer individuals, if follow-up has been over 1 year and poor. We empirically treat all women with VDRL titers of 1:4 or higher with a positive MHA-TP test, regardless of prior history of treatment. This will avoid missing latent syphilis relapses or reinfections, which, if untreated, might lead to a case of congenital syphilis.

If the duration of latent syphilis is less than 1 year, the gravida can be treated according to guidelines for early syphilis.[16] If the duration of latent syphilis is unknown or over 1 year, one must decide whether a lumbar puncture is necessary to rule out asymptomatic neurosyphilis. Although progression to symptomatic neurosyphilis is uncommon in healthy young women with early latent syphilis, it is wise to consider a cerebrospinal fluid (CSF) VDRL test, cell count, and protein determination in asymptomatic women likely to have disease of over 1 year's duration.[17,18] A CSF evaluation should be performed in all patients with any clinical signs or symptoms of neurosyphilis.[16] If a lumbar puncture is unavailable or refused with latent disease of unknown or over 1 year's duration, the patient should be treated for possible asymptomatic neurosyphilis.[16,18]

TREATMENT

The determining factor in the efficacy of treatment of syphilis during pregnancy is the detection of infection as early in pregnancy as possible. Serologic tests should be performed at the initial prenatal visit and repeated at 28 weeks and at delivery in high-risk populations.[3] Serologic screening is cost effective in pregnant women, even in populations with a low incidence of syphilis.[19]

Once the diagnosis of syphilis is made, the pregnant patient should be carefully exam-

TABLE 1. Recommendations for Treatment of Syphilis During Pregnancy

Early syphilis[a]
   Benzathine penicillin G 2.4 million units IM
   as a single injection

Syphilis of more than 1 year's duration[b]
   Benzathine penicillin G 2.4 million units IM
   weekly for 3 doses

Neurosyphilis
   Aqueous crystalline penicillin G 2–4 million units
   IV every 4 hours for at least 10 days, followed by
   benzathine penicillin G 2.4 million units IM
   weekly for 3 doses

   Aqueous procaine penicillin G 2.4 million units
   IM daily, plus probenecid 500 mg orally 4 times
   daily, both for 10 days, followed by benzathine
   penicillin G 2.4 million units IM weekly
   for 3 doses

   Benzathine penicillin G 2.4 million units IM
   weekly for 3 doses (not recommended for
   HIV-infected adults)

[a]Primary, secondary, and latent syphilis less than 1 year's duration.
[b]Latent syphilis of unknown or of more than 1 year's duration, cardiovascular or late benign syphilis.

ined to rule out other sexually transmitted diseases. Women with syphilis should be treated according to the CDC guidelines for pregnant women (Table 1).[10,16] The mainstay of treatment is long-acting benzathine penicillin G, as it is in the nonpregnant patient. Unfortunately, there is little prospectively collected data regarding the efficacy of these guidelines during pregnancy, especially with regard to prevention of fetal infection.[20–22] It is well documented that pregnancy is associated with decreased plasma levels of most antibiotics, especially the penicillins (see chapter 2); this may influence the efficacy of maternal and fetal treatment. Moreover, treatment during late pregnancy presents another significant problem, for most therapeutic failures occur during this time.[5,10,23]

Pregnant women with syphilis and who are allergic to penicillin present a therapeutic challenge, for the most appropriate therapy for them is penicillin. The CDC recommendations for the nonpregnant patient who is allergic to penicillin include either erythromycin or tetracycline.[16,22] Erythromycin, which has a high cure rate in the adult with early syphilis, may not prevent congenital syphilis.[3,5,10,21,22] Tetracycline, which is also effective in the nonpregnant patient,[22] is generally not recommended for pregnant women because of possible yellow-brown discoloration of fetal deciduous teeth when the drug is used in the latter half of pregnancy.[24] However, other than this well-known fetal effect, tetracycline has not been shown to be teratogenic or cause any other adverse fetal effect.[25] Thus, tetracycline may be a reasonable therapeutic choice for the treatment of pregnant women with syphilis who are allergic to penicillin,[21,22] if penicillin desensitization is not readily available. Various cephalosporins also may be effective in the treatment of pregnant women with syphilis,[21,22] although they may result in significant allergic reactions in penicillin-allergic patients.[26] Recent limited clinical experience shows that ceftriaxone, given intramuscularly 250 mg daily for 10 days or 500 mg every other day for 10 days, may be effective in treating early syphilis.[27] Unfortunately, there are few data about its transplacental pharmacokinetics to recommend its use during pregnancy to prevent congenital syphilis.

An alternative to using other antibiotics in the penicillin-allergic pregnant patient with syphilis is the technique of penicillin desensitization (Table 2).[28–30] First, the patient should be skin tested for the presence of IgE to both the major determinant antigen penicilloyl polylysine and to the minor determinant antigens benzylpenicillin G and benzylpenicilloic acid.[29,31] Patients with reactivity to any of these antigens can have an allergic reaction to penicillin and are candidates for penicillin desensitization. The penicillin desensitization protocol with the most clinical experience, and which also appears to be both efficacious and safe, is the oral phenoxymethyl penicillin regimen.[29,30,32] This regimen is based on gradually increasing

TABLE 2. Recommendations for Treatment of Pregnant Women With Syphilis Who Are Allergic to Penicillin

Skin testing to confirm penicillin sensitivity
Penicillin desensitization
   Requires hospitalization for at least 24 hours
   Intravenous access, resuscitation medications
     and equipment
   Oral protocol—graduated oral doses of
     phenoxymethyl penicillin (penicillin V
     suspension)
   Parenteral protocol—graduated intravenous doses of
     aqueous crystalline penicillin G
Other antibiotics
   Recommended only for early syphilis
   Erythromycin 500 mg orally 4 times daily
     for 15 days
   Tetracycline HCl 500 mg orally 4 times daily
     for 15 days
   Neonatal treatment with benzathine penicillin G,
     50,000 units/kg intramuscularly

doses of penicillin to an endpoint of temporary tolerance to parenteral therapy. Another protocol for use in pregnancy, although less tested, utilizes a graduated intravenous dose regimen of penicillin.[28] It must be pointed out that penicillin desensitization requires hospitalization with close observation for 24 hours for acute and delayed allergic reactions. An intravenous line is required with resuscitation equipment and medications nearby. Desensitization results in only a temporary tolerance and will not prevent future allergic reactions.

A significant complication of penicillin therapy in pregnant women with early syphilis is the Jarisch-Herxheimer reaction, which classically includes fever, myalgia, hypotension, and tachycardia.[33] In pregnancy, this reaction also may manifest uterine contractions, preterm labor, and premature delivery.[3] Patients with fever should take antipyretics and those with contractions should seek examination to rule out preterm labor. The value of prophylactic antipyretics in preventing fever and preterm delivery is unknown.

After treatment of the gravida, it is essential to refer her sexual partner(s) for investigation and treatment.[16] Many clinical maternal treatment failures are the result of reinfection from untreated sexual partners. As noted in the previous section, nontreponemal tests may be used to assess response to therapy. In pregnancy, quantitative RPR or VDRL titers should be repeated monthly until delivery.[10] Gravidas are retreated for a persistent high-titer RPR or VDRL after 3 months, a persistent fourfold increase in RPR or VDRL titer, or clinical lesions of primary or secondary syphilis.[10] VDRL titers generally are lower than RPR titers; clinicians should not interpret a change in titer with different testing techniques.[11,14]

HUMAN IMMUNODEFICIENCY VIRUS COINFECTION

Recent reports of adults with early syphilis who are human immunodeficiency virus (HIV) coinfected have questioned the effect of concurrent HIV infection on the natural course of syphilis.[34–36] HIV-infected individuals may present with unusual manifestations of syphilitic infection, sometimes with laboratory evidence of central nervous system involvement. Others have reported treatment failures or relapses in HIV-coinfected adults with subsequent progression to neurosyphilis.[35,37] These reports suggest that the impaired cellular and hormonal immune response in HIV-infected adults may alter the presentation of syphilis and its response to therapy.[35,38,39]

Currently, the CDC recommends no changes in the treatment of primary, secondary, or early latent syphilis in HIV-infected adults (Table 1),[16] but stresses the need for closer follow-up in this group.[18] The CDC advises a CSF analysis prior to treatment of all HIV-coinfected adults with latent syphilis of unknown or more than 1 year's duration. Benzathine penicillin G for treatment of asymptomatic neurosyphilis in HIV-infected adults should be avoided; parenteral aqueous

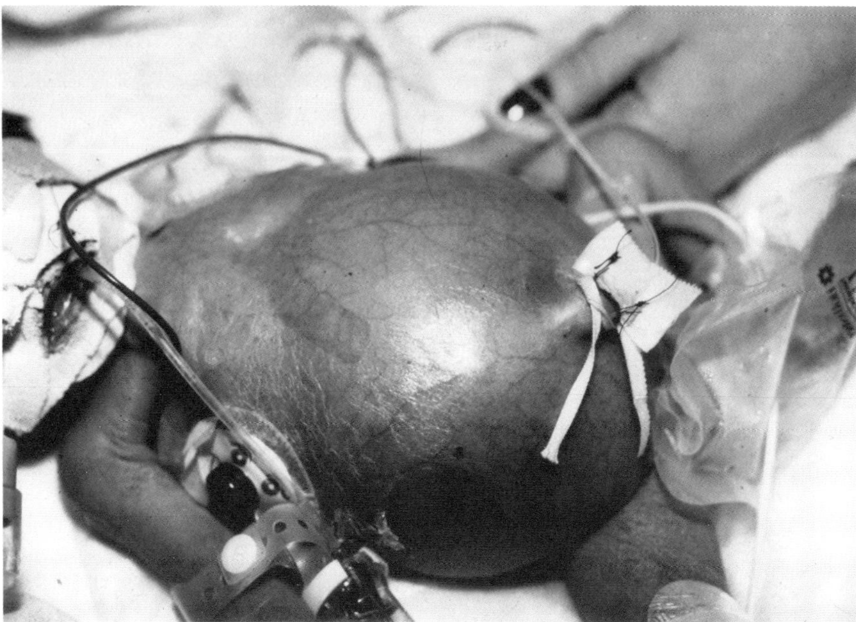

Fig. 2. Characteristic physical findings in an infant with congenital syphilis: prematurity; massive abdominal enlargment from hepatomegaly, splenomegaly, and ascites; jaundice; and petechiae.

penicillin G for at least 10 days is recommended (Table 1).[18]

CONGENITAL SYPHILIS

It is well established that *T. pallidum* readily crosses the placenta, infecting the fetus, and may result in congenital infection, preterm delivery, and stillbirth. Evidence of clinical disease in the fetus is generally not present prior to 18 weeks of gestation and probably is related to the relative immunoincompetence of the fetus at this age.[40] Mothers delivering with early syphilis, especially secondary syphilis, are at greatest risk of having a newborn with overt congenital syphilis.[1,10]

Since neonatal infection is systemic and usually without cutaneous lesions for darkfield microscopy, the diagnosis of congenital syphilis is based primarily on characteristic clinical signs (Fig. 2, Table 3) and laboratory tests (Table 4).[2,10,41] All newborns with a

TABLE 3. Characteristic Clinical Findings in Newborns With Congenital Syphilis

Hepatosplenomegaly
Osteochondritis or periostitis[a]
Jaundice[a]
Petechiae or purpuric skin lesions
Lymphadenopathy
Hydrops, edema, ascites
Rhinitis or "snuffles"
Pneumonia alba
Myocarditis
Nephrosis
Pseudoparalysis

[a]Most common findings.

suspected diagnosis of congenital syphilis should have a lumbar puncture for CSF analysis by VDRL, cell count, and protein determination,[10] as well as long-bone radiography.[42] Radiographic studies will reveal significant metaphyseal bone changes in over 95% of cases of infected infants less than 4 weeks of age.[41,42]

Serologic evaluation of either the cord

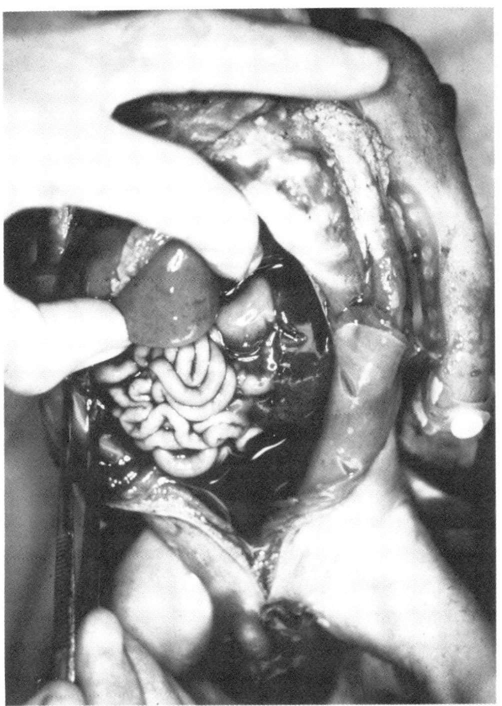

Fig. 3.   Autopsy findings in a stillborn with congenital syphilis: hepatomegaly, splenomegaly, and ascites.

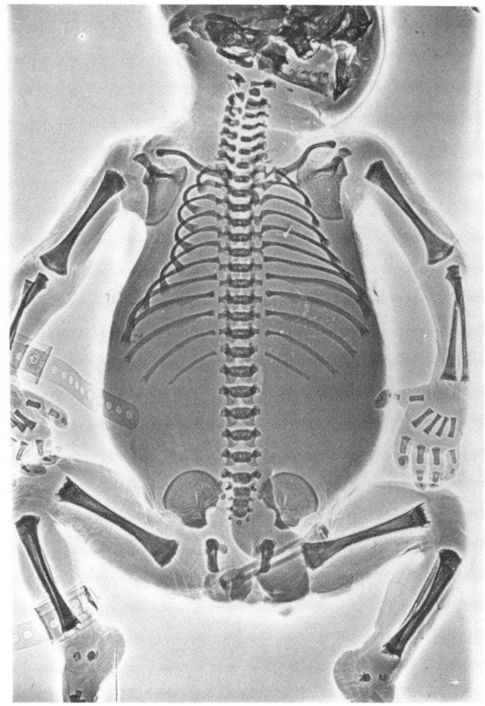

Fig. 4.   Xeroradiography in a stillborn with congenital syphilis that has diffuse osteochondritis.

TABLE 4. Common Laboratory Findings in Newborns With Congenital Syphilis

Reactive serologic test for syphilis
Anemia
Hyperbilirubinemia
Thrombocytopenia
Abnormal liver function tests
Elevated CSF cell count or protein
Reactive CSF VDRL test

blood or, preferably, blood from the neonate is difficult because of transplacental transfer of maternal IgG antibody. However, neonatal VDRL titers that are at least fourfold higher than maternal levels generally are indicative of fetal infection.[2,10] IgM does not cross the placenta, so elevated levels should reflect fetal/neonatal production. Unfortunately, in the past, antitreponemal IgM antibody testing was not proved clinically valuable.[43–45] Current research with monoclonal antitreponemal IgM tests with removal of rheumatoid factor may hold promise for improved diagnosis, especially in asymptomatic infants.[46,47]

The diagnosis of congenital syphilis in the stillborn infant can be difficult.[10,48] Whole-body radiographs followed by autopsy (Fig. 3) may be especially helpful.[42,49] Special staining with silver or immunofluorescence technique may be useful for identifying spirochetes in fetal tissue, the umbilical cord, or the placenta.[10,48,50] Demonstration of osteochondritis on x-ray is especially helpful in the stillborn that has undergone significant autolysis.[49,51] An example of xeroradiography findings in a stillborn with diffuse symmetric osteochondritis secondary to congenital syphilis is shown in Figure 4.

Treatment of neonatal infection consists primarily of parenteral aqueous crystalline penicillin G or procaine penicillin G given for at least 10 days.[10,16] Asymptomatic infants of women who were either treated late in pregnancy or treated with nonpenicillin regimens should be considered inadequately treated; these infants should be given 50,000 units/kg of benzathine penicillin G intramuscularly (Table 2).[10,16]

SUMMARY

There has been a recent significant increase in infectious syphilis in heterosexuals in the United States, especially in women. Approximately 80% of women with primary and secondary syphilis are between the ages of 15 and 35 years[52] and are thus in the peak childbearing years. Maternal infection may result in significant fetal morbidity, including prematurity, congenital infection, and even fetal/neonatal death. Most cases of congenital infection are related to a lack of or inadequate prenatal care. Serologic screening is cost effective in preventing congenital infection, and early prenatal care for women at risk for syphilis should be made readily accessible. Such patients should also be screened at 28 weeks of gestation and at delivery. The mainstay of therapy is early detection and treatment with benzathine penicillin G. In the penicillin- allergic patient, either penicillin desensitization followed by benzathine penicillin G therapy or, alternatively, erythromycin or tetracycline therapy should be utilized. The diagnosis of congenital syphilis may be difficult, especially in the asymptomatic neonate or stillborn infant who has undergone autolysis. Radiographic demonstration of osteochondritis may be especially helpful in the latter situation.

REFERENCES

1. Fiumara NJ, Fleming WL, Downing JG, et al.: The incidence of prenatal syphilis at the Boston City Hospital. N Engl J Med 247:48–52, 1952.

2. Kaufman RE, Jones OG, Blount JH, et al.: Questionnaire survey of reported early congenital syphilis: Problems of diagnosis, prevention, and treatment. Sex Transm Dis 4:135–139, 1977.

3. Wendel GD: Gestational and congenital syphilis. Clin Perinatol 15:287–303, 1988.

4. Centers for Disease Control: Syphilis and congenital syphilis—United States, 1985–1988. MMWR 37:486–489, 1988.

5. Centers for Disease Control: Congenital syphilis, United States, 1983–1985. MMWR 35:625–628, 1986.

6. Centers for Disease Control: Summary of notifiable diseases, United States, 1987. MMWR 36(54):39–40, 1988.

7. Centers for Disease Control: Increases in primary and secondary syphilis, United States. MMWR 36:393–397, 1987.

8. Centers for Disease Control: Relationship of syphilis to drug use and prostitution—Connecticut and Philadelphia, Pennsylvania. MMWR 37:755–764, 1988.

9. Mascola L, Pelosi R, Blount JH, et al.: Congenital syphilis: Why is it still occurring? JAMA 252:1719–1722, 1984.

10. Centers for Disease Control: Guidelines for the prevention and control of congenital syphilis. MMWR 37(S1):1–13, 1988.

11. Larsen SA, Hunter EF, McGrew BE: Syphilis. In Wentworth BB, Judson FN (eds): "Laboratory Methods for the Diagnosis of Sexually Transmitted Diseases." Washington, DC: American Public Health Association, 1984, pp 1–42.

12. Hart G: Syphilis tests in diagnostic and therapeutic decision making. Ann Intern Med 104:368–376, 1986.

13. Moore JE, Mohr CF: Biologically false-positive serologic tests for syphilis. JAMA 150:467–473, 1952.

14. Brown ST, Zaidi A, Larsen SA, et al.: Serological response to syphilis treatment. JAMA 253:1296–1299, 1985.

15. Fiumara NJ: Treatment of early latent syphilis of less than one year's duration. Sex Transm Dis 5:85–88, 1978.

16. Centers for Disease Control: 1985 Sexually transmitted disease treatment guidelines. MMWR 34(4S):21–25, 1985.

17. Wiesel J, Rose DN, Silver AL, et al.: Lumbar puncture in asymptomatic late syphilis. An analysis of the benefits and risks. Arch Intern Med 145:465–468, 1985.

18. Centers for Disease Control: Recommendations for diagnosing and treating syphilis in HIV-infected patients. MMWR 37:600–608, 1988.

19. Stray-Pederson B: Economic evaluation of maternal screening to prevent congenital syphilis. Sex Transm Dis 10:167–172, 1983.

20. Jackson FR, Vanderstoep EM, Knox JM, et al.: Use of aqueous benzathine penicillin G in the treatment of syphilis in pregnant women. Am J Obstet Gynecol 83:1389–1392, 1962.
21. Thompson SE: Treatment of syphilis in pregnancy. J Am Vener Dis Assoc 3:159–167, 1976.
22. Brown S: Update on recommendations for the treatment of syphilis. Rev Infect Dis 4(S): 837–841S, 1982.
23. Mascola L, Pelosi R, Alexander CE: Inadequate treatment of syphilis in pregnancy. Am J Obstet Gynecol 150:945–947, 1984.
24. Genot MT, Golan HP, Porter PJ, Kass EH: Effect of administration of tetracycline in pregnancy on the primary dentition of the offspring. J Oral Med 25:75–79, 1970.
25. Elder HA, Santamarina BA, Smith S, Kass EH: The natural history of asymptomatic bacteriuria during pregnancy: The effect on the clinical course and the outcome of pregnancy. Am J Obstet Gynecol 111:441–462, 1971.
26. Sullivan TJ: Pathogenesis and management of allergic reactions to penicillin and other betalactam antibiotics. Pediatr Infect Dis 1:344–350, 1982.
27. Hook EW, Roddy RE, Handsfield HH: Ceftriaxone therapy for incubating and early syphilis. J Infect Dis 158:881–884, 1988.
28. Ziaya PR, Hankins GDV, Gilstrap LC, Halsey AB: Intravenous penicillin desensitization and treatment during pregnancy. JAMA 256:2561–2562, 1986.
29. Wendel GD, Stark BJ, Jamison RB, et al.: Penicillin allergy and desensitization in serious maternal/fetal infections. N Engl J Med 312:1229–1232, 1985.
30. Stark BJ, Earl, HS, Gross GN, et al.: Acute and chronic desensitization of penicillin-allergic patients using oral penicillin. J Allergy Clin Immunol 79:523–532, 1987.
31. Sullivan TJ, Wedner HJ, Shatz GS, Parker CW, Wedner HJ: Skin testing to detect penicillin allergy. J Allergy Clin Immunol 68:171–180, 1981.
32. Sullivan TJ, Yecies LD, Shatz GS, Parker CW, Wedner HJ: Desensitization of patients allergic to penicillin using orally administered beta-lactam antibiotics. J Allergy Clin Immunol 69:275–282, 1982.
33. Brown ST: Adverse reactions in syphilis therapy. J Am Vener Dis Assoc 3:172–176 1976.
34. Johns DR, Tierney M, Felsenstein D: Alteration in the natural history of neurosyphilis by concurrent infection with the human immunodeficiency virus. N Engl J Med 316:1569–1572, 1987.
35. Lukehart SA, Hook EW, Baker-Zander SA, et al.: Invasion of the central nervous system by *Treponema pallidum*: Implications for diagnosis and treatment. Ann Intern Med 109:855–862, 1988.
36. Radolf JD, Kaplan RP: Unusual manifestations of secondary syphilis and abnormal humoral immune response to *Treponema pallidum* antigens in a homosexual man with asymptomatic human immunodeficiency virus infection. J Am Acad Dermatol 18:423–428, 1988.
37. Berry CD, Hooton TM, Collier AC, et al.: Neurologic relapse after benzathine penicillin therapy for secondary syphilis in a patient with HIV infection. N Engl J Med 316:1587, 1987.
38. Tramont EC: Treatment of syphilis in the AIDS era. N Engl J Med 316:1600–1601, 1988.
39. Musher DM: Editorial. How much penicillin cures early syphilis? Ann Intern Med 109:849–851, 1988.
40. Silverstein AM: Congenital syphilis and the timing of immunogenesis in the human fetus. Nature 194: 196–197, 1962.
41. Hira SK, Bhat GJ, Patel JB, et al.: Early congenital syphilis: Clinicoradiologic features in 202 patients. Sex Transm Dis 12:177–183, 1985.
42. Cremin BJ, Fisher RM: The lesions of congenital syphilis. Br J Radiol 43:333–341, 1970.
43. Alford CA, Polt SS, Cassady JV, et al.: Gamma M-fluorescent treponemal antibody in the diagnosis of congenital syphilis. N Engl J Med 280:1086–1091, 1969.
44. Kaufman RE, Olansky DC, Weisner PJ: The FTA-ABS (IgM) test for neonatal congenital syphilis: A critical review. J Am Vener Dis Assoc 1:79–84, 1974.
45. Mamunes P, Cave UG, Budell JW, et al.: Early diagnosis of neonatal syphilis: Evaluation of a gamma M-fluorescent treponemal antibody test. Am J Dis Child 120:17–21, 1970.
46. Dobson SRM, Taber LH, Baughn RE: Recognition of *Treponema pallidum* antigens in IgM and IgG antibodies in congenitally infected newborns and their mothers. J Infect Dis 157:903–909, 1988.
47. Sanchez PJ, McCracken GH, Wendel GD, et al.: Molecular analysis of the fetal IgM response to *Treponema pallidum* antigens: Implications for improved serodiagnosis of congenital syphilis. J Infect Dis 159:508–517, 1989.
48. Oppenheimer EH, Hardy JB: Congenital syphilis in the newborn infant: Clinical and pathological observations in recent cases. Johns Hopkins Med J 129:63–82, 1971.
49. Cremin BJ, Draper R: The value of radiography in perinatal deaths. Pediatr Radiol 11:143–145, 1981.
50. Epstein H, King CR: Diagnosis of congenital syphilis by immunofluorescence following fetal death *in utero*. Am J Obstet Gynecol 152:689–690, 1985.
51. Cox SM, Wendel GD: Xeroradiography and skeletal survey in the diagnosis of congenital syphilis following fetal death. Abstract 42, Society of Perinatal Obstetricians, February 1987.

52. Centers for Disease Control: Syphilis—United States, 1983. MMWR 33:433–441, 1984.

53. Cox SM, Wendel GD. Xeroradiography and skeletal survey in the diagnosis of congenital syphilis following fetal death. Abstract 42, Society of Perinatal Obstetricians. February, 1987.

54. Centers for Disease Control. Syphilis—United States, 1983. MMWR 1984;33:433–441.

12

Sexually Transmitted Diseases:
I. Gonorrhea and Chlamydia

Joseph J. Apuzzio, M.D., and George D. Wendel, Jr., M.D.

If one includes viruses, bacteria, parasites, and fungi, there are 18 to 20 diseases that could be categorized as sexually transmitted diseases (STDs). Two of the most common STDs are gonorrhea and chlamydia, and both will be discussed in this chapter.

GONORRHEA

Neisseria gonorrhoeae is a gram-negative diplococcus that may be acquired by sexual contact or by vertical transmission to the fetus during the birth process. The organism is fastidious and has specific temperature and carbon dioxide requirements. The gonococcus will not tolerate drying and is killed by heat of 42°C or higher in just a few hours. Room air is toxic to the gonococcus and a CO_2 concentration of 2 to 10% is needed for cultivation. It is important that the organism be plated on the appropriate selective culture media, such as Thayer-Martin media, and placed in a candle jar until it can be processed by the laboratory.

The total number of cases of gonorrhea reported in the United States to the Centers for Disease Control (CDC) for the year 1986 was approximately one million. However, because many cases are not reported, the true incidence of gonorrhea infections is probably much higher.[1] Recently, there has been a development of penicillin resistance among the gonococci, which was first identified in the late 1970s. It is currently recommended that all isolates of *N. gonorrhoeae* be studied for penicillinase or beta-lactamase production; if an isolate is penicillinase-producing *N. gonorrhoeae* (PPNG), penicillins cannot be used.

Clinical Manifestations

Asymptomatic infections. It is apparent from several studies that pregnant patients may harbor *N. gonorrhoeae* in an asymptomatic state in the endocervix.[2] Recent data from our own population of pregnant patients indicate an incidence of 7.4% of endocervical gonorrhea.[3] It has been estimated that 20 to 80% of infected women are asymptomatic. These patients, if not treated, would then serve as a means of transmitting the disease to their sexual partners and the fetus at delivery. Therefore, routine testing of pregnant patients in high-risk populations, usually at the time of their first prenatal visit and also in the third trimester, is recommended.

Infections in Pregnancy, pages 125–131

Proctitis. It has been estimated that up to 50% of women with gonorrhea also have rectal colonization of the organism. Furthermore, in approximately 7–10% of women with gonorrhea, the rectal site is the only area colonized (i.e., the only area that would yield a positive culture). Therefore, the workup of a patient with suspected gonorrhea should include rectal specimens for isolation of *N. gonorrhoeae* as well as culture specimens from other suspected sites.

Pharyngeal infection. Pharyngeal gonococcal infection is often asymptomatic. It may be the only site of gonorrheal infection. Therefore, this area should also be kept in mind when evaluating a patient with suspected gonorrhea of the genital tract or disseminated infection.

Other infections. The gonococcus is potentially responsible for many infections in the female. It may cause infection in the urethra, paraurethral (Skene's) glands, and paravaginal (Bartholin's) glands. It may cause cervicitis, chorioamnionitis, postpartum endometritis, and even peritonitis. Untreated endocervical gonorrhea may also lead to postabortal infection after spontaneous or elective abortions. In the neonate, *N. gonorrhoeae* may cause ophthalmic infections. A particular disease that appears to occur more often during pregnancy is disseminated gonococcal infection.

Disseminated gonococcal infection. Disseminated gonococcal infection consists of a triad of arthritis or tenosynovitis, skin lesions, and fever. The initial phase begins with hematogenous spread of the gonococcus, resulting in skin lesions and other constitutional signs. The arthritis can cause a purulent effusion of the joints and may progress to destruction of cartilage if not treated. Pregnancy seems to increase the risk of disseminated gonococcal infection; gravidas account for approximately half of the reported cases. Usually the presenting sign in a pregnant patient is migratory polyarthralgias. Approximately half of the patients will present with a vesicular and pustular rash

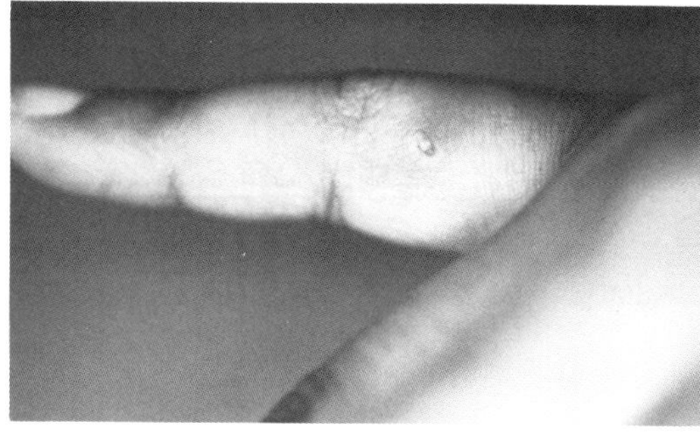

Fig. 1. Typical pustular rash of pregnant patient with disseminated gonococcal infection. (Photo courtesy of Dr. George Wendel, University of Texas Southwestern Medical Center, Dallas.)

that may overlay the affected distal joints (Fig. 1).[4] The upper limb joints are more commonly involved than the lower limbs; the wrists and hands are the most frequent sites. Since this phase is the gonococcemia phase, patients often have constitutional symptoms of malaise, fever, lassitude, and chills.[5,6] Acute gonococcal endocarditis may also occur.

Appropriate specimens for culture should be obtained from the blood, endocervix, pharynx, and rectum; purulent material from skin lesions or joints is often sterile. The treatment of disseminated gonococcal infection during pregnancy should consist of hospitalization and parenteral antibiotic therapy. If the beta-lactamase production is known to be negative, one may treat with aqueous penicillin G, 10 million units intravenously per day for at least 3 days followed by ampicillin or its equivalent, 500 mg four times a day for at least 7 days. As an alternative, or if the beta-lactamase activity is suspected or known to be present, cefoxitin, 1 g intravenously four times a day for 7 days, *or* cefotaxime, 500 mg intravenously four times a day for 7 days, *or* ceftriaxone, 1 g intravenously per day for 7 days, can be administered. Follow-up specimens for culture should be obtained to validate cure.

Pelvic inflammatory disease. The gonococcus is a common pathogen in acute salpingitis or acute pelvic inflammatory disease (PID). Pelvic inflammatory disease is not common in pregnancy, but should be considered in the differential diagnosis of women who have pelvic pain in the first trimester of pregnancy. The treatment includes admission to the hospital and parenteral antibiotics such as cefoxitin, 2 g intravenously every 6 hours, and erythromycin, 500 mg four times a day, rather than tetracycline. An alternative regimen is clindamycin, 900 mg every 8 hours, and an aminoglycoside such as gentamicin, 1.5 mg/kg every 8 hours. It is important to obtain serum peak and trough levels of the aminoglycoside to ascertain the proper dose. Erythromycin should provide adequate coverage for chlamydial coinfection.

Diagnosis

The diagnosis of gonococcal infection is based primarily on the isolation of the organism in culture. This is especially important because female patients are often asymptomatic carriers. Therefore, all sexually active females, especially those in younger age groups or those who have had several partners, should have a screening culture from the endocervix at the first prenatal clinic visit. The specimens should be plated directly onto selective media, such as Thayer-Martin media. The plate should then be placed in a candle jar or a commercially available system so that the environment can be enriched with carbon dioxide within minutes of plating the specimen. The plates may then be transported to the laboratory in the candle jar for appropriate processing and examination. Other sites that should be cultured as necessary include the pharynx, rectum, and urethra. As previously mentioned, studies have shown that the rectal area may be the only site of gonococcal infection.

A Gram stain from endocervical secretions may also be appropriate for those patients for whom an immediate diagnosis is necessary. The presence of gram-negative diplococci found in polymorphonuclear leukocytes is ev-

TABLE 1. Treatment of Uncomplicated Gonorrhea (PPNG Negative)

Amoxicillin 3.0 g orally
or ampicillin 3.5 g orally
or aqueous procaine penicillin G 4.8 million units IM

All given with 1.0 g probenecid orally
or ceftriaxone 250 mg IM

Coverage for *C. trachomatis*
  Erythromycin base or stearate 500 mg orally 4 times a day for 7 days
  or 250 mg orally 4 times daily for 14 days

idence that *N. gonorrhoeae* is present. Nonpathogenic *Neisseria* sp. are usually not cell associated.

An enzyme immunoassay (EIA) is a rapid technique available for the detection of gonococcal antigen in endocervical swabs. The test has a high specificity and sensitivity and is best used in patients who are asymptomatic but who have suspected gonorrhea. When used as a screening tool in an environment where the prevalence of gonorrhea is low, the positive predictive value of the test is poor. In this setting, it should be used as an indication for gonococcal culture, not presumptive treatment.

Treatment

The treatment of gonorrhea has been revised since the emergence of the penicillin-resistant *N. gonorrhoeae*.[7,8] Resistance may be plasmid-mediated, encoding for beta-lactamase or penicillinase, or chromosomally mediated, having broad-spectrum resistance to penicillins and other antimicrobials. In an area of the country where greater than 1% of gonococcal infections are resistant strains, one should select antibiotics that are effective against these strains. If the beta-lactamase production of gonorrhea is known to be negative, one can treat with penicillin as outlined in Table 1. If the beta-lactamase production is unknown or if the patient is from an area where greater than 1% of strains of *N. gonorrhoeae* are penicillinase-producing, one should use an antimicrobial

TABLE 2. Treatment of Uncomplicated Gonorrhea (PPNG Positive)

Ceftriaxone 250 mg IM (1 dose)
or spectinomycin[a] 2 g IM
Plus coverage for *C. trachomatis* as in Table 1

[a]Ineffective in pharyngeal infection and in prevention of syphilis.

as recommended in Table 2. As is true for any sexually transmitted disease, a repeat specimen for culture should be obtained to determine cure.

Pregnant women allergic to penicillin can be treated with spectinomycin (Table 2) or ceftriaxone, although cephalosporin cross-reactivity may well result in allergic reactions. It should be noted that patients treated for gonococcal infections should also receive antibiotic coverage for chlamydial infection (Table 1), because these infections are often associated. It is estimated that up to 50% of the women with gonorrhea also have chlamydial infection of the cervix.[9–11]

As is true for any sexually transmitted disease, tests for other STDs, including human immunodeficiency virus, should be ordered with appropriate consent. The sexual consort should also be evaluated and treated.

To prevent neonatal ophthalmia, ocular prophylaxis of 1% silver nitrate, 0.5% erythromycin, or 1% tetracycline ointment should be administered to all neonates. Each is effective in prevention of neonatal gonococcal and chlamydial ophthalmia, but probably none is as effective as screening and treating affected gravidas prior to delivery.[12] Neonates born to mothers with documented untreated endocervical gonorrhea should be prophylactically treated with aqueous penicillin G, 50,000 units intramuscularly,[13] or ceftriaxone, 125 mg intramuscularly.[7] Low-birth-weight infants should receive lower dosages. Gonococcal ophthalmia requires parenteral treatment with the previously mentioned drugs in higher doses for 7 days.[7,13]

CHLAMYDIA

Chlamydial organisms are common causes of genital tract disease in both males and females. Although there are no statistics as to the numbers of chlamydial infections in the United States, it has been suggested that *Chlamydia trachomatis* is the most common organism involved in acute pelvic inflammatory disease.[14] Chlamydia may also complicate pregnancy and be transmitted to the newborn through an infected endocervix during delivery, resulting in eye infections, pneumonia, and otitis media in the newborn.

Chlamydiae are obligate intracellular parasites. Although previously thought to be viruses, they are bacteria on the basis of their reproduction and their sensitivity to antibiotics. There are two species in the genus *Chlamydia*: *C. psittaci* and *C. trachomatis*, with 15 types of *C. trachomatis*. Types A, B, and C cause endemic trachoma, and serotypes D, E, F, G, H, I, J, and K cause oculogenital infections. Serotypes L1, L2, and L3 cause lymphogranuloma venereum, which is discussed in chapter 13.

Chlamydia is highly sensitive to temperature and will often be rapidly killed unless frozen below −40°C. Therefore, culture specimens must be obtained and processed very carefully in order to isolate the organism.

Epidemiology

The oculogenital types of *C. trachomatis* are probably the most prevalent sexually transmitted disease in the United States. *Chlamydia trachomatis* has been isolated from the endocervix in 20 to 30% of women attending sexually transmitted disease clinics and in many indigent-population prenatal clinics. At University Hospital in Newark, New Jersey, the carriage of chlamydia is 27% in our pregnant patients.[3] The majority of these patients are completely asymptomatic.

Some of the risk factors for chlamydial infection include young age of the patient, multiple sexual partners, unmarried marital status, and previous history of sexually transmitted disease.[15] These patients should be routinely screened for chlamydia from the endocervix at the first prenatal visit.[15]

Clinical Manifestations

Endometritis. Maternal chlamydia has been implicated as a cause of late endometritis after delivery. Wagner and colleagues described an increased infectious morbidity among women with prenatal endocervical chlamydial infection.[16] There is some evidence that chlamydia endometritis may occasionally cause such severe disease as to require hysterectomy. In one report, a patient developed endometritis after cesarean delivery and was initially treated with a cephalosporin.[17] She did not respond, and after several trials of various antibiotics, none of which covered chlamydia, she required hysterectomy for cure. Specimens for culture taken at the time of hysterectomy revealed *C. trachomatis.*[17]

Cervicitis. Mucopurulent cervicitis[18] is another infection that has been related to endocervical chlamydia as well as to other organisms. The cervix is usually eroded with discharge and appears hypertrophic.[19] Criteria for diagnosis include a yellow or green discharge, greater than 10 polymorphonuclear leukocytes per high-power field exam of the discharge, and bleeding or edema of the cervix.[18] If gonorrhea is also isolated from the endocervix, an antibiotic regimen against gonorrhea and chlamydia should be prescribed. If only chlamydia is isolated, either tetracycline, 500 mg orally four times a day for 7 days, or doxycycline, 100 mg twice a day for 7 days, should be prescribed. An alternative antibiotic when tetracycline is not indicated or during pregnancy is erythromycin base or stearate, 500 mg four times a day for 7 days.

Acute pelvic inflammatory disease. Acute PID is a clinical syndrome that includes endometritis, salpingitis, parametritis, and possibly peritonitis that is not related to recent surgery or pregnancy. Most cases are caused by several organisms, including *N. gonorrhoeae,*[3] *C. trachomatis,* anaerobic organisms, and facultative gram-negative organisms. The treatment of acute PID should include antibiotic coverage for chlamydia as well as other organisms. A useful method for making the clinical diagnosis of acute PID has been proposed by Hager and colleagues.[24]

Because this infection is a rare complication of pregnancy (with the possible exception of infected ectopic pregnancy) and beyond the scope of this text, it will not be discussed in further detail.

Premature labor. There is evidence that chlamydia may play a role in premature labor, but there are conflicting reports.[14,19–21] Martin and colleagues found the incidence of prematurity to be 4.5 times higher in women colonized by *C. trachomatis*[19]; Gravett et al. had similar findings.[20] However, Sweet and associates did not find a higher incidence of prematurity in colonized women,[21] and Harrison et al. found that a subgroup of women with recent evidence of chlamydia as defined by IgM antibodies had a higher risk of delivering prematurely.[14] In view of these conflicting reports, the role of chlamydia in prematurity remains to be determined by further study.

Acute urethral syndrome. Dysuria and frequency in a woman whose urine culture and sensitivity is negative may be due to chlamydial infection of the urethra. It should be remembered that *C. trachomatis* will not be recovered from the urine. If these patients also present with pyuria, they will usually benefit from antibiotic therapy directed against chlamydia.[22,23]

Fetal aspects. Vertical transmission of *C. trachomatis* to the fetus may occur during the second stage of labor by direct contact of the fetus with the infected endocervix. It is estimated that up to 50% of infants born to infected mothers will develop conjunctivitis 1 to 3 weeks after birth.[25] The major entry to the fetus is believed to be through the eye, and the nasopharynx is subsequently colonized. Also, the organism may extend into the middle ear by the eustachian tubes. Neonatal chlamydial conjunctivitis may be prevented by routine use of erythromycin ointment placed in the eyes of the newborn immediately after delivery. Many institutions, however, still use silver nitrate drops, which are not effective against chlamydia.

The usual course of chlamydial conjunctivitis is a healing process without sequelae, but nasopharyngeal infection may serve as a reservoir for otitis media and pneumonia. Topical erythromycin at the time of delivery will not prevent nasopharyngeal complications from developing. Chlamydial pneumonia is characteristically a late-onset pneumonia and occurs in up to 18% of infants born to infected mothers.[25] It begins roughly 1 to 4 weeks after delivery with a staccato-like cough; fever is often absent. A chest x-ray may be diagnostic for a focal or diffuse interstitial pattern. The disease is usually mild, although occasionally hospitalization is required.

Diagnosis

The diagnosis of chlamydial infection is best made by culturing the suspected area for chlamydia with appropriate culture material. The technique for obtaining and processing the organism must be fully understood because these cultures are expensive and often difficult to process. It is important to obtain infected cells, as the organism is an intracellular parasite. For example, obtaining a vaginal swab for chlamydia will not show the organism, because one is not obtaining the appropriate cells that harbor the organism. It has also been shown that swabs tipped with calcium alginate contained on an aluminum shaft yield better results than cotton swabs with wooden shafts. Specimens should be placed into appropriate chlamydia transport media and either processed immediately or frozen at −70°C. The specimens are then placed on tissue culture media (McCoy) and, after an appropriate incubation, stained with iodine, Giemsa stain, or fluorescein-labeled antibody to identify typical inclusions of C. trachomatis.

For conjunctival infection, one can obtain scrapings from infected tissue or eyelid and process them for inclusion bodies and culture.

Antigen tests for chlamydia are available and may be a less costly alternative for diagnosis. However, their reliability in a low-prevalence environment is questionable, especially as a screening tool. The ELISA technique (Chlamydiazyme) for detecting C. trachomatis antigen agrees with culture results in only 50% of cases when the prevalence of chlamydia in the population test is low (less than 3%). Therefore, in populations having a low prevalence of chlamydia infection, this test should be interpreted cautiously. A negative ELISA test agrees with culture results in 95% of cases.[26]

The other commonly used direct test uses monoclonal antibodies labeled with fluorescein to detect elementary bodies of chlamydia (MicroTrak). In one study in a population where the prevalence of chlamydia was 7%, a positive direct test correlated with a positive culture for chlamydia 93% of the time. A negative direct test agreed with the culture 99% of the time.[27]

Treatment

A patient who is asymptomatic but who has a positive culture for chlamydia or has symptomatic disease should be treated with either tetracycline or erythromycin. If the patient is pregnant, tetracycline should not be prescribed. Erythromycin base or stearate, 500 mg four times a day for 7 days should be prescribed.

It is important that patients be tested for cure after 3 or 4 weeks of initial treatment, and the sexual consorts of patients with chlamydia should also be evaluated and treated. Both patient and consort should be evaluated for other STDs.

The treatment of neonatal chlamydial infection involves either oral or parenteral erythromycin for a 2- to 3-week regimen.[13,15]

Application of erythromycin ointment for conjunctivitis is effective, but to eradicate potential nasopharyngeal colonization, oral or parenteral therapy is suggested. The parents of babies with chlamydial conjunctivitis should also be evaluated and treated for chlamydia.

REFERENCES

1. Centers for Disease Control: Summary of notifiable diseases, U.S. MMWR 35:51–57, 1986.
2. U.S. Dept. of Health & Human Services: STD Fact Sheet. Publication No. 81-8195, 1981.
3. Nichols R, Apuzzio J: Unpublished data.
4. Garcia-Kutzbach A, Dismuke S, Masi A: Gonococcal arthritis: Clinical features and results of penicillin therapy. J Rheumatol 1:210–220, 1974.
5. Holmes K, Counts G, Beaty H: Disseminated gonococcal infection. Ann Intern Med 74: 979–993, 1971.
6. Hanksfield H: Disseminated gonococcal infection. Clin Obstet Gynecol 18:131–142, 1975.
7. Centers for Disease Control: Antibiotic-resistant strains of *Neisseria gonorrhoeae.* Policy guidelines for detection, management and control. MMWR 36(5S):1, 1987.
8. Judson FM: Management of antibiotic-resistant *Neisseria gonorrhoeae* (Editorial). Ann Intern Med 110:5, 1989.
9. Thompson S, Washington A: Epidemiology of sexually transmitted chlamydia infections. Epidemiol Rev 5:96–123, 1983.
10. Stamm W, Guinan M, Johnson C, et al.: Effect of treatment regimens of *Neisseria gonorrhoeae* on simultaneous infection with *Chlamydia trachomatis.* N Engl J Med 310:545–549, 1984.
11. Brunham R, Kuo C, Steven C, et al.: Treatment of concomitant *Neisseria gonorrhoeae* and *Chlamydia trachomatis* infections in women. Rev Infect Dis 4:491–499, 1982.
12. Hammerschlag MR, Cummings C, Roblin PM, et al.: Efficacy of neonatal ocular prophylaxis for the prevention of chlamydial and gonococcal conjunctivitis. N Engl J Med 320:769, 1989.
13. Centers for Disease Control: 1985 STD Treatment Guidelines. MMWR 34(4S):81S–86S, 1985.
14. Harrison AR, Alexander E, Weinstein L, et al.: Cervical *Chlamydia trachomatis* and mycoplasma infections in pregnancy. JAMA 250:1721–1727, 1983.
15. Centers for Disease Control: *Chlamydia trachomatis* infections. MMWR 34:53S–74S, 1985.
16. Wagner GP, Martin D, Koutsky L, et al.: Puerperal infectious morbidity: Relationship to route of delivery and to antepartum *Chlamydia trachomatis* infection. Am J Obstet Gynecol 138:1028–1033, 1980.
17. Cutryn A, Sen P, Chung H, et al.: Severe pelvic infection from chlamydia after cesarean section. JAMA 247:1732–1734, 1982.
18. Brunham RC, Paavonen J, Stevens CE, et al.: Mucopurulent cervicitis—the ignored counterpart in women of urethritis in men. N Engl J Med 311: 1–6, 1984.
19. Martin D, Koutshep L, Eschenbach D, et al.: Prematurity and perinatal mortality in pregnancies complicated by maternal *Chlamydia trachomatis* infections. JAMA 247:1585–1588, 1982.
20. Gravett M, Nelson H, DeRoven T, et al.: Independent associations of bacterial vaginosis and *Chlamydia trachomatis* infections with adverse pregnancy outcome. JAMA 256:1899–1903, 1986.
21. Sweet R, Lander D, Walker C, et al.: *Chlamydia trachomatis* infection and pregnancy outcome. Am J Obstet Gynecol 156:824–833, 1987.
22. Paavonen J: *Chlamydia trachomatis* induced urethritis in female partners of men with NGU. Sex Transm Dis 6:69–71, 1979.
23. Stamm W, Wagner K, Ambet R, et al.: Cases of acute urethral syndrome in women. N Engl J Med 303:409–415, 1980.
24. Hager WD, Eschenbach D, Spence M, Sweet R: Criteria for diagnosis and grading of salpingitis. Obstet Gynecol 61:113–114, 1983.
25. Alexander ER, Harrison H: Role of *Chlamydia trachomatis* in perinatal infection. Rev Infect Dis 5: 713–719, 1983.
26. Chlamydiazyme Diagnostic Text: Enzyme immunoassay for the detection of *Chlamydia trachomatis.* Abbott Labs (package insert).
27. Allen M, Courter P: *Chlamydia trachomatis* direct specimen test. Microtract Silva Labs (package insert).

13

Sexually Transmitted Diseases:
II. Chancroid, Lymphogranuloma Venereum, Granuloma Inguinale, Molluscum Contagiosum, Pediculosis Pubis, and Scabies

Joseph J. Apuzzio, M.D., and Larry C. Gilstrap, III, M.D.

CHANCROID

Chancroid, also known as soft chancre, is an ulcerative sexually transmitted disease caused by *Hemophilus ducreyi*. This disease was first described by Ducrey in 1889. The organism is a small gram-negative bacillus found either singly or in clusters in pus obtained from ulcerations in infected patients. The disease usually involves genital tissues, including skin, mucosa, and associated lymphatics.

Epidemiology

Chancroid is more commonly found in tropical areas than in other parts of the world. The incidence of chancroid appeared to be decreasing in the United States until 1986, when over 3,700 cases were reported to the Centers for Disease Control.[1,2] The majority of the cases in males occur among men who frequent prostitutes.

Clinical Manifestations

Chancroid is transmitted by intimate sexual contact and has an incubation period of 1 to 14 days. The lesions are usually located on the genitalia, although they may occur at other sites, such as the mouth, fingers, and breast. Autoinoculation from the genital areas to other areas of the body is also possible. The genital lesions of chancroid are usually painful and ulcerative (Fig. 1). The lesions begin as pustules, which then enlarge and ulcerate. There is little or no induration of the ulcer, thus the name "soft chancre" was given. In contrast, the chancre from syphilis is usually indurated (hard). The ulcers from chancroid are often multiple, and when healing takes place, scarring usually occurs.

The inguinal lymph nodes draining the infected areas are involved in about 50% of the cases, usually unilaterally as a tender, swollen enlarged lymph node that may be fixed to the surrounding subcutaneous tissue and skin. The inguinal adenitis may spontaneously resolve or develop into a bubo (Fig. 2), which may rupture and drain for months if not treated with appropriate antibiotics. However, chancroid often heals spontaneously

Infections in Pregnancy, pages 133–141
© 1990 Alan R. Liss, Inc.

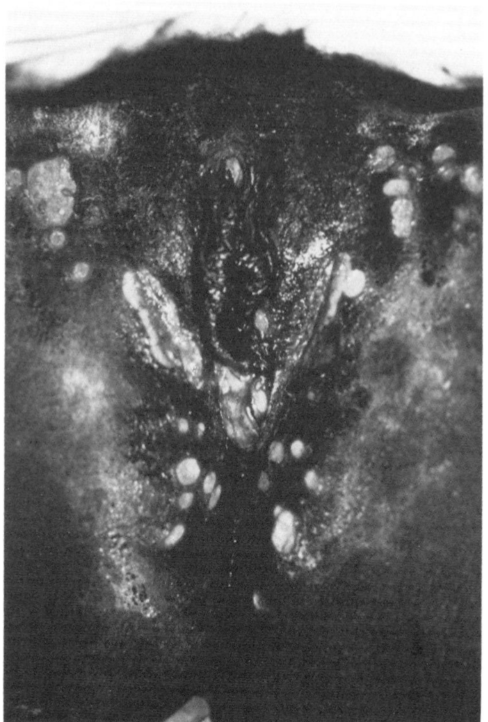

Fig. 1. "Typical" multiple ulcers in a pregnant woman with chancroid. (Photo courtesy of Dr. George Wendel, University of Texas Southwestern Medical Center, Dallas.)

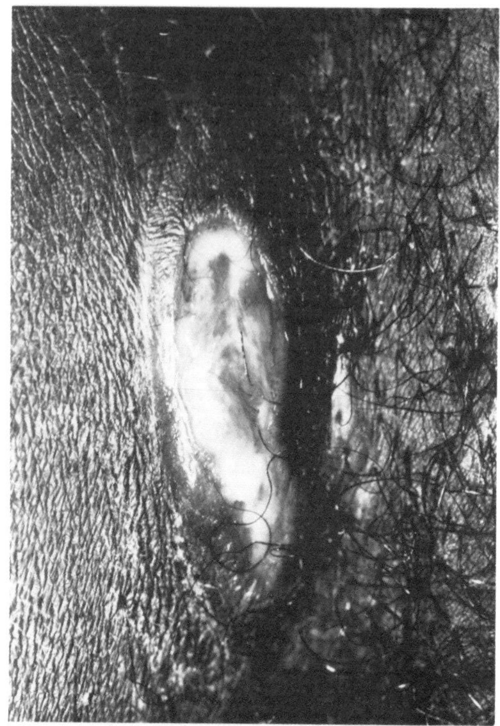

Fig. 2. Draining lymph node in patient with chancroid. (Photo courtesy of Dr. George Wendel, University of Texas Southwestern Medical Center, Dallas.)

even without treatment over a period of weeks. Occasionally, extensive scarring and fistula formation may occur in the anogenital region.

The fetal hazards of chancroid appear minimal but include one case report from 1976 when a newborn developed a *H. ducreyi* conjunctivitis presumably from the maternal genital tract during delivery.[3]

Diagnosis

The diagnosis of chancroid is made by clinical suspicion and isolation of the bacterum *H. ducreyi* from ulcers and buboes. A Gram stain of the material will usually reveal the gram-negative organisms, but other ulcerative diseases, including syphilis and herpes simplex, should be excluded by appropriate tests, such as dark-field examination and a herpes viral culture from the lesion. Unfortunately, neither Gram stain nor histopathology is specific for chancroid.

Treatment

Antibiotic therapy and the susceptibility patterns of *H. ducreyi* vary among geographic locations. Therefore, when the culture for the organism is performed, sensitivity should also be performed.

The recommended regimens from the Centers for Disease Control include the following:[4]

1. Erythromycin 500 mg orally four times a day for 7 days or
2. Ceftriaxone 250 mg intramuscularly as a single dose

Alternative regimens include:

1. Trimethoprim/sulfamethoxazole, one double-strength tablet orally twice a day for 7 days or
2. Trimethoprim/sulfamethoxazole, four double-dose or eight single-dose tablets orally in a single dose or
3. Amoxicillin 500 mg orally plus clavulanic acid 125 mg three times a day for 7 days

New information indicates that some of the quinolone group of antibiotics such as ciprofloxacin or enoxacin may also be effective,[5-8] but quinolones should not be prescribed for pregnant patients.

Successfully treated ulcers usually improve within a week after antibiotic therapy. If not, an alternative regimen should be selected and the susceptibility of the organism should be ascertained. Fluctuant lymph nodes may require aspiration, but incision or excision of the nodes through infected skin often delays healing and is not indicated.

LYMPHOGRANULOMA VENEREUM

Lymphogranuloma venereum (LGV) is a rare, sexually transmitted disease caused by *Chlamydia trachomatis* serotypes L1, L2, and L3. The Chlamydiaceae are a family of obligate intracellular parasites that are bacteria and produce by binary fission. They have an affinity for columnar epithelial cells lining mucus membranes. Further discussion of chlamydiae can be found in chapter 12. LGV can cause acute and chronic destruction of the anogenital region if not treated with appropriate antibiotics.

Epidemiology

LGV is a sexually transmitted disease that is mostly seen in warm or tropical climates such the third world countries and Southeast Asia. Males appear to be more commonly infected than females by a ratio of 3–9 to 1.[9] In the United States it is estimated that there are approximately 300 to 500 cases per year.

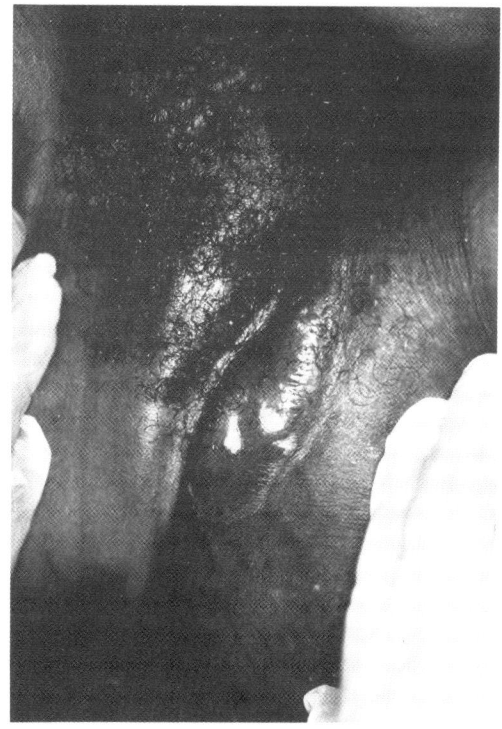

Fig. 3. Characteristic groove sign in a woman with LGV. (Photo courtesy of Dr. George Wendel, University of Texas Southwestern Medical Center, Dallas.)

Clinical Manifestations

The disease caused by LGV occurs in three phases after an incubation period of 1 to 3 weeks. During the first phase, a lesion may appear at the site of inoculation on the genital or anal area as a pimple or ulcer that usually heals quickly. Most patients are not even aware of the initial lesion. The second phase, which occurs several weeks after the initial phase, involves the regional lymphatics with edema and adenitis of the lymph nodes. The lymph nodes may be fluctuant and enlarged (buboes) and may spontaneously rupture and drain for weeks if untreated. The "groove sign" (Fig. 3) often associated with LGV is more apparent in men than in women and consists of enlarged inguinal and femoral nodes separated by the inguinal ligament. The inguinal ligament serves as the "groove" between the two enlarged lymph node areas. During this second phase of lymphadenitis, the patient commonly has constitutional symptoms such as fever, chills, myalgias, and headache, as well as leukocytosis.

The third phase of LGV occurs months to years after the initial infection and consists of chronic and destructive changes in the affected lymphatic areas. Untreated LGV may cause rectal, vaginal, urethral, and external genital destructive processes with fibrosis, strictures, and lymphedema. The lymphedema may be so massive as to cause "elephantiasis" of the genitalia. This scarring and deformity of the genital area may be quite severe and may preclude vaginal delivery for a pregnant patient. Also, it is suspected that the incidence of vulvar carcinoma is increased in women who have had LGV.

Diagnosis

The diagnosis of LGV is made by both clinical examination and appropriate laboratory studies. LGV should always be considered in the differential diagnosis in a patient with a genital ulcer, although the initial phase of the disease is so benign that a patient may not seek attention. One also needs to consider other STDs such as syphilis, chancroid, granuloma inguinale, and herpes genitalis.

The best method for diagnosis of LGV is to isolate the organism by tissue culture. However, chlamydial culture is often not readily available and can be technically difficult. Other tests such as the complement fixation test or Frei antigen test may be considered, but neither is definitive nor commonly used. A direct immunofluorescent test for diagnosis is also available.[10]

Treatment

The Centers for Disease Control recommends that nonpregnant patients with LGV be treated with tetracycline 500 mg four times a day for at least 2 weeks.[4] Alternative regimens include doxycycline 100 mg twice a day for at least 2 weeks or erythromycin 500 mg four times a day for at least 2 weeks. Sulfamethoxazole 1 g orally twice a day for at least 2 weeks or other appropriate sulfonamides may be prescribed.

Sexual partners of patients with LGV should be evaluated and treated as above. The patient management and follow-up should include aspiration of the fluctuant lymph nodes as needed through healthy adjacent normal skin. Incision and drainage of the nodes through infected areas usually delays healing and is not indicated.[3] Other sequelae such as strictures or fistula formation may require surgical intervention.

GRANULOMA INGUINALE

Granuloma inguinale is a rare ulcerative and granuloma-producing disease that affects primarily the genital and inguinal areas. It is most often seen in tropical regions such as India and the Caribbean, and fewer than 100 cases are reported annually in the United States.

Granuloma inguinale is a sexually transmitted disease, although autoinoculation and nonsexual transmission is possible. The organism response for the disease is *Calymmatobacterium granulomatis*, which is a nonmotile, gram-negative, pleomorphic bacillus.

Clinical Manifestations

The incubation period of granuloma inguinale is estimated to be between 8 and 80 days with an average of about 40 days. The lesion is usually a small, nontender nodule that may spontaneously regress and then reappear. Over a period of weeks the nodules may spread and coalesce, forming a "pseudobubo" when they infect the inguinal area. The painless ulcer has a beefy red velvety base with an indurated border. Other lesions may appear exophytic and resemble granulation tissue. The lesions continue to grow slowly and usually do not heal without therapy. There may be complete destruction and fibrosis of infected tissue and lymphedema-like change may occur.

Granuloma inguinale may also infect the endometrium with granulomatous involvement of the endometrium, parametrium, fallopian tubes, and ovaries. A case of granuloma inguinale involving the labia, cervix, and anus has been reported as a result of prior curettage of the endometrium.[11]

There is a suggestion from the literature that pregnant patients may have more extensive lesions than nonpregnant patients.[12] It appears that perinatal transmission may occur. The fetal effects from maternal granuloma inguinale are not completely understood because there are few cases reported in the literature. There have been intrauterine fetal deaths associated with granuloma inguinale.[13] Several case reports of infants being infected with granuloma inguinale after delivery have been reported. A 5-month-old infant had granuloma inguinale of the ear, skin, and umbilicus presumably from his mother who had granuloma inguinale at delivery.[14]

Diagnosis

The diagnosis of granuloma inguinale is based on clinical suspicion as well as isolation of the organism from lesions. Histologically, the appearance of the "Donovan body" is pathognomonic of granuloma inguinale. The large foamy cytoplasmic inclusions may be seen in white blood cells containing many of the darkly stained organisms. One can make a crush preparation on a microscope slide from a biopsy of granulation tissue and then stain the slide with Giemsa or Wright's stain to identify the monocytes with the Donovan bodies.

Treatment

Nonpregnant patients may be treated with oral tetracycline 500 mg four times a day for at least 2 to 4 weeks. In pregnancy, erythromycin, 500 mg four times a day, or co-trimoxazole, two tablets twice a day for at least 10 days, may be effective.[15] Usually lesions will regress within 1 to 2 weeks after treatment, but treatment should be continued for a minimum of 3 weeks. Treatment should be continued until all lesions are healed.[15]

MOLLUSCUM CONTAGIOSUM

Molluscum contagiosum virus (MCV) is a member of the double-stranded DNA poxviridae. It has a long incubation period of 2 weeks to 2 months before the typical skin lesions appear. It is essentially a benign epithelial virus that causes papulelike tumors to develop in the epithelium of the skin. The mode of transmission is through direct contact from an infected individual or from fomites. Epidemics have been known to occur in boarding schools where there is close proximity of pupils.

Molluscum contagiosum is being seen more frequently in patients who are infected by the human immunodeficiency virus, presumably because of immunosuppression.[16] However, even in private offices the incidence of MCV has increased 11-fold in the past 18 years. The age of the typical patient is the early twenties.[17]

Clinical Manifestations

The clinical manifestation of the lesion is an asymptomatic papule that is usually umbilicated and varies in size from 1 to 5 mm and occasionally up to 1 cm (Fig. 4). The lesions appear white, are often multiple, and may discharge a caseous material. They are usually not pruritic.

The sites affected are often the eyelids, trunk, face, and the anogenital region. Autoinoculation to other sites of the body with secondary bacterial infection of the area may occur.

There are no reports that pregnancy has exacerbated the disease or that the disease has affected pregnancy.

Diagnosis

As with most skin lesions, the differential diagnosis should exclude malignant and

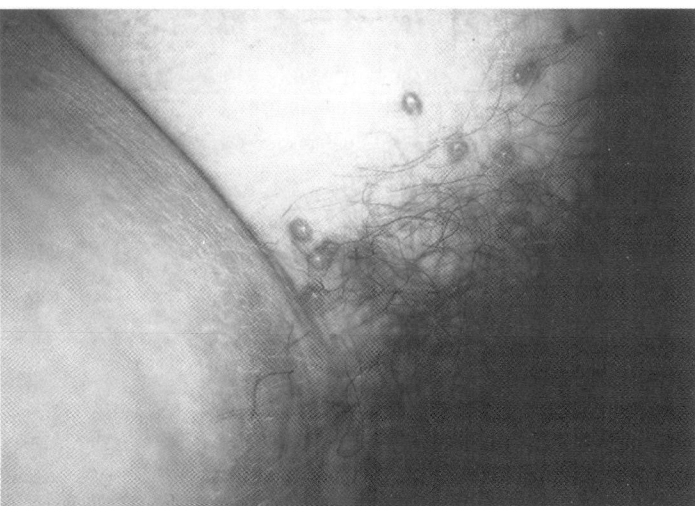

Fig. 4. Typical lesion of molluscum contagiosum. (Photo courtesy of Dr. George Wendel, University of Texas Southwestern Medical Center, Dallas.)

other nonmalignant lesions. The diagnosis of molluscum contagiosum is based on the typical clinical appearance of the white umbilical papule lesion that contains caseous material. Microscopic examination of the caseous material for the typical numerous hyaline intracytoplasmic inclusion bodies confirms the diagnosis. Recently, DNA restriction endonuclease analysis has been used to diagnose and classify the virus. This analysis indicates that there are two distinct types of MCV; however, lesions and sites of lesions were similar for both types.[18,19]

Treatment

Often the lesions persist for months and occasionally years, but the disease is usually self-limiting. Spontaneous regression without scarring is the usual course unless the patient is immunocompromised; these patients may have extensive disease.[20,21]

The patient may be observed for spontaneous regression of the lesions, but other modes of therapy, such as curettage of the lesion, desiccation, freezing, cautery, laser therapy, and chemical cautery can be used to enhance the process.

PEDICULOSIS PUBIS

Pediculosis pubis, or crab lice infection, is caused by the ectoparasite *Phthirus pubis*. The crab louse is relatively small, with the adult ranging from 0.8 to 1.2 mm in length.[22]

Epidemiology

The exact incidence of this infection is unknown, but it is frequently found in association with other sexually transmitted diseases. As many as one-third of patients with pediculosis pubis have other sexually transmitted diseases.[23] It is most often found in the 15–40 age group, with women more often infected than men in the younger ages (15 to 19 years).[22]

Clinical Manifestations

The pubic and perineal regions are the predominant sites of involvement. The characteristic "lesion" is produced by the attachment of numerous nits to the pubic hair (Fig. 5). There may be an associated dermatitis from scratching secondary to the often intense pruritis. It has been postulated that this intense pruritis may be immunologic instead

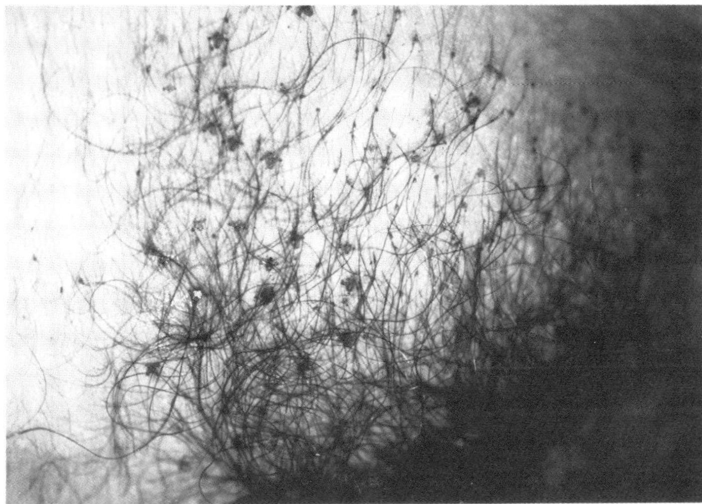

Fig. 5. Pregnant patient with pediculosis pubis infection. (Photo courtesy of Dr. George Wendel, University of Texas Southwestern Medical Center, Dallas.)

TABLE 1. Recommended Regimens for the Treatment of Pediculosis Pubis During Pregnancy

Initial therapy
   Pyrethrins and piperonyl butoxide (RID, A-200)
   Apply to infected and adjacent areas for 10 minutes
     and then wash off

Resistant or difficult cases
   Lindane cream or lotion (Kwell, Scabene)[a]
   Apply to infected areas and wash off after 8 hours

   Lindane shampoo[a]
   Apply for 4 minutes and wash off

[a]Use with caution during pregnancy (see text).

of mechanical.[22] The incubation period from exposure to onset of pruritis is approximately 30 days.[22]

Diagnosis

The diagnosis is based primarily on the identification of the characteristic nits attached to the hair shaft (usually with the aid of a hand lens) or by microscopic identification of the adult crab from a plucked hair.

Treatment

The most commonly used agent for the treatment of pediculosis pubis is lindane (Kwell, Scabene). Although it is generally not recommended for use during pregnancy,[4] it is listed as a pregnancy category B drug by two of its manufacturers. According to the manufacturers, lindane was not teratogenic in various laboratory animals given 10 times the human dose.[24] Although there have been no reports of teratogenic effects in humans, there are no adequate controlled studies. Approximately 10% of lindane may be absorbed systemically and may rarely cause central nervous system toxicity or convulsions.[22,25] For this reason, other agents such as the nonprescription pyrethrins and piperonyl butoxide combination (RID, A-200) probably should be used as the primary treatment for pediculosis pubis in the lactating and pregnant patient, reserving lindane for more serious or resistant infections. The recommended regimens for the treatment of pediculosis pubis during pregnancy are summarized in Table 1. It is important to remember to treat the sexual partner as well.

TABLE 2. Recommended Regimens for the Treatment of Scabies During Pregnancy

Initial therapy
  Crotamiton 10% cream or lotion (Eurax)
  Apply to entire body from neck down for 2 nights and wash off 24 hours after second application

  Sulfur (6%) in petrolatum
  Apply to entire body from neck down nightly for 3 nights. May bathe before applications and should bathe 24 hours after last application

Resistant or difficult cases
  Lindane cream or lotion (Kwell, Scabene)[a]
  Apply to entire skin surface from neck down and wash off after 8 hours

[a]Use with caution during pregnancy (see text).

SCABIES

Scabies is caused by the ectoparasite or mite *Sarcoptes scabiei*. It was first discovered by Bonomo in 1687.[22]

Epidemiology

Scabies classically occurs in 30-year cycles. It spreads primarily through close personal contact and sexual transmission is common. The usual age group is similar to that of pediculosis pubis (ages 15 to 40 years); however, infection is more common in men than in women and in whites as compared to blacks.[22]

Clinical Manifestations

The major manifestations include pruritis and an eczematous rash. There may also be a secondary neurodermatitis due to chronic scratching. The lesions are symmetrical and generally first appear on the hands (finger webs and side of the digits) and the flexor surface of the wrist.[22] Lesions may also appear on the elbows, axillae, breast, buttocks, and genital areas.[22] Lesions of the hands or other areas may be confused with secondary syphilis or other dermatologic conditions.

Diagnosis

The diagnosis is generally based on the characteristic skin lesions (burrows) and may be confirmed by microscopic identification of mites or fecal pellets.[22]

Treatment

The most effective treatment is probably achieved with the use of lindane lotion or cream applied to the affected areas for 8 hours. However, in the pregnant patient initial therapy should probably be with one of the alternate regimens, including crotamiton (Eurax) or sulfur in petrolatum (Table 2).

REFERENCES

1. Schmidt GP, Sanders LL, Blount JH, Alexander E: Chancroid in the United States: Re-establishment of an old disease. JAMA 258:3265–3268, 1987.
2. Centers for Disease Control: Summary of notifiable diseases, U.S. 1986. MMWR 35:51–57, 1986.
3. Ostler HB: Oculogenital disease. Surv Ophthalmol 20:233–246, 1976.
4. Centers for Disease Control: 1985 STD treatment guidelines. MMWR 34:76S–77S, 1985.
5. Naamara W, Kunimoto D, D'Costa L, et al.: Treating chancroid with Enoxacin. Genitourin Med 64:189–192, 1988.
6. Bodhidatta L, Taylor D, Chitwarakorn A, et al.: Evaluation of 500 and 1,000 mg doses of ciprofloxacin for the treatment of chancroid. Antimicrob Agents Chemother 32:723–725, 1988.
7. Naamara W, Plummer F, Greenblatt R, et al.: Treatment of chancroid with ciprofloxacin. Am J Med 82:317–320, 1987.
8. Dylewski J, D'Costa L, Nsanze H, Ronald AR: Single-dose therapy with trimethoprim-sulfamethoxazole for chancroid in females. Sex Transm Dis 13:166–168, 1986.
9. Schachter J: Lymphogranuloma venereum and other nonocular *Chlamydia trachomatis* infections. In Hobson D, Holmes K (eds): "Non-Gonococcal Urethritis and Related Infection." Washington, DC: American Society of Microbiologists, 1977, p 41.
10. Alacoque B, Cloppet H, Dumontel C, Moulin G: Histological, immunofluorescent and ultrastructural features of LGV. Br J Vener Dis 60:390–395, 1984.
11. Scrimgeour EM, Sengupta SK, McGoldrick IA: Primary endometrial and endocervical granuloma inguinale. Br J Vener Dis 59:198–201, 1983.
12. Latif A, Mason P, Paraiwa E: Treatment of donovanosis. Sex Transm Dis 15:27–29, 1988.
13. Wilson LA: Pregnancy and labor complicated by granuloma inguinale. JAMA 95:1093–1095, 1930.

14. Scott CW, Harper G, Jason R, et al.: Neonatal granuloma inguinale. Am J Dis Child 85:308–315, 1953.

15. Hart G: Donovanosis. In Holmes KK, Mardh P-A, Sparling PR, Weisner PJ (eds): "Sexually Transmitted Diseases." New York: McGraw-Hill, 1984, pp 393–397.

16. Miller S: Cutaneous cryptococcus resembling molluscum contagiosum in a patient with acquired immunodeficiency virus. Cutis 41:411–412, 1988.

17. Becker T, Blount J, Douglas J, Judson F: Trends in molluscum contagiosum in the U.S. Sex Transm Dis 13:88–92, 1986.

18. Porter CD, Muhleman MF, Cream JJ, Archard LC: Molluscum contagiosum—Characterization of viral DNA in clinical features. Epidemiol Infect 2:563–567, 1987.

19. Darai G, Reisner H, Scholz J, et al.: Analysis of genome of molluscum contagiosum virus by restriction endonuclease analysis and molecular cloning. J Med Virol 18:29–39, 1986.

20. Lynch PJ: Molluscum contagiosum venereum. Clin Obstet Gynecol 15:966–975, 1972.

21. Brown ST, Weinberger J: Molluscum contagiosum: Sexually transmitted disease—17 cases. J Am Dis Assoc 1:35–38, 1974.

22. Orkin M, Maibach HI: Scabies and pediculosis pubis. Dermatol Clin 1:111, 1983.

23. Chapel TA, Katta T, Kuszmar T, et al.: Pediculosis pubis in a clinic for treatment of sexually transmitted diseases. Sex Transm Dis 6:257, 1959.

24. Barnhart ER: "Physicians Desk Reference," 43rd edition. Oradell, NJ: Medical Economics Co., 1989, pp 1670, 2116.

25. Feldman RH, Maibach HI: Percutaneous penetration of some pesticides and herbicides in man. Toxicol Appl Pharmacol 28:126–132, 1974.

14

Herpes Simplex in Pregnancy

Mark G. Martens, M.D.

There has been a marked increase in reported cases of genital herpes simplex virus (HSV) infections over the past two decades. At one extreme, using current trends, forecasters have speculated that everyone in the world will have genital-tract herpes by the year 2030.[1] This increase has resulted in a heightened public awareness that has placed a tremendous pressure on physicians to act. The association of HSV infections with serious fetal morbidity, and sometimes mortality, has placed an even greater pressure on obstetricians and gynecologists to "do something."

That "something" was a repetitive testing regimen frequently followed by a cesarean section, resulting in over 50 cesarean sections performed to prevent one case of newborn herpes. This number is incongruous when one considers that HSV constitutes the lowest frequency of newborn infections among the TORCH pathogens (see Table 1), but is consistent with the public fascination and fear of an incurable venereal disease with infrequent, but serious fetal consequences. Obstetricians understandably rushed to develop protocols and methods in an attempt to prevent neonatal infection. However, the management protocols were based on a paucity of data because of the infrequency of neonatal infections. Well-designed prospective investigations have recently been completed; these strongly suggest that earlier preventive measures may have been excessive and did not provide truly effective measures to reduce the risk of neonatal herpes. With this recently gained knowledge a rational approach can now be formulated without increasing maternal morbidity, while still respecting the seriousness of fetal infections.

BIOLOGY AND EPIDEMIOLOGY

The herpes simplex virus belongs to the herpesvirus group, which also includes the varicella-zoster virus which causes chickenpox and shingles, cytomegalovirus, and the Epstein-Barr virus, which causes mononucleosis. They are all linear double-stranded DNA viruses enclosed in a lipid envelope, and they can be found in some form in all species of animals from invertebrates to vertebrates, such as oysters, fish, snakes, and all mammals.[2] Herpes simplex viruses can be separated into two types, HSV-1 and HSV-2, based on divergent antigenic and biologic characteristics. HSV-1 infection is usually acquired during the first 18 months of life.[3] It is often asymptomatic and is generally trans-

Infections in Pregnancy, pages 143–150

TABLE 1. Incidence of Maternal, Fetal, and Neonatal Infections Caused by Selected Microorganisms

Microorganism	Mother (per 1,000 pregnancies)	Fetus (per 1,000 livebirths)	Newborns (per 1,000 livebirths)
Cytomegalovirus	40–150	5–25	10–70
Rubella			
Epidemic	10–40	4–20	0
Interepidemic	0.1	0.5	0
Toxoplasma gondii	1.5–6.4	0.8–1	Unknown
Herpes simplex	10–15	Rare	0.1–0.5
Treponema pallidum	0.2	0.1	0
Group B streptococcus	10–250	—	—
Escherichia coli	Common	—	1–2

From Ledger,[1] with permission of the publisher.

mitted via the respiratory tract. The initial symptomatic manifestation is a gingivostomatitis characterized by vesicles in the oral cavity. Primary HSV-1 infection may rarely present as encephalitis or keratoconjunctivitis, often with serious consequences. After primary exposure in all HSV-1 infections, the virus appears to enter the cells of the trigeminal ganglion, where it usually remains latent.

HSV-2 infection generally follows puberty and is related to the onset of sexual activity. It is the most common cause of genital herpetic infection, and after primary infection also enters a state of latency, this time in the sacral dorsal root ganglia.

Although HSV-1 antibodies from a previous HSV-1 infection have several antigenic similarities to HSV-2 antibodies, they confer incomplete protection against HSV-2, and infections with the latter may still occur if the person is exposed.[4] HSV-2 is the most frequent cause of genital herpes infections; however, HSV-1 virus may be responsible for the first episodes of genital herpes infections in 10 to 40% of cases, and the numbers appear to be increasing.[5]

Perinatal transmission is usually due to genital transmission during the birthing process, and thus is often found to be HSV-2. HSV-1-infected neonates have been reported; however, careful consideration should be given to postnatal exposure from family members or hospital personnel if the maternal genital infection is HSV-2 in nature.

Genital HSV infection consultations in the private office rose 10-fold from 1966 to 1981.[6] Genital herpes infections are found in 1.6 to 8% of females attending sexually transmitted disease (STD) clinics[7,8] and in 0.25 to 3.0% of patients in non-STD clinic populations.[9] They are more prevalent in Caucasians than in non-Caucasians, contrary to most other STDs, such as *Neisseria gonorrhoeae*, which are usually seen 10 times more frequently in non-Caucasian populations. Pregnancy does not seem to affect the rate of recurrence, which has been found to be 0.01 to 4% in asymptomatic women.[10,11] This number may appear low, but it represents a significant total number of patients, and the incidence of neonatal HSV infections has been concomitantly increasing, from 2.6 cases per 100,000 livebirths in 1966–1969 to 28.2 cases per 100,000 livebirths in 1982.[12]

SPECTRUM OF DISEASE

Herpes simplex viruses are highly cytopathic, so much so that their culture and diagnosis are based upon this factor. Therefore, primary infection with the virus should cause serious cellular damage. Primary infections in the nonpregnant adult can cause the well-known and painful lesions of genital or oral herpes. Spread of the virus to the eye or brain can cause serious cellular destruction resulting in blindness or often fatal encephalitis. Disseminated infection can also result in widespread organ system involvement and failure.

Although the frequency of HSV infection is not increased during pregnancy, the severity of the disease may be increased. In animal models, the severity, duration of viral shedding, and mortality rate of HSV-2 infection in pregnant mice are significantly greater than in nonpregnant mice.[13] Also, increased levels of pregnancy hormones such as progesterone have been shown to enhance the spread of HSV in tissue culture.[14] These data are consistent with the fact that most cases of disseminated herpetic infections in non-immunocompromised adults occur in pregnant women, and all cases have occurred in the late second and third trimesters, when maternal T-cell function is partially compromised.[15]

Fetal infection can be serious, and while neonatal infection is the most publicized, there is probably a spectrum of adverse outcomes that can start as early as the first trimester. Infection of the first-trimester fetus would theoretically be devastating because of the smaller mass of rapidly proliferating tissue; therefore, the increased frequency of spontaneous abortion that has been documented with early primary infection is not surprising. Nahmias et al. found a 34% rate of spontaneous abortions in pregnant women with a diagnosis of HSV cervicitis in the first 20 weeks of gestation vs. a 10.6% rate ($P <$ .01) in their general population.[16] Other investigators have found up to a 300% increase in the spontaneous abortion rate with early HSV infection.[17,18] The etiology of the fetal wastage may be the result of hematogenous spread of the virus, but may also occur from ascending infection from primary cervical infection.[19] An increased rate of premature births has been found in infants whose mothers had primary genital infections after the 20th week of pregnancy.[16,17]

Transplacental infection of the fetus resulting in congenital infection is a rare sequel to maternal infection, but may result in morphologic alterations in organogenesis similar to congenital cytomegalovirus infections. These changes include microcephaly, often with intracranial calcifications, psychomotor retardation, and ocular abnormalities such as microphthalmia and retinal dysplasia.

The major perinatal problem is neonatal herpes infection. Because of the variety of its presentations, its exact incidence is not known for certain. It is estimated that neonatal herpes occurs in 1 of every 5,000 to 20,000 neonates in the United States.[20] Infection is usually associated with a lesion in the maternal genital tract, and the neonate acquires infection during vaginal delivery, unless prolonged rupture of membranes has occurred. Amstey and Monif found that infants delivered by cesarean section from mothers with vulvar herpes after 4 hours or more of ruptured amniotic membranes had an incidence of neonatal herpetic infections similar to that of vaginally delivered infants.[21] The risk of transmission has been documented to be approximately 40–60%, with the risk of death approximately 50%, and with another 15–25% of infants having residual CNS damage or ocular stigmata.[16,21]

The specifics of viral transmission are more complex, and its understanding is essential to the formulation of effective preventive protocols. Individuals who contract a primary infection during pregnancy pose the greatest risk to the infants for transmission of HSV. In fact, neonatal transmission appears to be approximately 10-fold less with recurrent disease.[22]

DIAGNOSIS

Tissue culture is the standard for diagnosis of HSV infections; however, the delay in obtaining results sometimes necessitates more immediate measures. Primary genital herpetic infection is of most concern and is manifested by 1) a systemic response that consists of fever, chills, and malaise; 2) inguinal lymphadenopathy; and 3) painful genital ulcerations (Fig. 1). Lesions often occur on the cervix and these may not be as easily

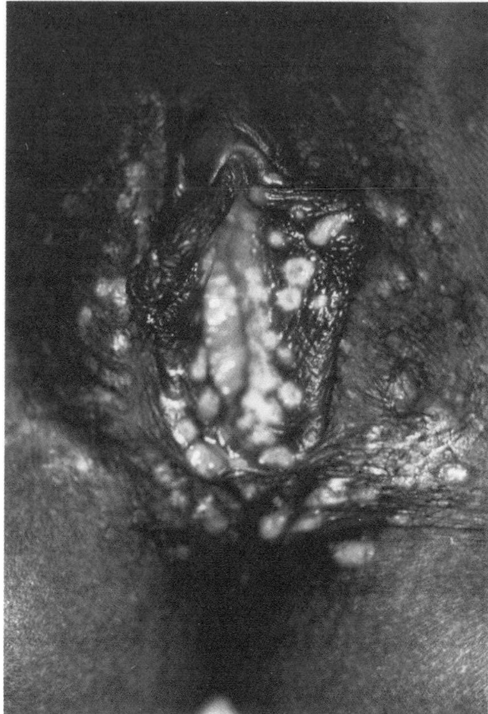

Fig. 1.   Pregnant patient with primary herpetic infection in addition to secondary syphilis. (Photo courtesy of Dr. George Wendel, University of Texas Southwestern Medical Center, Dallas.)

detected because of the presence of a less tender and poorly visualized lesion. These patients often present with a copious clear discharge or urinary incontinence or retention.

Systemic symptoms should not be overlooked in a patient with primary genital herpetic infection. Although dissemination is rare, it is more likely to occur in pregnancy as noted earlier, and the mortality of herpes encephalitis is close to 80% in untreated patients, with 90% of the survivors left with significant neurologic sequelae.

Cytologic diagnosis, such as with the Papanicolaou or Tzanck smear, is a more rapid method for diagnosis. However, it is less sensitive and specific than culture, with the sensitivity reported to be only 50 to 75%. A cytologic specimen is taken with a cotton-tipped applicator and spread on a glass slide. The specimen is fixed similar to that of a Pap smear and, after staining, is examined for the presence of an enlarged nucleus or nuclei in giant cells and the displacement of chromatin against the nuclear membrane, giving the nucleus the ground-glass appearance typically seen with viral infection.

All cells infected with a herpesvirus will have similar cytologic findings; therefore, varicella and cytomegalovirus infections should be ruled out, as the management of these infections is often quite different. While a primary herpetic lesion may necessitate immediate delivery by cesarean section, a varicella infection often requires delay of delivery and time for transplacental passive antibody formation.

Rapid diagnosis using immunofluourescent techniques has greater specificity; however, the sensitivity is still lacking when the seriousness of the infectious consequences are taken into account. Sensitivity in the most recent investigations using type-specific monoclonal antibodies has been found to be 78%, with a false-positive rate of 6%.[23]

Serologic diagnosis can help in establishing the diagnosis of a primary herpetic infection, but the delay necessary to obtain the convalescent sera to detect an antibody rise makes it an impractical test for decision making at the time of delivery. The absence of antibodies may have a place earlier in gestation, by documenting the patient's susceptibility to current or future exposure. Serologic testing will have an even greater role if herpes vaccine investigations currently underway demonstrate adequate protection, resulting in a vaccination program similar to that for rubella.

MANAGEMENT

Previous recommendations for the management of pregnant women suspected of having genital herpetic infections included a series of weekly cultures late in the third trimester, with cesarean section recommended for those with positive cultures at or near delivery. Unfortunately, this protocol not only failed to decrease the overall incidence of neonatal herpes,[24] but also resulted in an increase in the number of cesarean sections and in maternal morbidity and mortality associated with these additional cesarean sections. In fact, it has been estimated that by following the previously recommended culturing strategy, screening would have averted 11.3 neonatal deaths and 3.7 cases of severe retardation per year; however, 3.3 mothers would have died each year because of infection, anesthetic, or other complications of cesarean section.[25] The cost per case averted also would be greater than 1.8 million dollars per year.[25]

Reasons for the failure to affect the neonatal herpes infection rate are numerous. Positive antepartum maternal cultures correlated poorly with the probability of viral shedding at the time of labor and delivery.[26] Also, most women who deliver infants with neonatal HSV infections do not have a history of previous infections. Thus they would not have met the criteria for weekly culturing. Approximately one-third of infants who develop neonatal HSV infection are born prematurely, weigh less than 2,500 g, and are infected prior to the initiation of weekly culturing.[18]

It has been recommended that infants should be delivered by cesarean section if amniotic membranes have been ruptured for less than 6 hours, and if genital herpetic lesions are present on the gravida. Grossman reported that some infants have been spared infection even if amniotic membranes have been ruptured for more than 24 hours and delivery was by cesarean section.[27] Although there is not a large body of data to support this approach, some physicians elect to perform cesarean delivery when the amniotic membranes are ruptured for more than 12 hours. Some neonates have been found to be infected despite cesarean delivery within 2 hours of membrane rupture.[28] In one study, 12% of all reported cases of HSV infection occurred in infants delivered by cesarean section with intact membranes.[29] Despite the conflicting data, it is still well established that cesarean section in women with active infection at the time of delivery, especially primary infection, will significantly reduce the risk and incidence of neonatal HSV infection.

The difference in transmission rate between primary and recurrent HSV infections was first suspected following the demonstration of a 10-fold lower incidence of neonatal HSV infection than expected for the number of suspected infected mothers in the United States. A recent study demonstrated at least one documented symptomatic recurrence in 108 of 148 pregnant women with a history of recurrent herpes. The rate of those positive at delivery at term has been determined by Prober et al. to be 0.2% of 6,904 mothers.[30] If this is extrapolated to the number of infants born in the United States per year, an estimated 7,600 infants would be exposed per year. However, the number of reported neonatal HSV infections nowhere approaches this number if the classically quoted 50% infection rate is used. Prober et al. also supported the belief that primary maternal infection is the major risk factor in neonatal disease. In the study, only one infant developed neonatal HSV infection, and this was in one of the two mothers with primary infection. None of the infants born to mothers with recurrent disease developed herpes infection. Other studies have also documented the inconsistencies of maternal HSV shedding (0.1–0.4%) at delivery with the infrequency of neonatal infection (0.01–0.04%), supporting the difference in primary vs. recurrent maternal herpetic infection transmission rate.[29,31] Thus, the transmission rate of primary maternal infection to the exposed infant delivered vaginally is approximately 50%, while the transmission rate with recurrent maternal infection is approximately 0–4%.[32] Additional large studies have found a similar vertical transmission rate in primary infections with no infections in those infants born to mothers with documented recurrent infections.[33]

Theories explaining this discrepancy include 1) the presumed protective benefit of transplacental maternal IgG antibodies in infants born to mothers with recurrent disease and 2) the prolonged duration of viral shedding in primary maternal infections.[33] Explanation for the occurrence of neonatal HSV infection despite a documented previous positive herpes culture in the mother may be 1) a failure of maternal antibody formation due to maternal disease or immunosuppressive therapy such as steroid administration, 2) the higher incidence of neonatal HSV infections in preterm infants who have been demonstrated to have lower serum IgG levels than term infants[34], and 3) the prolongation of HSV shedding from a primary infection. Also, some of these infants born to mothers with a recurrent disease may not have vertical transmission as their source of infection, but a nosocomial infection. These infections are often HSV-1 and have been reported to occur at a rate of approximately 10%.[35] Thus, taking these data into consideration, the American College of Obstetricians and Gynecologists altered their protocol for pregnant women with HSV infections or a history of such infections to include the following[28]:

1. Cultures should be done when a women has active HSV lesions during pregnancy to confirm the diagnosis. If there are no visible lesions at the onset of labor, vaginal delivery is acceptable.

2. Weekly surveillance cultures of pregnant women with a history of HSV infection but no visible lesions are not necessary and vaginal delivery is acceptable.

3. Amniocentesis in an attempt to rule out intrauterine infection is not recommended for mothers with HSV infection at any stage of gestation.

Fear that omitting cultures would expose infants to active or asymptomatic shedders is unfounded, as a recent study found no positive cultures in 414 asymptomatic women cultured from 34 weeks until the onset of labor.[26] None of the 17 patients with asymptomatic shedding during the antepartum period did so at the onset of labor, and the five patients who were positive in labor had demonstrated positive antepartum culture. Also, patients with asymptomatic disease in labor rarely produce infected infants, presumably because of the low inoculum of virus.

The revised ACOG protocol is helpful for identifying active disease in the mother and hopefully avoiding exposure to infants, but it does little to aid pediatricians in assessing risk and treating potentially infected infants. The onset of neonatal herpes infection is sometimes insidious, with the demonstration of lethargy, poor feeding, irritability, apnea, and seizures, often in the absence of mucocutaneous lesions. Also, with disseminated HSV-1 infection, few infants demonstrate mucocutaneous lesions. Symptoms for HSV-1 and -2 often manifest only several days after birth, and the delay in diagnosis without lesions is a mean of 72 hours.

Maternal genital cultures taken at the time of delivery would be helpful to the pediatrician, especially in establishing a diagnosis in those infants presenting with the subtle findings described above. Results of cultures done at delivery would then be available prior to the onset of most symptoms, and antiviral therapy can then be instituted if deemed necessary.

Acyclovir is a nucleoside analogue whose highly selective activity inhibits the replication of HSV at concentrations that are mostly lower than those that inhibit mammalian cellular functions. Therefore, the drug is presumably safe for both mother and infant, and animal studies have failed to demonstrate fetal toxicity or teratogenicity even at extremely high doses.[36] Follow-up on fetal exposure is under way, but as yet unpublished, and therefore caution should still be used with its administration. Its presence in breast milk has been documented.[37] Acyclovir's use is indicated for life-threatening and disseminated HSV infections.

The use of acyclovir during pregnancy has

been demonstrated to be beneficial in cases of extreme prematurity, with rupture of membranes, or preterm labor in the presence of HSV lesions. Immediate delivery by cesarean section would be extremely detrimental to both mother and infant in such cases, and delay of delivery with concomitant use of acyclovir has resulted in good outcomes.[38] However, the effects of indiscriminate use of acyclovir are still unknown, as reports of the drug's effects on antibody response are under investigation.[39]

SUMMARY

Although old habits are hard to break, the necessity of abandoning the previous protocols for the management and prevention of neonatal HSV infection is essential in both the future prevention of HSV exposure and maternal morbidity and mortality from unnecessary surgery. The publication of several well-designed studies will give the obstetrician the information to make these changes for the protection of both mother and infant. However, even those changes will be altered in the future as more rapid diagnostic techniques and the potential of several HSV vaccines are further explored.

REFERENCES

1. Ledger WJ (ed): "Infection in the Female," Philadelphia: Lea and Febiger, 1986, p 215.
2. Rapp F: Herpes simplex viruses. In Holmes KK, Mardh PA, Sparling PF, Wiesner PJ (eds): "Sexually Transmitted Diseases." New York: McGraw-Hill, 1984, pp 438–449.
3. Plummer G: Serological comparison of the herpes viruses. Br J Exp Pathol 45:135–141, 1964.
4. Kawana T, Kawagol K, Takizawa K, Chen JG, Kawaguchi T, Sakamoto S: Clinical and virologic studies of female genital herpes. Obstet Gynecol 60:456–460, 1982.
5. Kalinyak JE, Feiagle G, Kocherty JJ: Incidence and distribution of herpes simplex virus 1 and 2 from genital lesions in college women. J Med Virol 1:175–180, 1979.
6. American College of Obstetricians and Gynecologists: Gynecologic Herpes Simplex Virus Infections (ACOG Technical Bulletin 119). Washington, DC: ACOG, 1988.
7. Jeansson S, Molin L: On the occurrence of genital herpes simplex virus infections. Acta Derm Venereol 54:479–482, 1974.
8. Venereal Disease Control Division, Bureau of State Services, Centers for Disease Control: Nonrepeated sexually transmissable disease—United States. MMWR 28:61, 1979.
9. Holmes KK, Mardh PA, Sparling PF, Wiesner PJ (eds): "Sexually Transmitted Diseases." New York: McGraw-Hill, 1984, pp 449–474.
10. Tejani N, Klein SW, Kaplan M: Subclinical herpes simplex genitalis infections in the perinatal period. Am J Obstet Gynecol 135:547, 1979.
11. Scher J, Bottone E, Desmond E, Simons W: The incidence and outcome of asymptomatic herpes simplex genitalis in an obstetric population. Am J Obstet Gynecol 144:906–909, 1982.
12. Sullivan-Balyai J, Hull HF, Wilson C, Corey L: Neonatal herpes simplex virus infection in Kings County, Washington. JAMA 250:3059–3062, 1983.
13. Young EJ, Gomez CI: Enhancement of herpes virus type 2 infection in pregnant mice. Proc Soc Exp Biol Med 160:416–420, 1979.
14. Amstey MS: Effect of pregnancy hormones on herpes virus and other DNA viruses. Am J Obstet Gynecol 129:159–163, 1977.
15. Monif GRG: Viruses. In Monif GRG (ed): "Infectious Diseases in Obstetrics and Gynecology," 2nd edition. Philadelphia: Harper and Row, 1982, pp 45–115.
16. Nahmias AJ, Josey WE, Naib ZM, et al.: Perinatal risk associated with maternal genital herpes simplex virus infection. Am J Obstet Gynecol 110:825–837, 1971.
17. Naib ZM, et al.: Association of maternal genital herpetic infection with spontaneous abortion. Obstet Gynecol 35:260–263, 1970.
18. Whitley RJ, Nahmias AJ, Visintine AM, et al.: The natural history of herpes simplex infection of mother and newborn. Pediatrics 66:489–494, 1980.
19. Hain J, et al.: Ascending transcervical herpes simplex infection with intact fetal membranes. Obstet Gynecol 56:106–109, 1980.
20. Sever JL, Larsen JW, Grossman JH: "Handbook of Perinatal Infections." Boston: Little Brown, 1979.
21. Amstey MS, Monif GRG: Genital HSV infection in pregnancy. Obstet Gynecol 44:394–397, 1974.
22. Nahmias AJ, Visintine AM: Herpes simplex. In Remington J (ed): "Infectious Disease of the Fetus and Newborn Infant." Philadelphia: W.B. Saunders, 1976, p 156.
23. Bell AM, Kingsley SR, Fiddian AP, Brigden WD: Sexually transmitted diseases in pregnancy. Br Med J 288:1456, 1984.

24. Chuange Ty: Neonatal herpes: Incidence, prevention, and consequences. Am J Prev Med 4(1):47–53, 1988.

25. Binkin NJ, Koplan JP, Cates W Jr: Preventing neonatal herpes. The value of weekly viral cultures in pregnant women with recurrent genital herpes. JAMA 251(21):2816–2821, 1984.

26. Arvin AM, Hensleigh PA, Prober CG, et al.: Failure of antepartum maternal cultures to predict the infant's risk of exposure to herpes simplex virus at delivery. N Engl J Med 315(13):796–800, 1986.

27. Grossman JH III: Herpes simplex virus (HSV) infections. Clin Obstet Gynecol 25(3):555–561, 1982.

28. American College of Obstetricians and Gynecologists: Technical Bulletin 122, Washington, DC: ACOG, 1988.

29. Stone KM, Brooks CA, Guinan ME, et al.: Neonatal herpes—Results of one year's surveillance. Abstracts of the 25th Interscience Conference on Antimicrobial Agents and Chemotherapy. Washington, DC: American Society for Microbiology, 1985, p 185, abstract 515.

30. Prober CG, Hensleigh PA, Bauchel FD, et al.: Use of routine viral cultures at delivery to identify neonates exposed to herpes simplex virus. N Engl J Med 318:882–891, 1988.

31. Brown ZA, Vontver LA, Benedetti J, et al.: Genital herpes in pregnancy: Risk factors associated with recurrence and asymptomatic viral shedding. Am J Obstet Gynecol 153(1):24–30, 1985.

32. Brown ZA, Vontver LA, Benedetti J, et al.: Effects on infants of a first episode of genital herpes during pregnancy. N Engl J Med 317(20):1246–1251, 1987.

33. Prober CG, Sullender WM, Yasukawa LL, et al.: Low risk of herpes simplex virus infections in neonates exposed to the virus at the time of vaginal delivery to mothers with recurrent genital herpes simplex virus infections. N Engl J Med 316(5):240–244, 1987.

34. Harris RE: Maternal and fetal immunology. Obstet Gynecol 51:733–739, 1978.

35. Yeager AS, Arvin AM: Reasons for the absence of a history of recurrent genital infections in mothers of neonates infected with herpes simplex virus. Pediatrics 73(2):188–193, 1984.

36. Moore HL, Szczech GM, Rodwell DE, et al.: Preclinical toxicology studies with acyclovir: Teratologic, reproductive and neonatal tests. Fund Appl Toxicol 3:560–568, 1983.

37. Meyer LJ, DeMiranda P, Sheth N, Spruana S: Acyclovir in breast milk. Am J Obstet Gynecol 158:586–588, 1988.

38. Utley K, Bromberger P, Wagner L, Schneider H: Management of primary herpes in pregnancy complicated by ruptured membranes and extreme prematurity; Case report. Obstet Gynecol 69(3):471–473, 1987.

39. Bernstein DI, Lovett MA, Bryson YJ: The effects of acyclovir on antibody response to herpes simplex virus in primary genital infections. J Infect Dis 150:7–13, 1984.

15

Cytomegalic Virus Infection in Pregnancy

Frederick E. Harlass, M.D., and Patrick Duff, M.D.

Cytomegalovirus infection is the most common perinatal infection in the United States. It affects approximately 1–2% of all newborns. The vast majority of infections are transmitted in utero by hematogenous dissemination across the placenta. A small percentage of infants acquire infection during passage through a contaminated birth canal. The most serious manifestations of in utero infection occur in association with a primary maternal infection. They include stillbirth, hepatosplenomegaly, jaundice, petechiae, thrombocytopenia, microcephaly, and chorioretinitis. In utero infections resulting from recurrent maternal infection are extremely uncommon. Cytomegalovirus infection may be diagnosed by culture of the virus, by demonstration of IgM antibody, or by confirmation of a significant increase in IgG antibody titer. There is no effective antiviral chemotherapy or vaccination for cytomegalovirus infection at the present time. Accordingly, every effort must be made to prevent acquisition of primary infection by susceptible pregnant women. Preventive measures include attention to the personal hygiene of young children in the home, reduction of occupational exposure, and avoidance of transfusion of infected blood products.

HISTORY

In 1881, Ribbert first described large, cytoplasmic inclusions in the cells of an infant who had died of syphilis.[1] Subsequently, Tietze (1905) and Lowenstein (1907) described similar inclusions in the cells of the parotid glands of children.[2,3] Initially, these inclusions were thought to be due to a protozoan infection. However, over the next several decades, the similarities of these cells to those infected by the varicella-zoster and herpes simplex viruses led to the recognition that the histologic changes were due to a viral infection. The exact nature of these inclusions finally was elucidated in 1926 when Kuttner and Cole confirmed the viral etiology of the disease.[4]

Farber and Wolbach (1932) were the first to use the term "salivary gland virus disease" because of the virus's ability to induce characteristic nuclear inclusions in the epithelial lining of the salivary ducts.[5] Smith (1954) was able to propagate the salivary gland virus in culture, utilizing mouse embryonic tissue.[6]

The opinions and assertions contained herein are the private views of the authors and are not to be construed as official or as reflecting the views of the Department of the Army or the Department of Defense.

Infections in Pregnancy, pages 151–163

TABLE 1. Maternal Serosusceptibility to Cytomegalovirus Within Various Socioeconomic Populations

Author	Year	No. of patients	Socioeconomic status	Seronegative (%)
Peckham et al.[17]	1983	14,789	Upper middle	44
Chandler et al.[14]	1985	1,129	Heterogeneous	43
Stagno et al.[16]	1986	16,218	Upper income	64
			Low income	23
Yow et al.[15]	1988	4,578	Upper middle	48

This technique led to the near-simultaneous recovery of human cytomegalovirus by Smith,[7] Rowe et al.,[8] and Weller and associates.[9] Because the term "salivary gland disease" was misleading, Weller et al. suggested that the term "cytomegalovirus" be used.[10] In 1962 Weller and Hanshaw were the first to identify the specific pathologic effects associated with perinatal cytomegalovirus infection.[11]

VIROLOGY

Cytomegalovirus is classified as a herpesvirus. Other members of this group include herpes simplex virus type 1, herpes simplex virus type 2, varicella-zoster virus, and the Epstein-Barr virus. Herpesviruses have an inner core that contains linear double-stranded DNA. The core is surrounded by an icosahedral capsid, which, in turn, is contained within an outer envelope. The overall diameter of the virus is about 200 nm.

The life cycle of the cytomegalovirus is typical of enveloped virions. The virus enters the host cell by fusion of its membrane with that of the cell. The nuclear capsid enters the cytoplasm, where the viral DNA is extruded. Viral DNA then enters the nucleus, where new viral particles are synthesized and reassembled. The complete viral particles attain an envelope by budding through the inner nuclear membrane and then subsequently migrate through the cytoplasm in a vacuole and exit the host cell. As is true with the other herpesviruses, cytomegalovirus can remain dormant in the host and reactivate at a future time. The virus has a predilection for epithelial cells, but can replicate in many different cells.

Throughout evolution, the antigenic structure of the various strains of cytomegalovirus has become species specific. Hence, human cytomegalovirus cannot infect any other animal species. This fact has limited the ability of scientists to study human strains of cytomegalovirus. Many of the initial investigations, therefore, were performed with murine and guinea pig cytomegalovirus. It now is possible, however, to culture human cytomegalovirus in fibroblasts, and tissue culture techniques have improved considerably in recent years.

EPIDEMIOLOGY

Cytomegalovirus infection can affect humans at any point in life beginning with conception. The infection occurs worldwide, and the highest prevalence rates are found in young children of low socioeconomic backgrounds. Cytomegalovirus infection is the most common congenital infection in the United States: approximately 1 to 2% of all infants are infected.[12,13]

The principal method of transmission of cytomegalovirus in the perinatal period is transplacental hematogenous dissemination. A very small proportion of neonates acquire infection as a result of passage through the maternal genital tract or from breast-feeding. The following sections will describe each of these modes of transmission in detail.

Transplacental Transmission

Prospective investigations of pregnant women have shown that approximately 40–

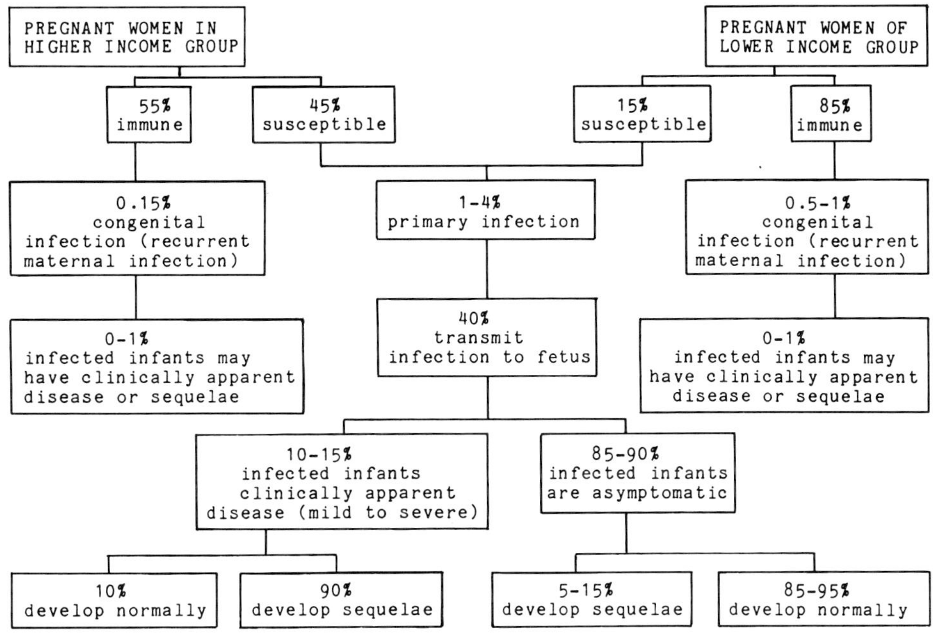

Fig. 1. Outcome of cytomegalovirus infection during pregnancy. (From Stagno and Whitley,[23] with permission of the publisher.)

50% of the adult population is susceptible to cytomegalovirus infection (Table 1). The rate of seroconversion during pregnancy ranges from 0.09 to 3.7%.[16,18,19] Risk factors for *primary* infection during pregnancy include maternal age less than 25 years,[15] young children in the home,[15,20] children in day-care centers,[21] and, paradoxically, upper socioeconomic status.[22] Of women who have a primary infection during pregnancy, 20 to 50% (mean: 40%) will transmit the virus to the fetus.[15,19,20,22] Primary maternal infection results in the most severe form of perinatal infection.[22] Figure 1 summarizes the expected consequences of primary maternal infection during pregnancy.

Unlike rubella, toxoplasmosis, and varicella, where acquired infection imparts permanent immunity, fetal infection still may occur even when a woman has apparent immunity to cytomegalovirus. Of women who develop recurrent infection, approximately 0.15–1% will transmit the virus to the fetus.[23]

However, although maternal immunity is an incomplete barrier to vertical transmission, it does appear to reduce the virulence of fetal infection. There are only three reported cases of a seroimmune mother who delivered a severely affected child (Table 2). In addition, Stagno (personal communication) now has followed approximately 30 children for up to 15 years who were known to be infected in utero following a recurrent maternal infection. Only two of these children have sequelae: one child has mild sensorineural hearing loss and another has chorioretinitis.

Recurrent infection appears to be secondary to reactivation of latent cytomegalovirus rather than reinfection with a different antigenic strain. Huang et al. used restriction endonucleases to investigate cytomegalovirus infections in mothers and their children.[24] Their intent was to determine whether recurrent infections were due to reinfection with a different antigenic strain or recurrence of an endogenous infection. They found that cy-

TABLE 2. Fetal Abnormalities Following Recurrent Cytomegalovirus Infection

Author	Year	Defect
Ahlfors et al.[25]	1982	Hepatosplenomegaly, petechiae, thrombocytopenia, severe sensorineural hearing loss
Peckham et al.[17]	1983	Severe neurological damage and bilateral sensorineural hearing loss
Rutter et al.[26]	1985	IUGR, microcephaly, splenomegaly, thrombocytopenia, hypotonia, motor delay, sensorineural hearing loss

tomegalovirus strains from congenitally infected babies were identical to strains isolated from their mothers. Strains in infected siblings also were concordant.

The data relating fetal damage to the gestational age at which maternal infection occurs are inconclusive. Some authors have been able to confirm a direct relationship between severity of fetal and neonatal disease and trimester of exposure.[16,25,27,28] Other investigators, however, have not been able to demonstrate this association.[15,19,22,30,31]

Transmission at the Time of Delivery

Cervical secretions are an important reservoir of cytomegalovirus.[32–34] The overall prevalence of cervical shedding in pregnant and nonpregnant women is approximately the same, 3 to 5%. However, there appears to be an increased rate of cervical shedding as pregnancy advances.[13] This observation may be related to the alterations in cell-mediated immunity that occur during pregnancy.[35]

Fortunately, infants are very unlikely to acquire infection as a result of passage through a contaminated birth canal. Should infection develop, it is most likely to be manifest as a mild interstitial pneumonitis.[36]

Postnatal Transmission Through Breast Milk

Stagno et al. have confirmed the importance of breast milk in transmission of the virus.[32] In a population of predominantly indigent black women, they isolated the virus from breast milk in 38 of 278 (13%) lactating mothers. Infected specimens were much less likely than uninfected ones to have detectable concentrations of IgA antibody directed against cytomegalovirus. Of those infants who were exposed to milk infected with cytomegalovirus, 58% became viruric between 4 weeks and 4 months of age.

Childhood Transmission

The age at acquisition of the virus has been found to be related to the socioeconomic status of the population examined.[13,16] When socioeconomic status has been controlled for, black and white children have similar rates of infection.[37] By the end of the first year of life, 8 to 60% of infants will excrete the virus.[38,39] The yearly rate of acquisition in the general population has been estimated at 5–10% up to age 4 and less than 5% between the ages of 4 and 15 years.[40]

The virus has been isolated from saliva, stool, tears, and urine. The principal risk factors for horizontal spread of cytomegalovirus among young children are poor personal hygiene and close personal contact. Accordingly, institutionalized children, as well as children from migratory families, have increased rates of transmission when compared to the general population.[41,42] Another important source of horizontal spread of cytomegalovirus is close personal contact in day-care centers.[20,21,43,44] Hutto et al. have shown that the highest rates of salivary excretion of cytomegalovirus occur in toddlers in the 12–24-month age group.[43] This group also has a very high frequency of hand-to-mouth or object-to-mouth contacts per hour. Additionally, Pass et al. have shown that there is a high seroconversion rate among the parents of children who in day care as compared to parents of children not attending day-care centers.[21] Thus these children may become the source of a primary maternal infection during a subsequent pregnancy.

Adult Transmission

Cytomegalovirus infection can be transmitted by sexual contact. Chretian et al. have reported transmission of cytomegalovirus mononucleosis between sexual partners, but not between individuals who had only casual household contact.[45] Lang and Kummer have demonstrated the presence of cytomegalovirus in semen.[29] Jordan et al. and Chandler and coworkers recovered the virus more frequently from the cervices of women attending a sexually transmitted disease clinic than from women having a routine gynecological or obstetric examination.[46,47]

Davis et al. demonstrated a significantly lower prevalence of cytomegalovirus antibody in nuns as compared to sexually active women.[48] An association between seropositivity, increased frequency of sexually transmitted disease, and an increased number of sexual partners has been confirmed.[41] Additionally, there is an increased rate of acquisition of antibody to cytomegalovirus in the general population at the peak of sexual activity—between adolescence and 35 years of age.[49,50]

Other documented forms of transmission of cytomegalovirus include blood transfusion, organ transplantation, and nosocomial sources. Conflicting evidence exists regarding the risk of transmission of cytomegalovirus in the health-care environment.[51–55] The overall risk of transmission appears to be quite small, but varying methodology and study design make it difficult to define the risk precisely.

CLINICAL MANIFESTATIONS OF CYTOMEGALOVIRUS INFECTION

Older Children and Adults

The overwhelming majority of cytomegalovirus infections in older children and adults are asymptomatic, and patients do not seek medical attention for their illness. In patients who do become clinically ill, the most common manifestations are those of a flulike illness, similar to mononucleosis. This syndrome was first described in 1965 by Klemola and Kaarrianen.[56] It is characterized by sudden abrupt spiking fevers to as high as 104°F, which typically persist for 2 to 3 weeks, but may last 8 to 9 weeks. Other common manifestations include headache, cervical lymphadenopathy, back and abdominal pain, sore throat, malaise, chills, myalgias, and arthralgias. Some patients have a transient morbilliform rash that lasts for 1 to 2 days. Others develop hepatitis, purpura, conjunctivitis, and splenomegaly.

Occasionally, these signs and symptoms may occur 2 to 3 weeks following a blood transfusion (the postperfusion syndrome). In this situation, the clinical illness usually resolves in 3 to 6 weeks. Based on these observations of blood transfusion recipients, the period of incubation has been estimated to be 20 to 50 days.

In a small percentage of patients, signs of central nervous infections such as encephalitis and aseptic meningitis become evident.[57,58] In addition, some patients develop Guillain-Barré syndrome.[59] Cytomegalovirus infection is particularly likely to be a cause of serious morbidity and mortality in immunosuppressed patients. In many bone marrow transplant units, cytomegalovirus pneumonitis now is the single most common cause of death.[60]

Infection in the Newborn

As noted in Figure 1, the severe manifestations of cytomegalovirus infection occur almost exclusively in infants born to mothers who have had a primary infection during pregnancy. Approximately 40% of mothers with primary infection will transmit infection to the fetus. Of these infants, 10–15% will have evidence of overt infection at birth. The most common findings in severely affected infants are hepatosplenomegaly, jaundice, thrombocytopenia, and petechiae (the "blueberry muffin baby"; Fig. 2a,b). Other manifestations include microcephaly, periventricular calcifications (Fig. 3), chorioret-

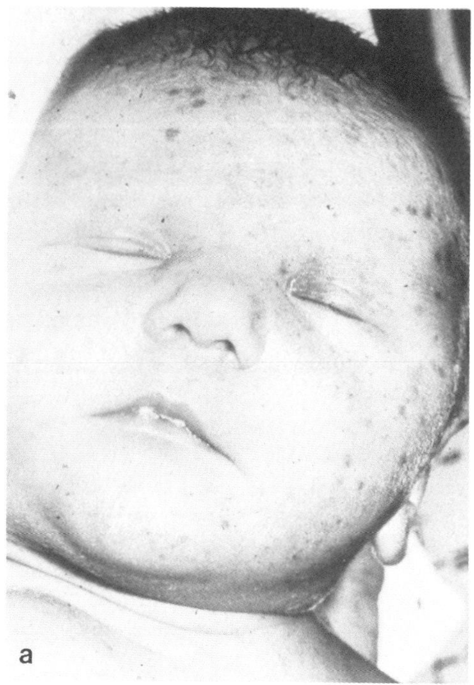

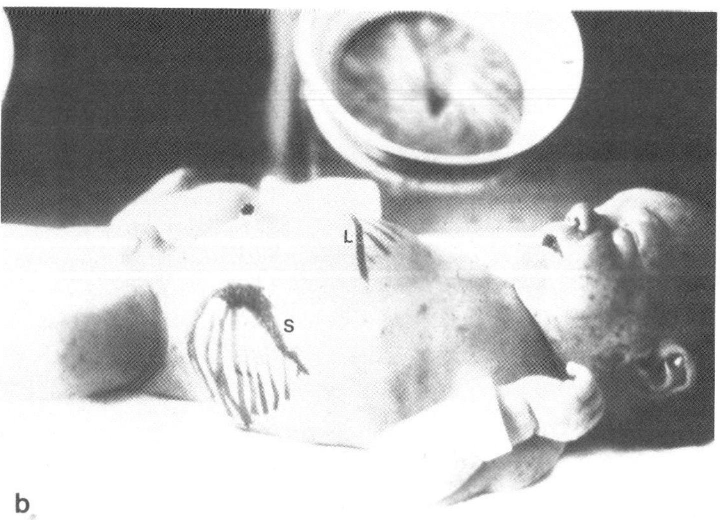

Fig. 2. a: An infected infant with multiple petechiae on the face. **b:** Prominent hepatomegaly (L) and splenomegaly (S) associated with severe cytomegalovirus infection. (Photos courtesy of Dr. Richard F. Jacobs, Division of Pediatric Infectious Disease, University of Arkansas for Medical Sciences, Little Rock.)

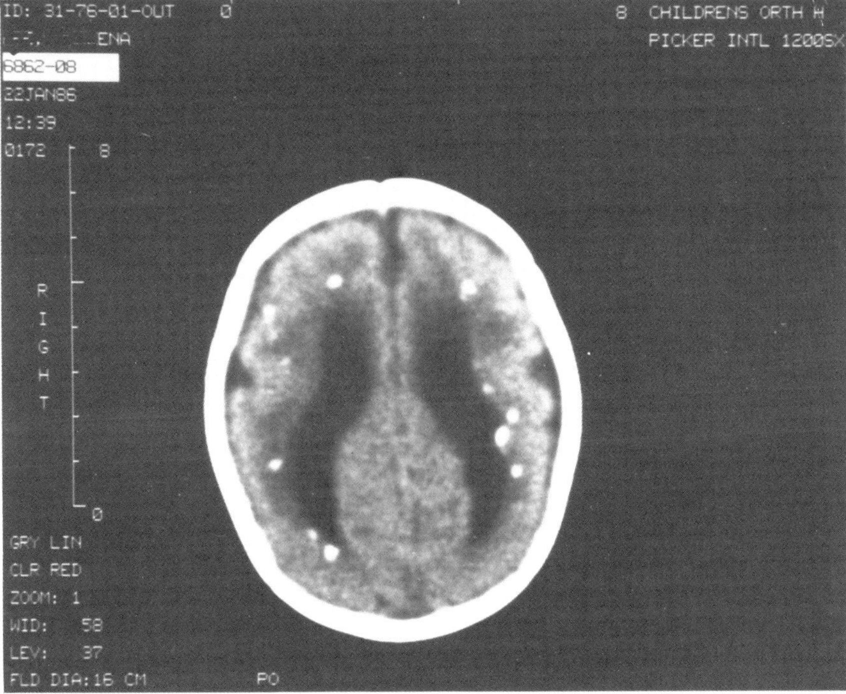

Fig. 3. Computed tomography scan of the head demonstrates characteristic periventricular calcifications. (CT scan courtesy of Dr. Janis Mercker, Department of Radiology, Children's Hospital and Medical Center, Seattle, WA.)

initis, seizures, and inguinal hernias. The approximate frequency with which these abnormalities occur is summarized in Table 3.

The mortality associated with severe cytomegalovirus infection may be as high as 30%.[61,62] Moreover, the long-term prognosis for surviving infants is guarded. Eighty to ninety percent of these infants subsequently experience developmental delays.[63,65] In addition, approximately 60% have hearing loss, 50% have neurologic deficits, 40% have IQs lower than 70, and 15% develop chorioretinitis.[66] Chorioretinitis may be progressive and may ultimately result in severe visual impairment and even complete blindness.

Eighty-five to ninety percent of infants who acquire infection in utero are asymptomatic in the immediate neonatal period. Subsequently, 5 to 15% of these infants develop complications. The most common manifestation of infection is progressive sensorineural hearing loss. Other sequelae include psychomotor retardation, learning disabilities, and defects in dentition.[12]

DIAGNOSIS

Tissue Culture

Cytomegalovirus can be isolated from a variety of body fluids, including blood, urine, tears, saliva, stool, and amniotic fluid.[67] It also can be cultured from tissue biopsies.[68] Urine has been the most consistent source of the virus. Human diploid cells (fibroblasts) are the most common tissue culture medium employed for isolation of the organism. Ideally, fresh specimens of body fluid or tissue should be transported immediately to the laboratory for processing. However, should a de-

TABLE 3. Clinical Findings Associated With Cytomegalovirus Infection Acquired In Utero

Affected system	Findings	Approximate frequency (%)
General	Intrauterine growth retardation	40
	Prematurity	35
Central nervous	Microcephaly	40
	Spasticity	22
	Cerebral calcification	3
	Chorioretinitis	10
	Deafness	8
	Mental retardation	55
	Seizures	12
	Optic atrophy	1
Respiratory	Interstitial pneumonitis	8
Reticuloendothelial	Hepatosplenomegaly	70
	Jaundice	55
Hematopoietic	Thrombocytopenia	60
	Petechiae	80
	Lymphadenopathy	7
Other	Inguinal hernia	26
	Dental defects	40

The data presented in this table are based upon information provided in Krech et al.,[49] Stagno,[63] and Stagno et al.[64]

lay be anticipated, samples of body fluid can be stored for up to 1 week at 4°C.

Depending upon the size of the viral inoculum, the organism produces a characteristic cytopathic effect within several days to weeks in standard tissue culture. Cultures should be maintained for a minimum of 21 days before being reported as negative. In the newborn, a positive culture within the first 2 weeks of life is compatible with an in utero infection. In infants with cytomegalovirus infection acquired during passage through an infected cervix, cultures obtained within the first 2 weeks of life typically are negative. Cultures then become positive 3 to 12 weeks after delivery.

A number of techniques have been developed to decrease the time necessary for detection of the virus in culture. Direct or indirect fluorescent monoclonal antibody techniques now are being used more commonly to detect cytomegalovirus antigens.[69,70] Gleaves and coworkers,[71,72] using a monoclonal antibody to early nuclear antigens, have shown that the shell vial cell culture assay is as specific, faster, and more sensitive than the standard tube culture method

(Fig. 4). This technique now is becoming the standard culture method for identification of cytomegalovirus. Chou and Merigan have extracted viral DNA from urine and detected it with a radiolabeled nucleic acid probe.[73] Additionally, electron microscopy has been used in virus identification.

Serologic Tests

Because the virus has been slow to grow in standard tissue culture, many physicians have relied upon serologic methods for diagnosis. At present, there are approximately 200 laboratories in the United States that provide serologic testing for cytomegalovirus.[74] These laboratories use several different methodologies for detecting antibody to cytomegalovirus, including enzyme-linked immunosorbant assay (ELISA), indirect immunofluorescence (IFF), complement fixation (CF), hemagglutination inhibition (HAI), fluoroimmunoassay (FIA), and radioimmunoassay (RIA).

Acute infections may be diagnosed by documenting a significant change in acute and convalescent IgG titers or by demonstrating

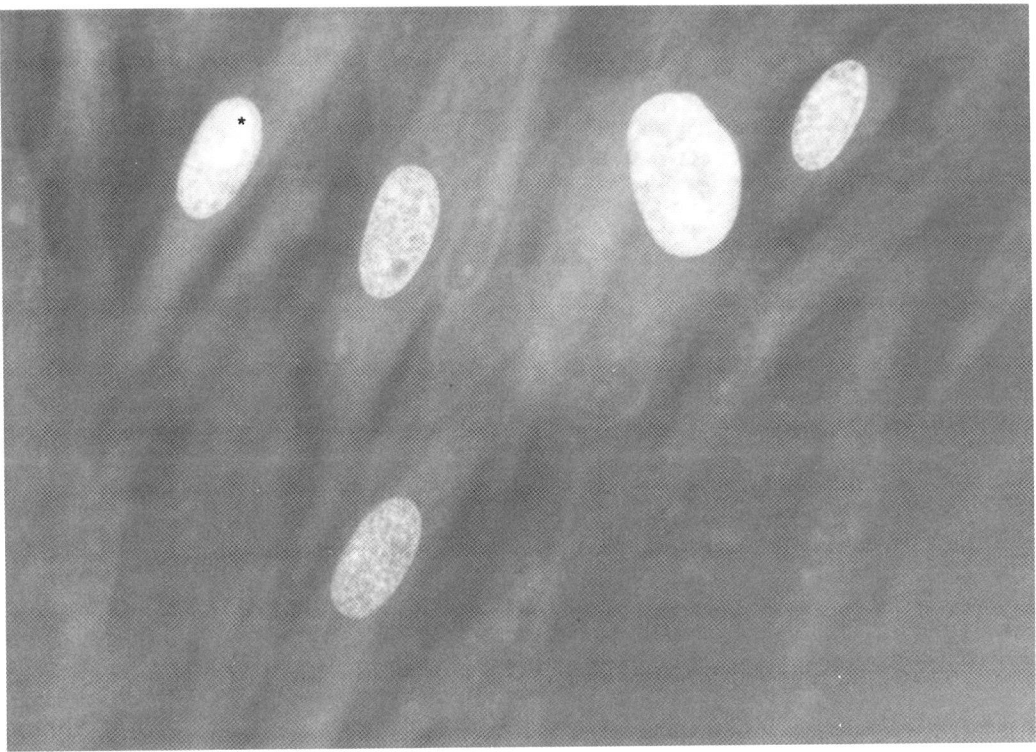

Fig. 4. MRC-5 shell vial monolayer with cytomegalovirus infected cells. One infected nucleus shows a clump of early antigen staining (*). This photograph demonstrates the variety of nuclear shapes seen in these infected monolayers. ×630. (Photo courtesy of Barbara Judson, Division of Clinical Trials, Microbiology, Syva Company, Palo Alto, CA.)

the presence of IgM-specific antibody. Congenital cytomegalovirus infection is best diagnosed serologically by demonstrating cytomegalovirus-specific IgM antibody in cord blood or neonatal serum.[63] The vast majority of infected neonates (>80%) have IgM-specific antibody in their serum.[61] Other laboratory findings include atypical lymphocytosis, thrombocytopenia, and alteration in liver function tests.

The best tests for identifying IgG antibody appear to be the ELISA and CF test. IgM may be identified by either ELISA or IIF. Rheumatoid factor and IgG must be removed from the patient's serum prior to testing for IgM in order to avoid confusing cross-reactions.

MANAGEMENT OF CYTOMEGALOVIRUS INFECTION

Antiviral Agents

Several antiviral agents have been evaluated for the treatment of cytomegalovirus infection, and a few have shown modest activity against the organism. These drugs include the purine and pyrimidine nucleoside analogues (idoxuridine, cytosine arabinoside, adenine arabinoside, fluorodeoxyuridine, acyclovir, and ganciclovir) and phosphonoformate (Foscarnet). Interferon and immunoglobulins also have been under investigation. None of the clinical trials to date, however, have included pregnant patients. Rather, they have focused attention primarily on treatment of immunocompromised patients, transplant recipients, and congenitally infected newborns.[75] Many of the medications have significant toxicity. Moreover, their teratogenic potential is unknown. Until there is a highly reliable method of confirming the presence of in utero infection, we cannot recommend any of these agents in the treatment of pregnant women.

Vaccination

The importance of a vaccine would lie in the prevention of primary cytomegalovirus infections in seronegative pregnant patients as well as immunocompromised individuals. Two different vaccine strains, AD169 and Towne 125, have now been developed and tested in human volunteers. These vaccines are attenuated live viruses; neither strain has been associated with clinical illness. Both vaccines show appropriate immunogenicity and result in production of complement-fixing and neutralizing antibodies.[76-80]

Despite the initial promising test results, two major concerns must be resolved before the widespread implementation of a vaccination program. The first concern is the issue of latency and possible future reactivation of infection. The second is the possible oncogenic potential of the virus.

Until a vaccine is licensed for use, we must emphasize prevention of transmission of the virus. Person-to-person transmission requires close contact with an infected host. Therefore, good personal hygiene, especially hand washing, and avoidance of contact with contaminated body fluids are the most effective means of preventing acquisition of cytomegalovirus.

Management During Pregnancy

It is doubtful that routine screening of the obstetric population for cytomegalovirus would be cost effective, in view of the fact that only 1 in 10,000 to 20,000 infants will develop severe cytomegalic inclusion disease.[81] However, screening of patients whose occupation or living environment exposes them to cytomegalovirus (e.g., women who work in day-care centers, mothers of children who attend day care) should be considered. In addition, should a pregnant woman require a blood transfusion prior to delivery, it is essential that she receive blood products that are negative for cytomegalovirus.

Because the majority of primary and recurrent cytomegalovirus infections in the adult are asymptomatic, it often is difficult to establish a diagnosis. Moreover, when a primary infection is confirmed, serological titers are not predictive of fetal infection or the extent of fetal injury. The patient should be counseled that approximately 40% of offspring will have either clinical or laboratory evidence of cytomegalovirus infection and that some neonates ($\leq 30\%$ of the total number infected) will be severely affected. Patients should be advised that pregnancy termination is an option that they may wish to consider. If they elect to continue the pregnancy, they should be followed with serial ultrasound examination to assess fetal growth and to identify possible anatomic abnormalities such as periventricular calcifications.

If a patient has a recurrent cytomegalovirus infection, the likelihood of severe fetal damage is minimal. Termination of pregnancy for fetal indications does not appear to be justified.

Mothers who are actively shedding cytomegalovirus in the third trimester should be delivered vaginally unless an obstetric indication for cesarean delivery is present. There is no evidence at present that cesarean delivery is effective in preventing either immediate or delayed manifestations of cytomegalovirus infection.

REFERENCES

1. Ribbert H: Veber protozoenartige Zellen in der Niereeines syphilitischen Negeborenenund in der Parotis von Kindern. Zentralbl Allg Pathol 15: 945–948, 1904.
2. Tietze A: Ein protozoenbefund in einer erkrankten parotis. Mitteilungen aus den grezgebieten der medizin und chirurgie 14.03–310, 1905.
3. Lowenstein C: Ueber protozoenartige gebilde in

den organen von kindern. Zentralbl Allg Pathol 18:513–518, 1907.

4. Kuttner AG, Cole R: Further evidence concerning the significance of nuclear inclusions as indicators of transmissible agents. Proc Soc Exp Biol Med 23:537–539, 1926.

5. Farber S, Wolbach SB: Intranuclear and cytoplasmic inclusions ("protozoan-like bodies") in the salivary glands and other organs of infants. Am J Pathol 8:123–125, 1932.

6. Smith MG: Propagation of salivary gland virus of the mouse in tissue culture. Proc Soc Exp Biol Med 86:435–440, 1954.

7. Smith MG: Propagation in tissue cultures of a cytopathogenic virus from human salivary gland virus (SGV) disease. Proc Soc Exp Biol Med 92:424–430, 1956.

8. Rowe WP, Hartley JW, Waterman S, Turner HC, Huebner RJ: Cytopathogenic agent resembling human salivary gland virus recovered from tissue cultures of human adenoids. Proc Soc Exp Biol Med 92:418–424, 1956.

9. Weller TH, Macauley JC, Craig JM, Wirth P: Isolation of intranuclear inclusion producing agents from infants with illnesses resembling cytomegalic inclusion disease. Proc Soc Exp Biol Med 94:4–12, 1957.

10. Weller TH, Hanshaw JB, Scott DE: Serological differentation of viruses responsible for cytomegalic inclusion disease. Virology 12:130–132, 1960.

11. Weller TH, Hanshaw JB: Virological and clinical observations of cytomegalic inclusion disease. N Engl J Med 266:1233–1244, 1962.

12. Stagno S, Pass RF, Dworsky ME, Britt WJ, Alford CA: Congenital and perinatal cytomegalovirus infections: Clinical characteristics and pathogenic factors. In Plotkin SA, Michelson S, Pagano JS, et al. (eds): "CMV: Pathogenesis and Prevention of Human Infection." March of Dimes Birth Defects Foundation, Birth Defects: Original Article Series. New York: Alan R. Liss, 1984.

13. Stagno S, Pass RF, Dworsky ME, Alford CA: Maternal cytomegalovirus infection and perinatal transmission. Clin Obstet Gynecol 25:563–576, 1982.

14. Chandler SH, Alexander R, Holms KK: Epidemiology of cytomegalovirus infection in a heterogenous population of pregnant women. J Infect Dis 152:249–256, 1985.

15. Yow MD, Williamson DW, Leeds LJ, et al.: Epidemiologic characteristics of cytomegalovirus infection in mothers and their infants. Am J Obstet Gynecol 158:1189–1195, 1988.

16. Stagno S, Pass RF, Cloud G, Britt WJ, Henderson RE, Walton PD, Veren DA, Page F, Alford CA: Primary cytomegalovirus infection in pregnancy: Incidence, transmission to fetus, and clinical outcome. JAMA 256:1904–1908, 1986.

17. Peckham CS, Chin KS, Coleman JC, Henderson K, Hurley R, Preece PM: Cytomegalovirus infection in pregnancy: Preliminary findings from a prospective study. Lancet 1:1352–1355, 1983.

18. Grant S, Edmond E, Syme J: A prospective study of cytomegalovirus infection in pregnancy: Laboratory evidence of congenital infection following maternal primary and reactivated infection. J Infect 3:24–31, 1981.

19. Griffiths PD, Campbell-Benzie A, Heath RB: A prospective study of primary cytomegalovirus infection in pregnancy women. Br J Obstet Gynaecol 87:308–314, 1980.

20. Pass RF, Little EA, Stango S, Britt WJ, Alford CA: Young children as a probable source of maternal and congenital cytomegalovirus infection. N Engl J Med 316:1366–1370, 1987.

21. Pass RF, Hutto C, Ricks R, Cloud GA: Increased rate of cytomegalovirus infection among parents of children attending day-care centers. N Engl J Med 314:1414–1418, 1986.

22. Stagno S, Pass RF, Dworsky ME, et al.: Congenital cytomegalovirus infection: The relative importance of primary and recurrent maternal infections. N Engl J Med 306:945–949, 1982.

23. Stagno S, Whitley RJ: Herpesvirus infection of pregnancy: Part 1: Cytomegalovirus and Epstein-Barr virus infection. N Engl J Med 313:1270–1274, 1985.

24. Huang E-S, Alford CA, Reynolds DW, Stagno S, Pass RF: Molecular epidemiology of cytomegalovirus infections in women and their infants. N Engl J Med 303:956–962, 1980.

25. Ahlfors K, Ivarsson SA, Johnson T, Svanberg L: Primary and secondary maternal cytomegalovirus infections and their relation to congenital infection. Acta Paediatr Scand 71:109–113, 1982.

26. Rutter D, Griffiths P, Trompeter RS: Cytomegalovirus inclusion disease after recurrent maternal infection. Lancet 2:1182, 1985.

27. Monif GRG, Egan EA II, Helch B, Eitzman DV: The correlation of maternal cytomegalovirus infection during varying stages in gestation with neonatal involvement. J Pediatr 80:17–20, 1972.

28. Stern H, Tucker SM: Prospective study of cytomegalovirus infections in pregnancy. Br Med J 2:268–270, 1973.

29. Lang DJ, Kummer JF: Demonstration of cytomegalovirus in semen. N Engl J Med 287:756–758, 1972.

30. Preece PM, Pearl KN, Peckham CS: Congenital cytomegalovirus infection. Arch Dis Child 59:1120–1126, 1984.

31. Nankervis GA, Kumar JL, Cox FE, Gold E: A prospective study of maternal cytomegalovirus in-

fection and its effect on the fetus. Am J Obstet Gynecol 149:435–440, 1984.

32. Stagno S, Reynolds DW, Pass RF, Alford CA: Breast milk and the risk of cytomegalovirus infection. N Engl J Med 302:1073–1076, 1980.

33. Reynolds DW, Stagno S, Hosty TS, Tiller M, Alford CA: Maternal cytomegalovirus excretion and perinatal infection. N Engl J Med 289:1–5, 1973.

34. Numazaki Y, Yano N, Morizuka T, Takai S, Ishida N: Primary infection with human cytomegalovirus: Virus isolation from healthy infants and pregnant women. Am J Epidemiol 91:410–417, 1970.

35. Gehrz RC, Marker SC, Knorr SO, Kalis JM, Balfour HH Jr: Specific cell-mediated immune defect in active cytomegalovirus infection of young children and their mothers. Lancet 2:844–847, 1977.

36. Stagno S, Brasfield DM, Brown MB, et al.: Infant pneumonitis associated with cytomegalovirus, chlamydia, pneumoncystis, and ureaplasma: A prospective study. Pediatrics 68:322–329, 1981.

37. Cabau N, Labadie MD, Vesin C, Feingold J, Boue A: Seroepidemiology of cytomegalovirus infections during the first years of life in urban communities. Arch Dis Child 54:286–290, 1979.

38. Levinsohn EM, Foy HM, Kenny GE, et al.: Isolation of cytomegalovirus from a cohort of 100 infants throughout the first year of life. Proc Soc Exp Biol Med 31:957–962, 1968.

39. Leinikki R, Heinonen K, Pettay O: Incidence of cytomegalovirus infections in early childhood. Scand J Infect Dis 4:1–5, 1972.

40. Stern H: Isolation of cytomegalovirus and clinical manifestations of infection at different ages. Br Med J 1:665–669, 1968.

41. Hanshaw JB, Betts RF, Simon G, Boynton R: Acquired cytomegalovirus infection: Association with hepatomegaly and abnormal liver function tests. N Engl J Med 272:602–609, 1965.

42. Li FP, Hanshaw JB: CMV infection among migrant children. Am J Epidemiol 86:137–147, 1967.

43. Hutto C, Little A, Ricks R, Lee JD, Pass RF: Isolation of cytomegalovirus from toys and hands in a day care center. J Infect Dis 154:527–530, 1986.

44. Nelson DB, Peckham CD, Pearl KN, Chin KS, Garrett AJ, Warren DE: Cytomegalovirus infection in day nurseries. Arch Dis Child 62:329–332, 1987.

45. Chretien JH, McGinnis CG, Muller A: Venereal causes of cytomegalovirus mononucleosis. JAMA 238:1644–1645, 1977.

46. Jordan MC, Rousseau WE, Noble GR, Stewart JA, Chin TOY: Association of cervical cytomegalovirus with venereal disease. N Engl J Med 288:932–934, 1973.

47. Chandler SH, Holmes KK, Wentworth BB, Gutman L, Weisner PJ, Alexander ER, Handsfield HH: The epidemiology of cytomegalovirus infec-

tion in women attending a sexually transmitted disease clinic. J Infect Dis 152:597–605, 1985.

48. Davis LE, Stewart JA, Garvin S: Cytomegalovirus infection: A seroepidemiologic comparison of nuns and women from a venereal disease clinic. Am J Epidemiol 102:327–330, 1973.

49. Krech U, Jung M, Jung F: "Cytomegalovirus Infections of Man." New York: Karger, 1971.

50. Weller TH: The cytomegaloviruses. Ubiquitous agents with protean clinical manifestations. N Engl J Med 285:203–214, 267–274, 1971.

51. Ahlfors K, Ivarsson S-A, Johnson T, Renmarker K: Risk of cytomegalovirus infection in nurses and congenital infection in their offspring. Acta Paediatr Scand 70:819–823, 1981.

52. Dworsky ME, Welch K, Cassidy G, Stagno S: Occupational risk for primary cytomegalovirus infection among pediatric health-care workers. N Engl J Med 309:950–953, 1983.

53. Friedman HM, Lewis MR, Nemerofsky DM, Plotkin A: Acquisition of cytomegalovirus infection among female employees at a pediatric hospital. Pediatr Infect Dis 3:233–235, 1984.

54. Adler SP, Baggett J, Wilson M, Lawrence L, McVoy M: Molecular epidemiology of cytomegalovirus in a nursery: Lack of evidence for nosocomial transmission. J Pediatr 208:117–134, 1986.

55. Gurevich I, Cunha BA: Non-parenteral transmission of cytomegalovirus in a neonatal intensive care unit. Lancet 2:222–224, 1981.

56. Klemola E, Kaarrianen L: Cytomegalovirus as a possible cause of a disease resembling infectious mononucleosis. Br Med J 2:1099–1102, 1965.

57. Phillips CA, Fanning WL, Gump DW, et al.: Cytomegalovirus encephalitis in immunologically normal adults. Successful treatment with vidarabine. JAMA 238:2299–2300, 1977.

58. Causey JQ: Spontaneous cytomegalovirus mononucleosis-like syndrome and aseptic meningitis. South Med J 69:1384–1387, 1976.

59. Kabins S, Keller R, Peitchel R, et al.: Idiopathic polyneuritis caused by cytomegalovirus. Arch Intern Med 136:100–101, 1976.

60. Neiman PE, Reeves W, Ray G, Flournoy N, et al.: Prospective analysis of interstitial pneumonitis and opportunistic viral infection among recipients of allogeneic bone marrow grafts. J Infect Dis 136:754–767, 1977.

61. Stagno S, Pass RF, Dworsky ME, Alford CA: Congenital and perinatal cytomegalovirus infections. Semin Perinatol 7:31–42, 1983.

62. Hanshaw JB: Cytomegalovirus. In Remmington JS, Klein JO (eds): "Infectious Diseases of the Fetus and Newborn Infant," 2nd edition. Philadelphia: W.B. Saunders, 1983, pp 104–142.

63. Stagno S: Cytomegalovirus infection: A pediatri-

cian's perspective. Curr Probl Pediatr 26:630–667, 1986.

64. Stagno S, Pan RF, Thomas JP, et al.: Defects of tooth structure in congenital CMV infection. Pediatrics 69:646–664, 1982.

65. Weller TH, Hanshaw JB: Virologic and clinical observations on cytomegalic inclusion disease. N Engl J Med 226:1233, 1962.

66. Conboy JJ, Pass RF, Myer GT, et al.: Symptomatic congenital cytomegalovirus infection and mental retardation. Program issue, APS/SPR. Pediatr Res 20:160A, 1986.

67. Yambo TJ, Clark D, Weiner L, Aubry RH: Isolation of cytomegalovirus from the amniotic fluid during the third trimester. Am J Obstet Gynecol 139:937, 1981.

68. Stagno S, Pass RF, Reynolds DW, et al.: Comparative study of diagnostic procedures for congenital cytomegalovirus infection. Pediatrics 65:251, 1980.

69. Sacks SL, Freeman HF: Cytomegalovirus hepatitis. Evidence for direct viral infection using monoclonal antibodies. Gastroenterology 86:346–350, 1984.

70. Volpi A, Whitley RJ, Ceballos R, et al.: Rapid diagnosis of pneumonia due to cytomegalovirus with specific monoclonal antibodies. J Infect Dis 147:1119–1120, 1983.

71. Gleaves CA, Smith TF, Shuster EA, Pearson GR: Rapid detection of cytomegalovirus in MRC-5 cells inoculated with urine specimens by using low-speed centrifugation and monoclonal antibody to an early antigen. J Clin Microbiol 917–919, 1984.

72. Gleaves CA, Smith TF, Shuster EA, Pearson GR: Comparison of standard tube and shell vial cell culture techniques for the detection of cytomegalovirus in clinical specimens. J Clin Microbiol 217–221, 1985.

73. Chou W, Merigan TC: Rapid detection and quantitation of human cytomegalovirus in urine through DNA hybridization. N Engl J Med 308:921–925, 1983.

74. Taylor RN, Przybyszewski VA: "Proficiency Testing Summary Analysis—Public Health Immunology 1984-I." Atlanta: Centers for Disease Control, 1984.

75. Dworsky M, Pass RF, Stagno S, Whitley RJ: Therapeutic approaches to the control of cytomegalovirus infections. In Plotkin SA, Michelson S, Pagano JS, et al. (eds): "CMV: Pathogenesis and Prevention of Human Infection." March of Dimes Birth Defects Foundation, Birth Defects: Original Article Series. New York: Alan R. Liss, 1984.

76. Elek SD, Stern H: Development of a vaccine against mental retardation caused by cytomegalovirus infection in utero. Lancet 1:1–5, 1974.

77. Plotkin SA, Farquhar J, Hornberger E: Clinical trials of immunization with the Towne 125 strain of human cytomegalovirus. J Infect Dis 134:470–475, 1976.

78. Glazer JP, Friedman HM, Grossman RA, et al.: Vaccination of pediatric nurses with live attenuated cytomegalovirus. Am J Dis Child 136:294–296, 1982.

79. Osborn JE: Cytomegalovirus: Pathogenicity, immunology and vaccine initiatives. J Infect Dis 143:618–630, 1981.

80. Lang DJ: Cytomegalovirus immunization. Status, prospects and problems. Rev Infect Dis 23:449–458, 1980.

81. Gibbs RS, Sweet RL: Maternal and fetal infections. In Creasy RK, Resnick R (eds): "Maternal-Fetal Medicine: Principles and Practice." Philadelphia: W.B. Saunders, 1984, pp 636–639.

16

Hepatitis Complicating Pregnancy

Edward R. Yeomans, M.D.

More than ever before, those who assume the responsibility of caring for pregnant women must be knowledgeable about hepatitis complicating pregnancy. Devastating diseases such as cirrhosis and hepatocellular carcinoma that affect adults have been traced to perinatally transmitted hepatitis B virus (HBV). Reliable methods of interrupting perinatal transmission are available, but they require antenatal diagnosis for their implementation. Obstetricians have been called upon to screen all pregnant women for HBV, but details of when and how to screen are still being evaluated. There are a number of other ways in which hepatitis may complicate pregnancy:

1. It may present as hyperemesis gravidarum.
2. It may complicate transfusion of blood products.
3. Acute hepatitis may cause jaundice during pregnancy.
4. Fulminant hepatic failure in pregnancy may be due to hepatitis.
5. It may cause abnormalities in liver function tests in the asymptomatic patient.

The focus of this chapter is on those forms of viral hepatitis that result from infection with hepatotropic viruses (viruses with relative or absolute predilection for the hepatocyte) and particularly hepatitis B for the reasons noted above. Other types of hepatitis, both infectious and noninfectious, are considered briefly in the section on differential diagnosis.

ETIOLOGY

Rather than being virus specific, viral hepatitis can result from infection with four,[1] five,[2] six,[3] or possibly an even greater number of hepatotropic viruses. Included among these viruses are some that have been isolated, characterized, and classified as either RNA or DNA viruses, and others whose existence at present is only inferred from clinical and epidemiologic data (Table 1). Historically, a viral etiology for hepatitis was not firmly established until World War II, when outbreaks of hepatitis followed immunization of U.S. troops against yellow fever. The vaccine was stabilized with pooled human se-

The opinions expressed in this chapter are those of the author and not necessarily those of the United States Air Force or the Department of Defense.

Infections in Pregnancy, pages 165–176
Published 1990 by Alan R. Liss, Inc.

TABLE 1. The Hepatotropic Viruses

Hepatitis type	Viral agent	Antigen	Antibody	Comments
A	27 nm RNA virus	Whole virus (HAV)	Anti-HAV IgG, IgM	1. Fecal oral transmission 2. No chronic carrier state
B	42 nm DNA virus (Dane particle)	Surface (HBsAg)	Anti-HBs	1. Parenteral transmission 2. HBeAg correlatedwith infectivity 3. HBcAg not found in serum
		Core (HBcAg)	Anti-HBc	4. Viral DNA and DNA polymerase are contained in the core
		Core-associated (HBeAg)	Anti-HBe	5. Chronic carrier state 5–10%
D (delta)	Defective 35 nm virus requires concomitant HBV infection	Delta virus (HDV)	Anti-HDV IgG, IgM	1. Chronic infection possible 2. Increased risk of fulminant hepatitis
NANB (2 or 3 or more types)	Not isolated	?	?	1. Chronic infection possible 2. Leading cause of posttransfusion hepatitis

rum, and 14 weeks after vaccination jaundice appeared. Thus, this type of hepatitis was designated serum hepatitis or long-incubation hepatitis and contrasted with infectious (an obviously imprecise term) or short-incubation hepatitis. When the terminology proliferated to include nearly 50 terms for the two basic diseases,[4] the World Health Organization finally adopted the current terminology of hepatitis A for infectious and hepatitis B for serum hepatitis. In 1976 Blumberg won the Nobel Prize for his discovery of the Australia antigen, now referred to as hepatitis B surface antigen (HBsAg).[5] Using serologic techniques to identify HBsAg, Seeff et al. were able to confirm that the 1942 outbreak that followed yellow fever vaccination was a result of hepatitis B virus infection.[6] Gradually, as the sciences of virology and serology advanced, it became apparent that not all infectious or epidemic hepatitis was due to type A and not all serum hepatitis was due to type B, prompting introduction of the term "non-A, non-B" (NANB) hepatitis. This term, a succinct concession to our lack of knowledge in this area, certainly includes several different viruses (Table 1) and will

doubtlessly be altered as specific etiologic agents are identified.

Hepatitis A is caused by a 27 nm RNA virus classified in the family Picornaviridae, genus *Enterovirus*.[7] Hepatitis A virus (HAV) lacks a lipid envelope. Its entire genome has been cloned and characterized and the virus has been grown in tissue culture.

Hepatitis B is caused by a 42 nm DNA virus classified most recently as a hepadnavirus. It has a lipid envelope and has not yet been grown in cell culture. HBV, like HAV, has been cloned and sequenced.

Hepatitis D refers to infection with the delta agent, an incomplete viral particle that requires concomitant infection with HBV to supply its coat or envelope. Hepatitis D is not well described in pregnancy, but data from nonpregnant individuals would suggest that, in comparison with hepatitis B, it is usually more severe and has a greater tendency to become a chronic infection.

Finally, several types of NANB hepatitis have been described in pregnancy. One type is epidemic[8] (analogous to HAV infection) and two are due to blood-borne NANB viruses.[3] At this writing, none of the viral

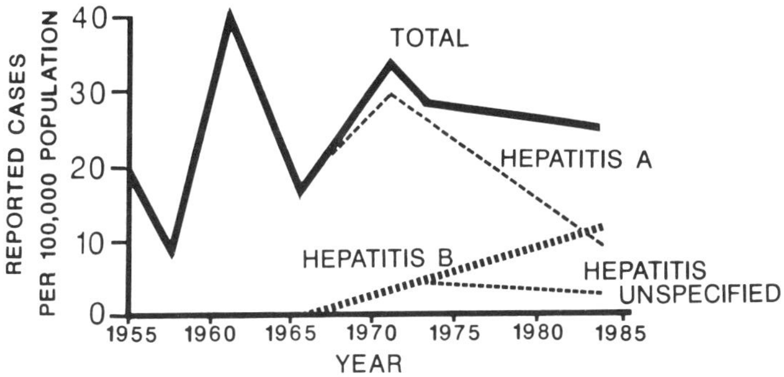

Fig. 1. Trends in viral hepatitis. (Modified from CDC data.)

agents responsible has been isolated, cloned, or sequenced.

EPIDEMIOLOGY

The incidence of hepatitis A is declining in developed countries (Fig. 1). The fecal-oral route is the predominant mode of transmission. The source of infection may be contaminated food or water or contact with an infected individual in a household, institutional, or intimate setting. Parenteral transmission does occur through transfusion or needle puncture, but only infrequently.

In contrast, hepatitis B is on the rise, as also shown in Figure 1. Transmission is usually parenteral and can be influenced by a number of factors, including route of infection, frequency of exposure, and size of inoculum (needle puncture vs. transfusion). Vertical transmission from mother to fetus/infant is of paramount concern for obstetricians and is influenced significantly by the presence of the hepatitis B "e" antigen. In one study, "e" antigen positivity was associated with vertical transmission in 85% of cases, whereas "e" antibody reduced transmission to 25% and surface antigen positivity only (without "e" markers) resulted in only a 10%, but not zero, vertical transmission rate. The important conclusion to be reached is that vertical transmission is possible irrespective of "e" antigen status if the mother is surface-antigen positive. In general, maternal-neonatal trans-

mission varies directly with the prevalence of HBV in the population.

NANB hepatitis can be transmitted either via the fecal-oral route or parenterally, depending on the subtype. Our knowledge of the epidemiology of the NANB agents has thus far outstripped our ability to identify and characterize the agents themselves. Now that serologic screening of blood donors for HBV is routine, NANB accounts for 90% of cases of posttransfusion hepatitis.

DIAGNOSIS/DIFFERENTIAL DIAGNOSIS

Serologic techniques are indispensable in making the diagnosis of viral hepatitis and identifying the viral agent. Such techniques also aid in defining the time course of infection (recent, remote; acute, chronic). For all forms of hepatitis caused by hepatotropic viruses, the most frequent clinical presentation is the patient who is asymptomatic. Moreover, the chronic carrier of HBV is most commonly asymptomatic. This further emphasizes the importance of serodiagnosis, since reliance on clinical symptoms or even on membership in high-risk groups (to be discussed later in this chapter) will leave cases undiagnosed and make prevention impossible.

Because no serologic markers have yet been identified for NANB hepatitis, it remains a diagnosis of exclusion. Acute hepa-

TABLE 2. Serologic Profiles for Hepatitis B*

Pattern	HBsAg	HBeAg	Anti HBc-IgM	Anti HBc-IgG	Anti HBe	Anti HBs
Usual						
Early acute infection	+	+	−	−	−	−
Ongoing acute infection	+	+	+	+	−	−
Chronic infection	+	−	−	+	±	±
Persistent carrier	+	±	−	±	±	−
Recovery (window period)	−	−	+	+	±	−
Complete recovery	−	−	−	+	±	+
Vaccinated	−	−	−	−	−	+
Unusual[a]						
1	+	−	−	+	−	+
2	+	−	−	−	−	−
3	−	+	−	−	−	−

*Usual and unusual (discordant) patterns arranged according to time sequence of appearance of antigens/antibodies in serum from L to R.

[a]Other unusual patterns are possible; repeat testing is recommended.

titis A can be ruled out by requesting an IgM anti-HAV, since IgM is the predominant early antibody formed against HAV and persists only for 1 to several months. Of note, an IgG anti-HAV is an indicator of past infection and does not aid in determining the agent responsible for acute hepatitis.

Therefore, the complexity of serodiagnosis of hepatitis is attributable only to hepatitis B. As is frequently the case, terminology is somewhat confusing because Blumberg's Australia antigen (AAg), hepatitis-associated antigen (HAA), and hepatitis B surface antigen (HBsAg) are all synonymous. The last, HBsAg, is the currently accepted abbreviation. This antigen is a surface protein; subtypes (adw, adr, ayw, ayr) have been described but are of interest only to the epidemiologist since they have no impact on the clinical course. The envelope that contains HBsAg is mainly composed of lipid and surrounds a core element consisting of double-stranded DNA, DNA polymerase, a core antigen, c, and an antigen e that is associated with the core antigen. The e antigen is found in serum and is correlated with infectivity. The c antigen is *not* found in serum but is only located in the hepatocyte or hidden beneath the envelope of whole viral particles. The three antigens s, e, and c each have

corresponding antibodies, anti-s, anti-e, and anti-c. Anti-c antibody may be of either IgM or IgG class, and this distinction has significance with regard to the temporal nature of the infection.

This bewildering array of immunologic responses to infection with the hepatitis B virus becomes even more confusing when it is realized that 1) a particular serologic profile may be capable of differentiating acute from chronic infection, 2) antibody detection is dependent on laboratory methodology, 3) some patients positive for hepatitis B surface antigen may be chronic carriers and have a superinfection with either delta or NANB viruses, and 4) as with all laboratory tests, unusual or discordant results do occur. Such results should be questioned by the clinician and in most instances repeated. Table 2 contains three examples of discordant serologic profiles.[9]

A reasonable diagnostic strategy for the obstetrician faced with either a jaundiced patient or a patient with abnormal liver enzymes is outlined in Table 3. A similar algorithm for screening appears later in the chapter.

The differential diagnosis of acute viral hepatitis due to hepatotropic viruses is summarized in Table 4, with emphasis on those

TABLE 3. Algorithm for Evaluation of Jaundice or Hepatocellular Enzyme Abnormalities

Request anti-HAV IgM[a] and HBsAg			
Anti-HAV IgM		HBsAg	
(+)	(−)	(−)	(+)
Recent HAV infection	No evidence for acute hepatitis A	Request anti-HBcIgG	Request anti-HBcIgM

(−)	(+)	(−)	(+)
No evidence for hepatitis B Pursue evidence for NANB hepatitis or other liver disease	Request full hepatitis profile and refer to Table 2	Suspect chronic infection or chronic carrier May have HDV or NANB superimposed on chronic carrier state	Recent acute infection with HBV

[a]Anti-HAV IgG is not the proper test to request. If positive, it would imply past infection and current immunity.

entities of greatest concern for obstetricians. Under the heading of "drug-induced hepatitis," a few representative drugs likely to be used to treat pregnant women are listed. The evidence implicating betamimetic drugs as a cause of hepatitis is meager,[10,11] but because of their wide use in the treatment of preterm labor, they are included. According to Sherlock, liver disease in pregnancy may be generally classified into three groups: unique to pregnancy, incidental to pregnancy, and complicated by pregnancy.[12] Acute viral hepatitis is incidental to pregnancy and represents the single most common cause of jaundice in the pregnant woman. Two disorders classified as unique to pregnancy, preeclampsia/eclampsia and acute fatty liver of pregnancy (AFLP), are associated with hepatocellular enzyme abnormalities and need to be distinguished from acute viral hepatitis (Table 5). There is some evidence that preeclampsia and AFLP may be part of the same spectrum;[13] however, this debate is beyond the scope of this chapter. The interested reader is referred to some recent reports.[14,15]

Several of the systemic viral infections listed in Table 4 can incite hepatitis as a prominent manifestation. Detailed information pertaining to these viral agents is provided in other chapters of this book, but a few are of sufficient importance to warrant consideration briefly here. In particular, herpes hepatitis is frequently anicteric[16] yet devastating in its effects: both fetal and maternal mortality are in excess of 50%. The potential effectiveness of antiviral agents such as acyclovir remains to be evaluated. Cytomegalovirus, another virus in the herpes family, also causes hepatitis as one aspect of systemic infection. As noted in Table 4, other members of the herpes family, Epstein-Barr virus and varicella, along with rubella, coxsackie, adenovirus, echovirus, and mumps—in short, almost all viruses—have the capability of producing a hepatitis-like picture. Clearly, it is not feasible to rule out each one of these viruses prior to assuming that hepatitis is likely to be NANB. It is sufficient simply to look for evidence of multisystem involvement suggestive of infection with one of these agents.

CLINICAL COURSE

Two maxims should be borne in mind at the outset:

1. Asymptomatic infection occurs more frequently than symptomatic infection. This

TABLE 4. Differential Diagnosis of Acute Viral Hepatitis Due to Hepatotropic Viruses

Hepatitis complicating systemic viral infection
  Herpes—frequently anicteric infection
  Cytomegalovirus—can be associated with mononucleosis-like illness
  Epstein-Barr virus
  Varicella
  Rubella
  Coxsackie
  Adenovirus
  Echovirus
  Mumps
  Numerous other less common viral infections

Liver disease unique to pregnancy
  Preeclampsia/eclampsia (see Table 5)
  Acute fatty liver of pregnancy (AFLP) (see Table 5)
  Intrahepatic cholestasis of pregnancy
  Hyperemesis gravidarum—may actually be caused by viral hepatitis in some cases

Liver disease incidental to pregnancy
  Drug-induced hepatitis
    Halothane   Sulfa drugs
    Isoniazid (INH)   Erythromycin estolate
    Ketoconazole   Phenytoin
    Methyldopa   Oral contraceptives
    Acetaminophen   Betamimetics—Ritodrine, Terbutaline (see text)
  Gall bladder disease
  Parasitic infection (amebiasis)
  Budd-Chiari syndrome

Liver disease complicated by pregnancy
  Chronic hepatitis
  Cirrhosis
  Hyperbilirubinemic states—Dubin-Johnson, Gilbert's, Rotor syndromes

TABLE 5. Three Conditions in Pregnancy Associated With Hepatocellular Enzyme Elevation

	Acute viral hepatitis	Preeclampsia/eclampsia (includes HELLP syndrome)	AFLP
Trimester of occurrence	Any	Late second, third	Usually third
Abdominal pain	Uncommon	+	+
Hypertension	Absent	Present, maybe severe	Usually mild
Jaundice	Common	Relatively uncommon	Common
Aminotransferase	400–5,000 IU/liter	Usually <500	>100, <1,000
Serology	(+) unless NANB	Negative	Negative
Thrombocytopenia	Rare	Common	Relatively common
DIC	Rare unless fulminant	Possible	Common

fact highlights the importance of serodiagnosis as outlined in the previous section.

2. No agent is associated with a pathognomonic clinical course. Rather, most agents produce a very similar clinical picture.

History and physical exam, coupled with judicious ordering of laboratory tests, should lead to the correct etiologic diagnosis in the symptomatic patient. The importance of etiologic diagnosis will be emphasized in the section dealing with prevention. In the approach to the patient with suspected hepatitis, the clinician must be cognizant of the

```
HAV   IP  P  CLIN   RECOVERY
      HAV          ANTI-HAV IGM              ANTI HAV IGG
```

```
      IP         P  CLIN   RECOVERY
                 HBS AG     ANTI HBS
HBV
                 HBE AG     ANTI HBE
                    ANTI HBC IGM
                        ANTI-HBC IGG
```

```
      IP         P  CLIN   RECOVERY
HDV
         HDV            ANTI HDV IGM   ANTI HDV IGG
```

```
      IP       P  CLIN   RECOVERY
NANB
      NO SEROLOGY
```

```
   1  2  3  4  5  6         1  2  3
       MONTHS                 YEARS
```

Fig. 2. Time line: acute viral hepatitis. IP, incubation period; P, prodrome; CLIN, clinical.

crucial importance of time, that is, the temporal evolution of the disease process. Not only will symptoms and signs vary according to when the patient is first seen, but interpretation of serologic results and aminotransferase values will be markedly influenced by the time at which they are assayed. These considerations are shown diagrammatically in a time-line format in Figure 2. Infection with HAV, HBV, and NANB agents all can be subdivided into an incubation period, a variable (but usually brief) prodrome, an icteric or clinical stage, and a recovery (convalescent) period, as shown in the figure. In developed countries the clinical course of hepatitis in pregnant women is no different from that in nonpregnant individuals.

During the incubation period the virus invades the hepatocyte (thus the term "hepatotropic"). Specific laboratory tests may detect viral presence but it is not until the prodromal stage that the infection becomes clinically manifest. The prodrome often consists of fatigue, headache, myalgia, arthralgia, and occasionally upper respiratory symptoms, thereby making hepatitis indistinguishable from any other flulike syndrome. It is the appearance of icterus (from the Greek meaning golden thrush) or jaundice (from the French jaune meaning yellow) that prompted Dr. Osler to remark that "jaundice is the disease your friends diagnose."[17] Acute viral hepatitis is the most common cause of jaundice during pregnancy. Scleral icterus is first evident when the serum bilirubin rises to 2–3 mg/dl. Higher levels are required before staining of skin and mucous membranes is apparent. Associated symptoms in the icteric phase include nausea, vomiting, diarrhea, anorexia, dark urine, and light stools. Loss of taste for cigarettes is a classic occurrence in smokers and diminished sense of smell is sometimes present. Weight loss may be noted. With regard to the impact of hepatitis on pregnancy, there is no demonstrable increase in abortions, stillbirths, malformations, or growth retardation. An association with preterm delivery has been noted. The most significant impact is the potential for vertical transmission of hepatitis B.

The severity of clinical infection is dependent on the size of the inoculum (needle puncture vs. transfusion) and the immune response of the host. If the host cannot mount an effective immune response to the viral invader, chronic infection for all but HAV may result. This logic explains why the relatively immunoincompetent newborn is so likely to develop a chronic infection when exposed at delivery to a mother who is surface-antigen positive for hepatitis B.

The most characteristic laboratory abnormality in acute viral hepatitis is aminotransferase elevation, varying from 400 to more than 5,000 IU/liter. Alanine aminotransferase (ALT) is the most liver specific, and this accounts for its use in the "surrogate screening" of potential blood donors for NANB hepatitis, described below in the section on prevention. Bilirubin is variably elevated and may exceed 20 mg/dl in severe cases, with roughly equal direct- and indirect-reacting fractions: Figure 2 illustrates the time sequence of serologic findings for hepatitis B. For hepatitis A, IgM forms early and disappears in 1 to 6 months; IgG anti-HAV persists and usually confers life-long immunity. No serologic markers have yet been discovered for NANB hepatitis. This breakthrough may be soon and holds the promise of vaccine development as has occurred for hepatitis B. For the uncommon delta agent, an antidelta IgM and IgG have been characterized in a manner analogous to HAV.

COMPLICATIONS

For each of the hepatotropic viruses an uncommon but life-threatening complication is the development of fulminant hepatitis. This eventuates in about 1% of cases of hepatitis A and B and, with vertical transmission of the latter, occurs in about 1% of infected newborns. NANB hepatitis, especially in pregnant women in underdeveloped countries, has a higher rate of development of fulminant hepatitis, as does infection with the delta agent (which demands coinfection

with hepatitis B virus for its existence). About half of the patients with fulminant hepatitis die, and many of these develop severe coagulopathy and hepatic encephalopathy. It is worth noting that in those cases of fulminant hepatitis due to HBV, the individual may be surface-antigen negative. A positive test for IgM anti-HBc will clarify this unusual situation. Fulminant hepatitis requires the provision of intensive-care support; no specific treatment is available.

Another complication is the failure of acute viral hepatitis to resolve, leading to the development of a chronic infected state. Five to ten percent of hepatitis B infections become chronic. Infection with the delta agent increases the likelihood of chronic hepatitis, and a percentage of NANB hepatitis will also evolve to a chronic state. Chronic infection does not complicate infection with HAV.

Of the individuals who develop chronic hepatitis B, 75% will be asymptomatic carriers, detectable only by screening for HBsAg. Especially in high-prevalence areas, HBeAg will also be positive. Pregnant women who are both surface and e-antigen positive will give birth to infected infants 85% of the time unless steps are taken to interrupt this vertical transmission.

The remaining 25% of chronically infected patients will have either chronic persistent or chronic active hepatitis. This distinction can only be made histopathologically from a liver biopsy specimen. Chronic active hepatitis frequently progresses to cirrhosis. Chronic infection of any sort may lead to integration of viral DNA into the host's genome and ultimately result in hepatocellular carcinoma. This integration process has been well detailed.[18] Prevention of transmission of HBV infection is therefore a significant public health goal and is discussed below.

TREATMENT/PREVENTION

Specific treatment of acute viral hepatitis is not available. Hospitalization of pregnant

TABLE 6. Hepatitis B Vaccine Regimens*

	HBIG	Plasma-derived vaccine	Recombinant vaccine
Neonate	0.5 ml within 12 hours	10 μg IM 0, 1, 6 months	5 μg IM 0, 1, 6 months
Nonimmune adult	0.06 ml/kg within 24 hours	20 μg IM 0, 1, 6 months	10 μg IM 0, 1, 6 months

*These are current recommendations and are subject to change.

women with hepatitis can be either routine or selective. If selective, it must be remembered that nausea and vomiting may be severe and liver function may significantly deteriorate with prolongation of the prothrombin time. Admission may also be necessary to sort out the differential diagnosis of jaundice in pregnancy. Increased rest and a low-fat, high-carbohydrate diet are recommended, but the definitive value of these recommendations has not been demonstrated.

Because there is no effective treatment, prevention becomes exceedingly important. Measures to prevent HAV and NANB infection will be considered first, followed by a more detailed elaboration of the current recommendations for prevention of hepatitis B.

A pregnant woman exposed to hepatitis A should receive immune serum globulin (ISG) in a dose of 0.02 ml/kg intramuscularly. For prolonged exposures, three times that dose should be used. A vaccine for hepatitis A is in development. No vaccine exists for NANB, but several preventive measures have been investigated to lower the risk of development of posttransfusion hepatitis. Once routine screening of blood products for HBsAg was established, NANB quickly became the leading offender, accounting for 90 to 95% of cases of posttransfusion hepatitis in the United States today. Because the chance of hepatitis is increased in individuals with ALT elevation, donor blood can be screened for ALT, and those units with abnormal enzyme concentrations can be discarded. Immune serum globulin should be given to infants born to women with acute or chronic NANB hepatitis.

Prevention of mother-to-infant transmission of hepatitis B infection is highly successful when it is employed. However, successful prevention is dependent on detection of women at risk (for further details see the next section on screening).

The current recommendation for prevention of vertical transmission is to administer hepatitis B immune globulin (HBIG) 0.5 ml IM to the neonate as soon as possible after birth (within the first 12 hours is strongly advised).[19] Hepatitis B vaccine should be given concomitantly, 10 μg IM, but here the time element is less important (within 7 days of birth). Additional doses of the vaccine should be given at 1 and 6 months of age. It is noteworthy that these recommendations have changed several times in the recent past and may change again soon. Knowing the proper regimen is perhaps of greater significance to our pediatric colleagues; the role of the obstetrician is twofold: first, to identify the mother at risk of perinatal transmission and second, to communicate that information to the pediatrician in a timely manner.

The plasma-derived vaccine for hepatitis B became available in June of 1982.[19] Unfortunately, the threat of AIDS reached the public conscience at about the same time. Fear of contamination of the vaccine with the AIDS virus might have prevented a more widespread voluntary immunization of health-care workers at risk than has occurred to date. A recombinant vaccine produced in yeast became available in the summer of 1986.[19] As shown in Table 6, the correct vaccine dose is determined by age of the recipient and type of vaccine administered. Victims of accidental needle punctures should receive the three-dose immunization series.

TABLE 7. Routine Screening for Hepatitis B

Author	No. screened	No. HBs Ag +	Population prevalence	No risk factors (%)
Malecki[28]	741	8	1.1	62
Cruz et al.[25]	7,962	43	0.54	67
Wetzel[29]	585	8	1.37	—
Summers et al.[24]	15,399	136	0.88	50
Kumar et al.[22]	4,399	23	0.52	55
Jonas et al.[23]	5,356	64	1.2	47
Friedman[30]	505	19	3.5	47
Christian and Duff[27]	1,520	10	0.66	0

TABLE 8. Algorithm for Screening Pregnant Women to Reduce the Incidence of Perinatal Transmission of Hepatitis B

HBsAg at 34 weeks[a]	
(+)	(−)
1. Notify pediatricians of need to treat the neonate	No further action necessary (remember to screen on admission to labor those with no prenatal care)
2. Test household contacts	
3. Full profile to assess whether disease in mother is acute or chronic[b]	

[a]The CDC recommends that this screen be done at entry into OB care. This would result in missing acute hepatitis cases in the third trimester.

[b]This step is deemed unnecessary by the CDC. However, e antigen is correlated with infectivity and some HBsAg + individuals will not be chronic carriers but will have either acute hepatitis or chronic active hepatitis. A full profile should include HBeAg, HBeAb, anti-HBcIgM, anti-HBcIgG, and liver function tests.

There is preliminary evidence that the type of vaccine used may affect immunogenicity. The Recombivax lacks the pre-S region of the viral genome and, as a result, may be less immunogenic.[20]

SCREENING

There can be no doubt that the success of a hepatitis B prevention program depends on the positive identification of the patient at risk. Until recently, selective screening of pregnant women was advocated by the Centers for Disease Control (CDC). However, a number of studies have challenged the effectiveness of such a screening protocol.[21–25] Roughly half of the women found to be surface-antigen positive were not identified using recommended historical/ethnic/behavioral risk factors (Table 7). This finding has led to a revised recommendation for *routine* prenatal screening for hepatitis B surface antigen.

Thus far, the cost-effectiveness of such an approach is uncertain. Arevalo and Washington found routine screening to be cost effective.[21] The CDC has recommended that screening be done early in pregnancy in conjunction with other prenatal testing.[26] Because more than 90% of women found to be HBsAg positive on routine screening will be carriers, CDC chose to recommend against retesting later in pregnancy those who had positive tests early on. However, additional testing is recommended when 1) the mother may have acute hepatitis, 2) there is a history of exposure during pregnancy, or 3) particularly high-risk maternal behavior is evident.

It should be noted that, although routine testing is almost certain to become widely adopted, the prevalence of HBsAg+ individuals in the United States is quite low (1–3/1,000). At least one author has reported no improved yield of routine vs. selective screening.[27] Obstetricians have been laboring under an increasing "screening burden" (MSAFP, glucose intolerance, sexually transmitted diseases, rubella, etc.), and new suggestions for screening may meet with some resistance, especially when the yield is low. However, it must be conceded that the public health impact of preventing not only a chronic disease but a form of cancer as well is enormous. False positives for HBsAg are relatively few and the methodology using either RIA or ELISA is readily available and reliable. An algorithm for HBsAg screening is shown in Table 8.

SUMMARY AND CONCLUSIONS

Acute viral hepatitis during pregnancy is not a single disease. Although the clinical picture for all types is similar, epidemiologic and serologic data will usually lead to a type-specific diagnosis of hepatitis. Hepatitis B is by far the most important type for obstetricians, since prevention of perinatal transmission is possible. Routine screening may lead to increased identification of the patient at risk for vertical transmission of hepatitis B. Management of the acutely infected patient is limited to supportive care. Identification of NANB viral agents may lead to breakthroughs comparable to those for hepatitis B. Advances in all areas of viral hepatitis continue; as a result, the practicing clinician must closely monitor the changing recommendations.

REFERENCES

1. Stevens CE: Viral hepatitis in pregnancy: The obstetricians's role. Clin Obstet Gynecol 25:577–584, 1982.
2. Syndman DR: Hepatitis in pregnancy. N Engl J Med 313:1398–1401, 1985.
3. Koff RS: Hepatitis in pregnancy. N Engl J Med 314:1581–1582, 1986.
4. Zuckerman AJ: The history of viral hepatitis from antiquity to the present. In Deinhardt F, Deinhardt J, (eds): "Viral Hepatitis: Laboratory and Clinical Science." New York: Marcel Dekker, 1983, p 13.
5. Blumberg BS: Australia antigen and the biology of hepatitis B. Science 197:17–25, 1977.
6. Seeff LB, Beebe GW, Hoofnagle JH, et al.: A serologic follow-up of the 1942 epidemic of post-vaccination hepatitis in the United States Army. N Engl J Med 316:965–970, 1987.
7. Lemon SM: Type A viral hepatitis. New developments in an old disease. N Engl J Med 313:1059–1067, 1985.
8. Khuroo MS: Study of an epidemic of non-A, non-B hepatitis. Possibility of another human hepatitis virus distinct from post-transfusion non-A, non-B type. Am J Med 68:818–824, 1980.
9. Hollinger FB: Serologic evaluation of viral hepatitis. Hosp Pract 22:101–114, 1987.
10. Alcena V: Severe hemolytic anemia, leukemoid reaction, acidosis, hypokalemia, and transient hepatitis associated with the administration of ritodrine hydrochloride (Yutopar). Am J Obstet Gynecol 144:852–854, 1982.
11. Suzuki M, Inagaki K, Kihira M, Matsuzawa K, Ishikawa K, Ishizuka T: Maternal liver impairment associated with prolonged high-dose administration of terbutaline for premature labor. Obstet Gynecol 66:14S–15S, 1985.
12. Sherlock S: Jaundice in pregnancy. Br Med Bull 24:39–43, 1968.
13. Minakami H, Oka N, Sato T, Tamada T, Yasuda Y, Hirota N: Preeclampsia: A microvesicular fat disease of the liver? Am J Obstet Gynecol 159:1043–1047, 1988.
14. Snyder RR, Hankins GDV: Etiology and management of acute fatty liver of pregnancy. Clin Perinatol 13:813–825, 1986.
15. Riely CA: Acute fatty liver of pregnancy. Semin Liver Dis 7:47–54, 1987.
16. Goyert GL, Bottoms SF, Sokol RJ: Anicteric presentation of fatal herpetic hepatitis in pregnancy. Obstet Gynecol 65:585–588, 1985.
17. Lemmer JH: Hepatitis B as an occupational disease of surgeons. Surg Gynecol Obstet 159:91–98, 1984.
18. Shafritz DA, Shouval D, Sherman HI, Hadziyannis SJ, Kew MC: Integration of hepatitis B virus DNA into the genome of liver cells in chronic liver disease and hepatocellular carcinoma. N Engl J Med 305:1067–1073, 1981.
19. Centers for Disease Control: Recommendation of the Immunization Practices Advisory Committee: Update on hepatitis B prevention. Ann Intern Med 107:353–357, 1987.
20. Sherlock S: Viral hepatitis. Dig Dis Sci 31:122S–132S, 1986.

21. Arevalo JA, Washington E: Cost-effectiveness of prenatal screening and immunization for hepatitis B virus. JAMA 259:365–369, 1988.
22. Kumar ML, Dawson NV, McCullough AJ, et al.: Should all pregnant women be screened for hepatitis B? Ann Intern Med 107:273–277, 1987.
23. Jonas MM, Schiff ER, O'Sullivan MJ, et al.: Failure of Centers for Disease Control criteria to identify hepatitis B infection in a large municipal obstetrical population. Ann Intern Med 107:335–337, 1987.
24. Summers PR, Biswas MK, Pastorek JG, Pernoll ML, Smith LG, Bean BE: The pregnant hepatitis B carrier: Evidence favoring comprehensive antepartum screening. Obstet Gynecol 69:701–704, 1987.
25. Cruz AC, Frentzen BH, Behnke M: Hepatitis B: A case for prenatal screening of all patients. Am J Obstet Gynecol 156:1180–1183, 1987.
26. Centers for Disease Control: Prevention of perinatal transmission of hepatitis B virus: Prenatal screening of all pregnant women for hepatitis B surface antigen. MMWR 37:341–346, 1988.
27. Christian SS, Duff P: Is universal screening for hepatitis B infection warranted in all prenatal populations? Obstet Gynecol 74:259–261, 1989.
28. Malecki JM, Guarin O, Hulbert A, Brumback C: Prevalence of hepatitis B surface antigen among women receiving prenatal care at the Palm Beach County health department. Am J Obstet Gynecol 154:625–626, 1986.
29. Wetzel AM, Kirz DS: Routine hepatitis screening in adolescent pregnancies: Is it cost effective? Am J Obstet Gynecol 156:166–169, 1987.
30. Friedman SM, DeSilva LP, Fox HE, Bernard G: Hepatitis B screening in a New York City obstetrics service. Am J Public Health 78:308–310, 1988.

17

Varicella-Zoster Infections in Pregnancy

Mark G. Martens, M.D.

Varicella-zoster infections during pregnancy are a serious concern because of the potential for profound fetal effects. However, it differs from other viruses in pregnancy because of its potential to cause serious or fatal maternal consequences. Therefore, management of varicella-zoster infection needs to address both the mother and fetus.

VARICELLA-ZOSTER VIRUS

The varicella-zoster (VZ) virus is a member of the herpesvirus family, along with the herpes simplex viruses, cytomegalovirus, and Epstein-Barr virus. It consists of a linear double-stranded molecular core surrounded by an icosahedral capsid and lipid envelope. The capsid is composed of 162 hexagonal prisms, called capsomeres. The outer envelope is derived from the inner nucleus membrane of the infected cell. The site of biosynthesis of viral DNA is primarily in the host cell nucleus, which results in intranuclear inclusion bodies. However, assembly of viral particles can also occur in the cytoplasm.

Primary infection with VZ virus results in varicella (chickenpox). Chickenpox is a common childhood disease that presents with typical skin lesions. It is highly contagious and usually is acquired prior to the reproductive years in most persons in the United States. Among children it is generally self-limited; however, if the disease is acquired in adulthood, severe constitutional and pulmonary symptoms can occur.

Zoster (shingles) is a reactivation of the latent VZ virus. It usually occurs in older adults or immunocompromised patients and occurs only rarely during pregnancy. It is characterized by painful vesicular lesions in a pattern of distribution that follows one to three dermatomes. The intense pain is a result of sensorineural ganglion involvement and follows similar dermatomes. Because zoster is a reactivation of latent VZ virus and maternal antibodies are present in normal healthy women, zoster usually poses no threat to the fetus or neonate.

EPIDEMIOLOGY AND CLINICAL PRESENTATION

It is estimated that 2–3 million cases of chickenpox occur annually in the United States, and because of its extreme contagiousness, greater than 90% of cases occur before adulthood. Therefore, the occurrence of chickenpox among reproductive age

Infections in Pregnancy, pages 177–184

women is uncommon, amounting for only 2% of all chickenpox cases. The attack rate in pregnancy is infrequent, with approximately 1–5 cases of VZ infection per 10,000 pregnancies. While rare, this is still significant, as VZ infection carries with it both serious maternal and fetal consequences.

Varicella is contracted easily by way of the respiratory portal, and following an incubation period of 10 to 21 days, infection results with the development of crops of intensely pruritic vesicles in association with constitutional symptoms. Lesions at all stages may be seen simultaneously in a single infected area of the body. In children, fever and rash occur simultaneously, whereas in adults, fever and malaise generally precede the rash by one to several days. The rash usually begins on the face and scalp and then spreads to the trunk. Extremities are often less involved. The skin lesions start as macules and progress to vesicles, pustules, crusts, and then scabs. The lesions occur in crops, consistent with intermittent viremia, and persist for approximately 4 days, coincident with the production of measurable amounts of circulating antibody. Individual lesions progress rapidly, from small red macules to pustules to crusts within 12 to 24 hours. The crusts usually persist for approximately 1 week; they then fall off, leaving shallow pink depigmented depressions that disappear over several months. Fever persists as long as new lesions occur, but rarely exceeds 100–101°F, unless secondary bacterial infection occurs. Encephalitis, meningitis, myocarditis, glomerulonephritis, and arthritis are possible, but are rare occurrences. Varicella pneumonia, however, is not uncommon in the adult and is associated with significant morbidity and mortality, especially in the pregnant patient.

MATERNAL VARICELLA INFECTION

Varicella infection, while an infrequent occurrence in the adult, tends to be much more severe than in childhood. However, despite earlier claims, varicella does not appear to occur at a greater frequency in pregnant women.[1–3]

Much of the increased morbidity and mortality associated with adult varicella infections is due to varicella pneumonia. Although it is uncommon in children, 11 to 33% of adults with chickenpox show clinical or roentgenographic evidence of pneumonia.[4,5] Harris and Rhoades, in a review of 173 cases of varicella pneumonia, found an overall mortality rate of 17%.[6] Of those cases of pneumonia in pregnancy, a 41% mortality rate was identified.[6] Young and Gershon found that 29% of 77 patients with varicella in pregnancy developed pneumonia, of which 45% died.[7] Mortality did not occur independent of varicella pneumonia. Thus it appears that if the patient is spared the development of pneumonia, chickenpox will usually rapidly resolve.

Pulmonary symptoms begin 2 days before to 6 days after the onset of the rash. Up to one-third of patients will have only a mild, nonproductive cough. However, severe cases will begin or rapidly progress with additional symptoms, including high fevers (often with chills), inspiratory chest pain, cough, hemoptysis, dyspnea, and cyanosis. Physical examination usually reveals rales, wheezes, and an increased expiratory phase. Patients will often complain of headaches, and if cerebral spinal fluid is obtained, a lymphocytic pleocytosis is often found.

Recovery is rapid and usually occurs within 7 days in mild cases. Moderately ill patients have a prolonged course lasting 1 to 2 weeks, with resolution of the patient's shortness of breath usually occurring 2 to 3 days after the rash fades. If the infection persists, progressive deterioration with increasing dyspnea, tachypnea, cyanosis, and sometimes eventual death due to respiratory insufficiency may occur. Pleural effusions occur in 5–10% of cases because of focal lesions of the pleura. Other complications include pulmonary edema, subcutaneous emphysema, secondary bacterial infections, and pulmonary abscesses. If the patient survives, persistent

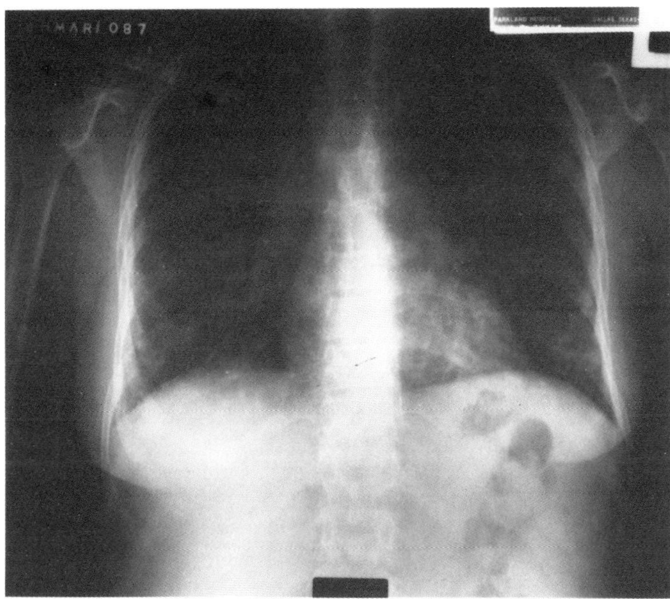

Fig. 1. Characteristic x-ray of a pregnant woman with varicella pneumonia. (Photo courtesy of Dr. Susan Ramin, University of Texas Southwestern Medical Center, Dallas.)

pulmonary fibrosis and diffusion abnormalities may occur.

The etiology of maternal hypoxia is due to an interstitial pneumonitis caused by an alveolar-capillary block that is created by an intraalveolar hemorrhage. Therefore, hemoptysis is a very serious sign that cannot be dismissed. Confirmation of the pneumonitis is made by x-ray (Fig. 1). Roentgenographic changes are usually more prominent than either symptoms or physical findings. The typical picture shows diffuse nodular densities that range in size from 2 to 20 mm scattered throughout both lung fields with a tendency to concentrate at the bases and hilum. Nodules in a given area may disappear on serial examinations, and others may coalesce to form discrete infiltrates and areas of consolidation. Whereas the roentgenographic changes will improve in 5 to 10 days in patients with mild disease, these changes may persist for 6 to 12 weeks in survivors of severe disease. Also, residual scarring and focal necrosis may persist for years, often calcifying and resembling healed miliary tuberculosis.

Successful treatment of maternal varicella infection focuses mainly on the early diagnosis of maternal pulmonary involvement. Without pulmonary infection, varicella usually resolves without complication. However, varicella pneumonia can be life threatening, and prompt identification and hospitalization are imperative. Patients exposed to or presenting with signs of varicella infection with any pulmonary symptoms should be seen and examined as soon as possible. Chest x-rays should be performed, and if changes consistent with pulmonary involvement are identified, the patient should be hospitalized and placed under observation. Respiratory isolation should be instituted to prevent transmission to susceptible personnel and nosocomial spread. Progressive pulmonary disease involves intensive monitoring of the patient's respiratory status, often requiring intensive care. Oxygen supplementation is determined by serial arterial blood gas measurements. Endotracheal intubation may become necessary. While supportive care was all that could be done in the past, several reports have now demonstrated excellent results with antiviral therapy. Acyclovir, a DNA-polymerase inhibitor, is well known for its use in treating herpes simplex infections. However, as varicella is a member of the herpesvirus family, it too responds to acyclovir administration, and has been used successfully by Landsberger et al.,[8] Eder et al.,[9] and Hankins et al.[10] A maternal dose of 10 mg/kg intravenously every 8 hours was used by Landsberger and colleagues. Acyclovir may also be helpful for other rare, but serious maternal complications of herpesvirus family infections in pregnancy such as encephalitis, myocarditis, and pericarditis; however, data are limited.[11–13]

Although these treatment options are now available, preventive or at least ameliorative measures may also be beneficial. Zoster immune globulin (ZIG) and varicella-zoster immune globulin (VZIG) have been demonstrated to substantially decrease the symptoms of susceptible women exposed to chickenpox.[14,15] The dose of VZIG is 1.25 ml administered intramuscularly; it should be administered within 72 hours of exposure for maximum effectiveness. Studies with ZIG have demonstrated activity when 0.2 to 0.4 ml/kg was administered within 96 hours of exposure. If ZIG was administered from the 3rd to 10th day after contact, a modified varicella syndrome occured.[16]

VZIG is now in greater supply than only a few years ago; however, routine administration upon exposure is often not necessary, as a majority of women have already had the disease and are seropositive. Enders found that 93.1% of women exposed to VZ while pregnant were seropositive.[16] Even if a woman denies or is uncertain of having had varicella infection in childhood, 81 to 95% of these women were seropositive, and therefore not candidates for VZIG.[4,17,18] Thus, with expeditious determination of VZ virus membrane antigen or equivalent antivaricella antibody status in pregnant women exposed to varicella, those in need of VZ immunoglobulin passive immunization can be identified.

Although not currently available, a live attenuated varicella vaccine has been tested with excellent results.[19,20] Weibel and associates demonstrated a 94% seroconversion rate, and the vaccine was 100% effective in preventing varicella.[19] If approved, vaccination of susceptible children could all but eliminate the serious consequences of adult varicella infection and the fetal sequelae, which are discussed below.

VARICELLA-ZOSTER INFECTION IN THE INFANT

VZ infections during pregnancy can result in two separate entities. A constellation of malformations associated with maternal VZ virus infection early in pregnancy was first described by LaForet and Lynch in 1947.[21] However, more frequently encountered with VZ virus is an infection of the newborn that is devoid of the aforementioned congenital abnormalities.

Brunell separates these two distinct VZ virus infections of the infant into varicella embryopathy (VE) for the congenital infection associated with fetal malformations and varicella of the newborn (VON), which is reserved for infection of the newborn in the early weeks of life.[22] These two entities, while caused by the VZ virus, are the results of two separate situations and require different management plans.

Varicella Embryopathy

As noted above, VE is a result of maternal infection early in pregnancy. This syndrome of multiple congenital anomalies includes fetal growth retardation, aplasia of a single limb with cicatrization of the skin, neurologic damage, and ocular changes (Table 1). The ophthalmologic lesions include chorioretinitis, microphthalmia, cataracts, and nystagmus. Rarely, optic atrophia, a Horner-like syndrome, or anisocoria can occur. Neurologic defects include motor and sensory deficits, overt paralysis, and dysphagia. Some of the virus's adverse effects are not detected

TABLE 1. Major Anomalies Seen With the Varicella Embryopathy Syndrome

Fetal growth retardation
Limb aplasia
Cicatrization of the skin
Neurologic defects
Motor and sensory deficits
Paralysis
Dysphagia
Ophthalmologic defects
Chorioretinitis
Microphthalmia
Cataracts
Nystagmus

at birth, especially the ocular changes, and may also include psychomotor retardation and seizure activity.

Postmortem examination of these infants reveal extensive damage to the nervous system, including cerebellar and cortical atrophy[21,23,24] and focal calcification.[25]

Unilateral aplasia may include a leg, an arm, the mandible, or a hemithorax.[21,24,26–29] As the child grows, hemiatrophy or facial asymmetry may occur.[22] Because of laryngeal and swallowing changes and persistent dyspnea, aspiration and recurrent pneumonia often cause the early death of some infants.[23,28] Intestinal obstruction in the newborn period resolving without surgical intervention may represent autonomic innervation involvement.[22]

A variety of skin manifestations have been observed in VE and are most commonly represented by linear cicatricial lesions involving the aplastic limb, with extension often onto the trunk. Discrete lesions at other sites may be seen and have been described as crusted, papular, and hyper- or hypopigmented.[21,28,30,31]

Necropsy analysis of affected neonates supports the hypothesis that the observed embryopathy is a result of viral cytopathic effects, which are magnified by incomplete organogenesis. A recent analysis of 52 infants whose mothers had contracted varicella in pregnancy revealed 27 infants with congenital malformations.[32] All these mothers had contracted varicella during the first 20 weeks of pregnancy, whereas the remaining 25 infants, whose mothers had varicella after 20 weeks of gestation, developed herpes zoster infection after birth. Close analysis of the congenital anomalies demonstrated segmented malformations with similar spinal cord innervation, with the remaining changes attributed to an encephalitis. Higa et al. therefore ascribe the mechanism of congenital malformations caused by VZ virus infection not to fetal varicella but to the development of herpes zoster in utero and to an encephalitis associated with herpes zoster.[32]

The frequency of VE in mothers contracting varicella during the first trimester of pregnancy is unknown. However, in a recent study on the outcome of 20 pregnancies complicated by varicella, 11 healthy and 6 defective offspring were reported.[33] Two pregnancies were voluntarily terminated, and one multifetal pregnancy resulted in a spontaneous abortion. Another review found 1 of 11 infants developed VE following VZ infection in the mother during the first trimester.[34]

Diagnosis of VE is made by the observation of the anomalies associated with the syndrome along with the historical information of a first-trimester maternal varicella infection. Serologic or culture diagnosis is often inconclusive, because evidence of transplacental transfer of VZ virus is usually lacking. Trlifajova et al. found no such transfer in 81% of infected mothers.[33] Supportive evidence of fetal infection includes declining maternal VZ virus antibody titers in the face of high neonatal titers, VZ virus antigen detected by indirect immunofluorescence, or IgM antibody to VZ virus at birth.[22] Attempts to isolate the virus at birth have been unsuccessful.[24]

As VE is a consequence of an early infection, treatment options are limited. All pregnant women exposed to VZ virus in early pregnancy without evidence of prior infection and protective antibodies should be immunized with VZIG. However, this strategy is primarily used in an attempt to modify maternal disease, and little is known regarding its effect on fetal disease.

Antiviral therapy with acyclovir, while effective in treating serious maternal complications of varicella, has not been studied with regard to VE. However, some of the anomalies associated with VE are not detected at birth, and some, such as the ocular changes, appear to manifest themselves progressively after birth. Antiviral therapy may help prevent this additional damage and prospective studies will be necessary to confirm this theoretical benefit. Regardless, close and long-term observation of infants born to mothers infected with VZ virus in early pregnancy is strongly recommended.

Varicella-Zoster Infection of the Newborn

VZ infections acquired by the neonate near the time of delivery can be serious, resulting in up to a 31% mortality rate.[35] The risk is highly variable though, and is related to specific factors. Most important of these is the acquisition of maternal antibody by the fetus, which results in protection of the infant. However, if the infant is born after the maternal viremia occurs, but before the mother has developed serum antibodies, the risk to the fetus will be high and often life threatening. Maternal viremia occurs approximately 12 to 48 hours prior to the onset of the maternal rash (10–17 days postexposure), with the subsequent development of detectable maternal antibody usually 4 to 5 days after the maternal rash appears. Therefore, infants born from 2 days prior to 5 days after the development of the maternal rash have the highest risk of being seriously affected, as they are born after exposure to the virus but prior to the development of a significant amount of protective antibody. Infants so exposed will then develop their viremia and rash between days 5 and 10 of life, after a similar but slightly abbreviated period. In fact, most, if not all, case fatalities occur during this time period, with no infant fatalities being reported prior to 5 or after 10 days

of life.[22,35] For reasons unknown, female infants appear to be at much greater risk of dying of VON.[36,37]

If infants do develop disease after 10 days of life, it is often mild.[38–41] Similarly, if the mother developed her rash 2 weeks prior to delivery, the infant should be exposed to little or none of the maternal viremia. Brunell, in a review of 37 such pregnancies, found only one death and one case of pneumonia in this group.[22]

The clinical course of neonatal varicella may vary in its progression as well as in its severity. Infants who escape with only a mild illness will have only a few macules and papules, which may develop into vesicles in the following 3 to 5 days. This usually is not accompanied by fever or other systemic signs.

Some infants will have a biphasic course with a few lesions followed by a few days of improvement, after which a more generalized eruption occurs. This resembles the clinical course of disseminated zoster, and may be related.[42] Those infants with a prolonged course of the infection, with the continual eruption of new lesions into the second week of life, often have a fatal outcome. Sudden and extensive lesions often signal visceral involvement with the probable development of pneumonia, leading to the infant's death.

Management and prevention of VON is based primarily upon the relationship of the onset of the maternal disease and delivery of the infant. Susceptible mothers exposed to varicella should receive VZIG, as noted earlier, to prevent or ameliorate maternal disease. Maternally administered VZIG does not affect the rate of neonatal infection, which was found to be approximately 50% in a study of 95 mothers receiving prophylaxis.[43] But maternal treatment did seem to influence the course of the disease for newborns at high risk (i.e., infants born within 2 days prior to 4 days after development of maternal rash). Forty-one (51%) such infants developed varicella with a mean incubation of 11 days; however, 13 had only mild chickenpox, 6 had mild to normal disease, and 2 had severe disease. No infants died or developed long-term sequelae.[40] Regardless of maternal treatment, and especially in cases where maternal exposure was not known and therefore without prophylaxis, the infants should receive VZIG at birth as passive immunization, at a dose of 1.25 ml.

Another strategy is to delay delivery for at least 4 to 5 days in mothers at term or in labor who present with varicella infections to allow transplacental transfer of protective maternal antibody. However, maternal complications of VZ and fetal well-being need to be closely observed, and may necessitate delivery within the high-risk period, before detectable levels of antibodies are noted.

In addition to passive immunization, antiviral therapy with agents such as vidarabine[44] and acyclovir[45] may be helpful in treating the complications of VZ infections in infants. However, the data are limited and more studies are necessary.

Infants born during the incubation period of an exposed mother (prior to onset of maternal viremia and rash) need to be isolated from the mother until 5 days following the onset of the maternal rash and should not be breast-fed. Isolation from other infants is also necessary, at least for 1 week after development of the rash or until the disease abates, or at least 20 days after exposure.[46]

As noted earlier, studies on immunization of susceptible infants and adolescents are promising.[19,20] Ninety-four percent of vaccinated patients seroconverted with 100% effectiveness in preventing varicella. The placebo control group had 39 of 446 children developing varicella. If further investigation provides equally good results, a vaccination program similar to that for rubella could well eliminate a large percentage of the morbidity and mortality in pregnant women and their offspring.

HERPES ZOSTER IN PREGNANCY

Herpes zoster is caused by the VZ virus. Because it is a reactivation of a previous varicella infection, protective maternal antibodies are usually present, and thus the virus does not pose a threat to the fetus. Herpes zoster infections do occur in neonates and, as mentioned earlier, possibly in the fetus. However, this is the result of a primary maternal varicella infection and not an isolated maternal herpes zoster infection.

REFERENCES

1. Hermann KL: Congenital and perinatal varicella. Clin Obstet Gynecol 25:605–609, 1982.
2. Pearson HE: Parturition varicella-zoster. Obstet Gynecol 32:21–27, 1964.
3. Brunell PA: Varicella-zoster infections in pregnancy. JAMA 199:315, 1967.
4. Hoeprich PD (ed): "Infectious Diseases," 2nd edition. Hagerstown, MD: Harper and Row, 1977, pp 744–758.
5. Paryani SG, Arvin AM: Intrauterine infection with varicella-zoster virus after maternal varicella. N Engl J Med 314(24):1542–1546, 1986.
6. Harris RE, Rhoades ER: Varicella pneumonia complicating pregnancy: Report of a case and review of literature. Obstet Gynecol 25:734, 1965.
7. Young NA, Gershon AA: Chicken pox, measles, and mumps. In Remington JS, Klein JO (eds): "Infectious Disease of the Fetus and Newborn." Philadelphia: W.B. Saunders, 1983, pp 375–402.
8. Landsberger EJ, Hager WD, Grossman JH: Successful management of varicella pneumonia complicating pregnancy. J Reprod Med 31(5):311–314, 1986.
9. Eder SE, Apuzzio JJ, Weiss G: Varicella pneumonia during pregnancy. Treatment of two cases with acyclovir. Am J Perinatol 5(1):16–18, 1988.
10. Hankins GD, Gilstrap LC, Patterson AR: Acyclovir treatment of varicella pneumonia in pregnancy. Crit Care Med 15(4):336–337, 1987.
11. Bernuau J, Caujolle B, Rouzioux C, Degott C, Rueff B, Benhamou JP: Severe acute hepatitis due to herpes-simplex in the 3rd trimester of pregnancy: Combatting with acyclovir. Gastroenterol Clin Biol 11(1):79, 1987.
12. Cox SM, Phillips LE, DePaolo HD, Faro S: Treatment of disseminated herpes simplex virus in pregnancy with parenteral acyclovir: A case report. J Reprod Med 31(10):1005–1007, 1986.
13. Hankey GJ, Bucens MR, Chamber JSW: Herpes simplex encephalitis in third trimester of pregnancy: Successful outcome for mother and child. Neurology 37(9):1534–1537, 1987.
14. Brunnell PA, Roxx A, Miller L, Kuo B: Prevention

of varicella by zoster immune globulin. N Engl J Med 280:1191, 1969.

15. Ross AH: Modification of chicken pox in family contacts by administration of gamma globulin. N Engl J Med 267:369, 1962.

16. Enders G: Management of varicella zoster contact and infection in pregnancy using a standardized varicella-zoster ELISA test. Postgrad Med J 61(Suppl 4):23–30, 1985.

17. Monif GRG: "Infectious Diseases in Obstetrics and Gynecology," 2nd edition. Philadelphia: Harper and Row, 1982, pp 81–89.

18. McGregor JA, Mark S, Crawford GP, Levin MJ: Varicella zoster antibody testing in the care of pregnant women exposed to varicella. Am J Obstet Gynecol 157(2):281–284, 1987.

19. Weibel RE, Neff MJ, Kuter BJ, et al.: Live attenuated varicella virus vaccine. Efficacy trial in healthy children. N Engl J Med 310:1409–1415, 1984.

20. Heath RB: Prevention of varicella by vaccination. J Hosp Infect 11(Suppl A):90–95, 1988.

21. LaForet E, Lynch CL: Multiple congenital defects following maternal varicella. N Engl J Med 126: 534–537, 1947.

22. Brunell PA: Varicella-zoster infections. In Amstey MS (ed): "Virus Infection in Pregnancy." Orlando, FL: Grune and Stratton, 1984, pp 131–145.

23. McKendry JBJ, Bailey JD: Congenital varicella associated with multiple defects. Can Med Assoc J 108:66–67, 1973.

24. Rinvik R: Congenital varicella encephalomyelitis in surviving newborn. Am J Dis Child 117:231–235, 1969.

25. Srabstein JC, Morrin N, Larke RPB, et al.: Is there a congenital varicella syndrome? J Pediatr 84:239–243, 1974.

26. Alexander I: Congenital varicella. Br Med J 2: 1074, 1979.

27. Dodion-Fransen S, Dekegel D, Thirty L: Congenital varicella-zoster infection related to maternal disease in early pregnancy. Scand J Infect Dis 5: 149–153, 1973.

28. Savage MO, Moosa A, Gordon RR: Maternal varicella infection as a cause of fetal malformations. Lancet 1:352–354, 1973.

29. Siegel M: Congenital malformations following chickenpox, measles, mumps, and hepatitis. JAMA 226:1521–1524, 1973.

30. Pettay O: Intrauterine and perinatal viral infections. A review of experiences and remaining problems. Ann Clin Res 11:258–266, 1979.

31. Frey HM, Bialkin G, Gershon AA: Congenital varicella: Case report of a serologically proved long-term survivor. Pediatrics 59:110–112, 1977.

32. Higa K, Dan K, Manabe H: Varicella-zoster virus infections during pregnancy: Hypothesis concerning the mechanisms of congenital malformations. Obstet Gynecol 69(2):214–222, 1987.

33. Trlifajova J, Benda R, Benes C: Effect of maternal varicella-zoster virus infection on the outcome of pregnancy and the analysis of transplacental virus transmission. Acta Virol 30(3):249–255, 1986.

34. Paryani SG, Arvin AM: Intrauterine infection with varicella-zoster virus after maternal varicella. N Engl J Med 314(24):1542–1546, 1986.

35. Meyers JD: Congenital varicella in term infants: Risk considered. J Infect Dis 129:215–217, 1974.

36. Raine DN: Varicella infection contracted in utero: Sex incidence and incubation period. Am J Obstet Gynecol 94:1144–1145, 1966.

37. Steen J, Pedersen RB: Varicella in a newborn girl. J Oslo City Hosp 9:36–45, 1959.

38. Brunell PA: Placental transfer of VZ antibody. Pediatrics 38:1034–1037, 1966.

39. Newman CGH: Perinatal varicella. Lancet 2: 1159–1161, 1965.

40. Readett MD, McGibbon C: Neonatal varicella. Lancet 1:644–645, 1961.

41. Schleubing-Dusseldorf HH: Nekrosen in leber, milz, und tebernieren bei nicht vereiteiten varizellen. Verh Dtsch Ges Pathol 22:288–293, 1927.

42. Stevens DA, Jordan GW, Waddell TF, et al.: Adverse effect of cytosine arabinoside on disseminated zoster in a controlled trial. N Engl J Med 289: 873–878, 1973.

43. Hanngren K, Grandien M, Granstrom G: Effect of zoster immunoglobulin for varicella prophylaxis in the newborn. Scand J Infect Dis 17(4):343–347, 1985.

44. Webster MH, Smith CS: Congenital abnormalities and maternal herpes zoster. Br Med J 2:1193, 1977.

45. Prober CG, Kirk LE, Keeney RE: Acyclovir therapy of chickenpox in immunosuppressed children—A collaborative study. J Pediatr 101:622–625, 1982.

46. Music SI, Fine EM, Togo Y: Zoster-like disease in the newborn due to herpes simplex virus. N Engl J Med 284:24–26, 1971.

18

Human Immunodeficiency Virus Infection in Pregnancy

Hunter A. Hammill, M.D., and Larry C. Gilstrap, III, M.D.

The first cases of acquired immune deficiency syndrome (AIDS) in the United States were recognized in 1981 among homosexual men. Since that time there have been over 85,000 cases reported in the United States.[1] It is somewhat ominous to note that there are 20 to 30 asymptomatic carriers estimated for every case identified. There have also been over 1,400 cases of AIDS in children under the age of 13, 80% of these acquired through perinatal transmission.[2]

The experience in the United States for heterosexual transmission is different from the African experience, where AIDS has been primarily a heterosexual bidirectional infection. The male-to-female case ratio in Africa is 1:1; in the United States it is 14:1.[3] The reasons for this difference are unknown; the African experience may predict future U.S. experience.

AIDS is caused by a retrovirus, currently termed the human immunodeficiency virus (HIV), which was first isolated in 1983.[4] It is estimated that 1.5 million persons may be infected with this virus in the United States.[5] Infection with this virus during pregnancy presents the clinician with a unique therapeutic dilemma. The major reason for

this dilemma is that there is very little available data regarding AIDS during pregnancy. Specific questions that must be addressed include the risk of infection to the mother and whether termination should be encouraged for all women, the attack rate on the fetus, and appropriate therapy, especially for opportunistic infections.

EPIDEMIOLOGY

It is estimated that by 1991, there will be 2.5 million HIV-infected persons in the United States with a cumulative quarter of a million deaths. In order to understand perinatal transmission, it is important to first consider the frequency of AIDS in the heterosexual population and, more specifically, in women. The United States Armed Forces routinely performs screening in all active-duty men and women, and as of August 1987, had tested over 3 million individuals.[6] From this screening program 4,800 infected individuals were identified, for an incidence of 1.6 positive tests per 1,000 males and 0.6 per 1,000 females. Additional studies, although small, have involved evaluation of female prostitutes, and these studies have re-

Infections in Pregnancy, pages 185–191

TABLE 1. Frequency of AIDS in Women in the United States

Total number of cases of AIDS	>82,000
Number of cases reported in women	6,900
Percent of cases reported in women	8.4%
Estimated percent of cases in women by 1991	10%
Percent of cases in women of reproductive age	80%
Percent of cases in women associated with IV drug abuse	53%

Data from Koonin et al.,[1] CDC,[8] Weinberg and Murray,[9] and Morgan and Curran.[10]

vealed that 19 to 86% of the women tested had antibodies to HIV.[7] Additional data have been acquired from wives or known sexual partners of HIV-positive hemophiliacs. In a study of 772 hemophiliacs, HIV antibodies were detected in 10% of their partners.[2]

Recently, the Centers for Disease Control (CDC) reported that there had been 6,900 cases of AIDS in women in the United States from 1981 through 1988.[8] As pointed out in Table 1, approximately 8.5% of all cases of AIDS occur in women and approximately 80% of these are in women of reproductive age.[1,8–10] Landesman and colleagues very aptly have pointed out that "the era when human immunodeficiency virus (HIV) disease will pose a major threat to women's reproductive health no longer looms in the future."[11] Thus, it is of paramount importance that clinicians providing care for pregnant women be cognizant of these facts. This is further underscored by the fact that approximately three-fourths of cases of AIDS in children were due to perinatal transmission. As of January 1989, there had been 1,087 cases of perinatally acquired AIDS reported in the United States.[13,14] Of these children, 53% were born to mothers who were intravenous (IV) drug abusers and 20% were born to sexual partners of drug abusers.[14] In other words, almost three-fourths of the cases of perinatally acquired AIDS involved exposure from IV drug-abusing parents.

The risk of perinatal transmission from mother to child is unknown. The major reason is that passively acquired maternal antibodies may persist in the newborn for up to 15 months.[15] However, it has been estimated that 20 to 50% of newborns of HIV-positive mothers will acquire the virus.[12,16]

The primary modes of transmission of the AIDS virus include use of contaminated needles, contaminated blood products, sexual intercourse (anally or vaginally), and transplacental passage. At present there is no evidence of HIV transmission through casual contact, food, or surface contact.[15] Transmission has also been reported from artificial insemination with donor sperm.[17]

EFFECTS OF AIDS IN PREGNANCY

There is little data regarding the effects of HIV infection on short-term pregnancy outcome. An increased frequency of spontaneous abortions, premature deliveries, premature rupture of the membranes, and low-birth-weight infants has been reported in a few uncontrolled studies.[18–20] However, in a recent prospective study of pregnancy outcome in intravenous drug abusers who were HIV infected, there were no differences in the frequency of abortions, stillbirths, preterm infants, or low-birth-weight infants compared to HIV-antibody-negative drug abusers.[13] None of the HIV-infected women in this study had advanced disease during pregnancy.

Although there is little evidence that asymptomatic HIV infection has any significant effect on pregnancy complications or immediate newborn outcome, it does present a significant risk to long-term neonatal outcome. As previously mentioned, 20 to 50% of the offspring of HIV-positive mothers will become infected, and the prognosis for these infants is poor.[15] In the recent report of the European Collaborative Study, which involved 271 children born to HIV-infected mothers, the estimated vertical transmission rate was 24%.[21] The authors of this report point out that although their estimate of perinatally acquired HIV infection may be an underestimate (secondary to the insensitivity of the test used), the higher rates reported by many other studies were actually overestimates.[21] They further postulate that these higher rates were based on antibody tests performed at less than 15 months of age when maternal passively acquired antibody was still present. Thus, it would appear that the rate of perinatally acquired HIV infection is at least 24% but probably less than 50%.

EFFECTS OF PREGNANCY ON HIV INFECTION

There has been significant concern that pregnant women with HIV infection may have a more rapid progression to AIDS.[15,22,23] For example, it has been reported that 45 to 75% of asymptomatic pregnant women developed symptoms of AIDS by 28–30 months postpartum.[22,23] It has been postulated that this "acceleration of disease" may be secondary to depression of cell-mediated immunity during pregnancy.[24] Although this progression in pregnant women is higher than that reported for HIV-infected homosexuals, hemophiliacs, and intravenous drug abusers,[22,23] there are several problems with these studies, including the small numbers of patients, lack of controls, and the fact that these women were identified after giving birth to infected children.[1,15] Moreover, preliminary data from two prospective studies indicate that pregnancy per se does not accelerate the occurrence of overt disease among asymptomatic HIV-infected women.[1]

Koonin and associates have recently reported a summary of 20 cases of maternal deaths from AIDS within one year of pregnancy.[1] Of these 20 women, 75% were either black or Hispanic, 50% were IV drug abusers, and 75% died of *Pneumocystis carinii* pneumonia.

In summary, there is not yet enough data to ascertain whether pregnancy per se accelerates the HIV disease state. It is also not

TABLE 2. Tests for the Detection of HIV Infection

Antibody tests (IgG)
ELISA
Western blot
Radioimmunoassay
Antigen test
ELISA for p24 antigen
Gene amplification techniques
Polymerase chain reaction
HIV culture

Adapted from Nicholas et al.[26]

known whether therapeutic abortion will improve a patient's condition or delay the progression to AIDS. However, it does appear that women in general have a shorter survival time from diagnosis than do men.[1,25]

DIAGNOSIS OF HIV INFECTION

The various tests for the detection of HIV infection are listed in Table 2. The standard screening test currently used is the enzyme-linked immunosorbent assay (ELISA). This test is used primarily to detect HIV-specific IgG antibodies.[26] All positive tests should be confirmed with a Western blot assay. At present there is no reliable test to detect HIV-specific IgM in acute or congenital infections.[26]

The most commonly used antigen test is the ELISA for the detection of the p24 antigen.[26] This test, which should be widely available in the near future, requires large amounts of serum, and detection of this antigen may actually be a poor prognostic sign.[26]

Two other tests for detection of HIV infection include culture and gene amplification. Both tests appear to be sensitive but neither is widely available at this time.[26]

One of the major dilemmas regarding testing is whether to screen select populations or to screen entire populations. With the application of universal precautions, there should be no difference in management of patients whether they are identified as seropositive or not. However, misconception has arisen with the predictive value of the negative ELISA test in a high-risk population. For groups at high risk of AIDS, such as IV drug abusers, hemophiliacs, and partners of IV drug abusers, the prevalence of HIV antibody positivity is high. The predictive value of a negative ELISA test may be as low as 77%. Conversely, in a low-risk population, the predictive value of a positive test is less than 3%, so that at least 97% of the positive tests in the general population when tested by a screening ELISA procedure, will be false positives and not indicative of HIV infection.[27]

Additional concern has arisen regarding indeterminate Western blot tests in the low-risk population. Currently, it is recommended to repeat these tests in 6 months. It is estimated that with repeat testing the rate of false-positive Western blots would be 0.001%.[28] New tests such as the p24 antigen test may help clarify these equivocal tests in the future.

Current recommendations are that all patients with a high-risk history be offered HIV antibody testing after appropriate counseling. This includes patients who are IV drug abusers, partners of IV drug abusers, hemophiliacs and their partners, individuals with a history of multiple sexual partners, and individuals who received blood products from 1978 to 1985.

When the mother is identified as the index case, it has been suggested that additional children also be tested. It is well established that not every child will be affected. Once a patient or child is identified, it is important to maintain the confidentiality of the patient's condition.

ANTEPARTUM MANAGEMENT

One of the biggest dilemmas facing the clinician caring for the pregnant woman who is HIV positive is how to counsel her. Although the exact incidence of perinatal transmission is not known, it appears to be

TABLE 3. Opportunistic Infections That May Be Associated With AIDS in Pregnant Women

Pneumocystis carinii pneumonia
Persistent herpes simplex infections
Toxoplasmosis
Cytomegalovirus
Candidiasis

somewhere in the 25–50% range. The prognosis for children who are HIV positive is bleak to say the least. Thus, the subject of pregnancy termination must at least be broached. If the patient elects to continue the pregnancy, she will need specialized care, which involves a team approach. This team is generally made up of an obstetrician to monitor pregnancy complications, someone to provide necessary psychological support, a neonatologist to provide evaluation and follow-up of the newborn, and an infectious-disease specialist for monitoring the immune status of the patient and treating possible opportunistic infections.

The obstetrician must be cognizant of the various signs and symptoms associated with progression of AIDS, such as weight loss, fatigue, persistent fever, diarrhea, anorexia, and night sweats. Although fatigue, weight loss, and anorexia are common symptoms in the first trimester of pregnancy, they may also be early manifestations of AIDS and must be evaluated.[16] The more common opportunistic infections that may be associated with AIDS in pregnant women are listed in Table 3. In addition to these infections, the pregnant woman who is HIV infected or who has AIDS should be screened for sexually transmitted diseases such as syphilis, chlamydia, and hepatitis B.[16] Patients should also be skin tested for tuberculosis. All patients who have a positive skin test for tuberculosis should then undergo a chest x-ray.

The treatment of pregnant women who are HIV positive is mainly supportive. In addition, a CBC with differential and platelet count, helper (CD4+) and suppressor (CD8+) T-lymphocyte counts and ratio,

TABLE 4. Drugs That May Be Used in the Treatment of Pregnant Women With AIDS

Drug	Indication	FDA category
Zidovudine	Symptomatic HIV	C
Pentamidine	*Pneumocystis carinii* pneumonia	C
Sulfamethoxazole/trimethoprim	*Pneumocystis carinii* pneumonia	C
Acyclovir	Herpes simplex infections	C
Ketoconazole	Candidiasis	C
Miconazole or clotrimazole	Candidiasis	B
Nystatin	Candidiasis	B
Sulfadiazine	Toxoplasmosis	C
Pyrimethamine	Toxoplasmosis	C

Adapted from Minkoff.[16]

and immunoglobulin status should be performed every trimester. Pregnant patients who actually have AIDS or one of the various opportunistic infections present a special problem, since a drug given to the mother may have effects on the fetus. Zidovudine (Retrovir, Burroughs-Wellcome), formerly called AZT, is the major antiviral agent used to treat patients with symptomatic HIV infections.[29] This drug is a thymidine analogue and inhibits reverse transcriptase. There is little information regarding either the efficacy or safety of this drug during pregnancy, thus it is an FDA category C drug. However, recent animal and human data would suggest that zidovudine does cross the placenta rapidly and in large amounts.[30,31] Although there are no human teratology studies, zidovudine was shown to be neither teratogenic nor embryocidal in a recent animal study.[32] Other drugs that may be used in the treatment of pregnant women with HIV infections are listed in Table 4. All are pregnancy category C drugs, and there is little or no information regarding either their safety or efficacy during pregnancy.

INTRAPARTUM MANAGEMENT

Obviously, a major concern to health-care providers during labor and delivery of women who are HIV positive is the risk of infection from exposure to body secretions. In 1987, the CDC published guidelines for the prevention of HIV infection in a health-care setting.[33] In this document it was emphasized and recommended that blood and body fluid precautions be considered in *all* patients. This concept of "universal precautions" mandates that all patients, including all pregnant women, be considered potentially infectious for HIV and other blood-borne pathogens.[33] Thus, precautions to prevent exposure to blood, amniotic fluid, or other body fluids should be instituted for all deliveries. Specifically, gloves, water-repellent gowns, masks, and protective eyewear should be used for all vaginal and cesarean deliveries.[16] Gloves should also be worn when handling the neonate, and frequent hand washing should be encouraged.[16]

POSTPARTUM CARE

Universal precautions must also be maintained throughout the postpartum period. Pediatricians should be made aware in advance of all known HIV-infected women so they also can institute blood and body fluid precautions in the nursery after the baby arrives. Serologic testing in the newborn generally provides little useful information since maternal antibodies will interfere with any testing in the infant.[16]

Breast-feeding is presently not recommended because of the fear of transmission of the virus to the fetus.[16] In fact, there has been a report of transmission of HIV infection to the infant, presumably through breast milk.[34] Patients should be counseled during the postpartum period regarding birth control and permanent sterilization.

SUMMARY

Acquired immune deficiency syndrome is a significant and serious health-care problem in the United States, and it is estimated that there have been over 82,000 cases to date. There have been approximately 7,000 cases reported in women, 80% of whom are of reproductive age.[8-10] Because there is very little information regarding either the treatment or outcomes of pregnancies in women with HIV infections, the clinician providing care for women is faced with difficult therapeutic decisions. Pregnancy termination should be discussed with all pregnant women who are HIV positive. Although it is unknown whether pregnancy per se alters the course of HIV infection, it is well documented that a significant number of newborns will acquire the infection perinatally. Precautions to avoid exposure to blood and other body fluids should be undertaken in all deliveries, either vaginal or cesarean section.

REFERENCES

1. Koonin LM, Ellerbrock TV, Atrash HK, et al.: Pregnancy-associated deaths due to AIDS in the United States. JAMA 261:1306–1309, 1989.

2. Centers for Disease Control: Human immunodeficiency virus infection in the United States. MMWR(S-6):1–28, 1987.

3. Padian N: Heterosexual transmission of acquired immunodeficiency syndrome: International perspectives and national projections. Rev Infect Dis 6:947–958, 1987.

4. Webber DJ, Redfield RR, Lemon SM: Acquired immunodeficiency syndrome: Epidemiology and significance for the obstetrician and gynecologist. Am J Obstet Gynecol 155:235–240, 1986.

5. Centers for Disease Control: Human immunodeficiency in the United States. MMWR 36(49):801–804, 1987.

6. Centers for Disease Control: Trends in HIV among civilian applicants to military service in the United States. MMWR 36(18):273–276, 1987.

7. Bakerman S: "Undertaking AIDS." Greenville, North Carolina: Interpretive Lab Data Inc., 1988, p 3.

8. Centers for Disease Control: AIDS Weekly Surveillance Report—United States. December 26, 1988, pp 1–5.

9. Weinberg DS, Murray HW: Coping with AIDS: The special problem of New York City. N Engl J Med 317:1469–1472, 1987.

10. Morgan WM, Curran JW: Acquired immunodeficiency syndrome: Current and future trends. Public Health Rep 101:459–465, 1986.

11. Landesman SH, Minkoff HL, Willoughby A: HIV disease in reproductive age women: A problem of the present. JAMA 261:1326–1327, 1989.

12. Adler M, Weber UJ, Gold J (eds): WHO statistics—AIDS. AIDS 2:145, 1989.

13. Selwyn PA, Schoenbaum EE, Davenny D, et al.: Prospective study of human immunodeficiency virus infection and pregnancy outcomes in intravenous drug users. JAMA 261:1289–1294, 1989.

14. Centers for Disease Control: Weekly Surveillance Report. January 16, 1989.

15. American College of Obstetricians and Gynecologists: Human Immune Deficiency Virus Infections. Technical Bulletin 123, December 1988.

16. Minkoff HL: Care of pregnant women infected with human immunodeficiency virus. JAMA 258:2714–2717, 1987.

17. Stewart G, Cunningham A, Driscoll A, et al.: Transmission of human T-cell lymphotropic virus type III by artificial insemination by donor. Lancet 2:581–584, 1985.

18. Minkoff HL, Deepak N, Menez R, et al.: Pregnancy resulting in infants with acquired immunodeficiency syndrome or AIDS-related complex. Obstet Gynecol 69:285–287, 1987.

19. Rubenstein A, Sicklick M, Gupta A, et al.: Acquired immunodeficiency with reversed T_4/T_8 ratios in infants born to promiscuous and drug-addicted mothers. JAMA 249:2350–2356, 1983.

20. Johnstone FD, MacCullum L, Brettle R, et al.: Does infection with HIV affect the outcome of pregnancy? Br Med J 296:467, 1988.

21. Peckham CS, Senturia AE, Newell ML, et al.: Mother-to-child transmission of HIV infection: European Collaborative study. Lancet 2:1039–1042, 1988.

22. Minkoff HL, Nanda D, Menez R, et al.: Follow-up of mothers of children with AIDS. Obstet Gynecol 87:288–291, 1987.

23. Scott GB, Fischl MA, Kalimas N, et al.: Mothers of infants with the acquired immunodeficiency syndrome: Evidence for both symptomatic and asymptomatic carriers. JAMA 253:363–366, 1984.

24. Peckham CS, Senturia YD, Ades AE: Obstetric and perinatal consequences of human immunodeficiency virus (HIV) infection: A review. Br J Obstet Gynaecol 94:403–407, 1987.

25. Rothenberg R, Woelfel N, Stonebumer R, et al.:

Survival with the acquired immunodeficiency syndrome. N Engl J Med 317:1297–1302, 1987.

26. Nicholas SW, Sondheimer DL, Willoughby AD, et al.: Human immunodeficiency virus infection in childhood, adolescence, and pregnancy: A status report and national research agenda. Pediatrics 83: 293–308, 1989.

27. Sivak SL, Wormser GP: Predictive value of a screening test for antibodies to HTLV-III. Am J Clin Pathol 85:700–703, 1986.

28. Centers for Disease Control: Update on serologic testing for antibodies to human immunodeficiency virus. MMWR 37(52):834–840, 1988.

29. Landesman S, Dehovitz J: "Management of HIV: Disease Treatment Handbook." New York: World Health Communications, 1988, p 20.

30. Fortunato SJ, Bawdon RE, Swank F, et al.: Transfer of azothymidine (AZT) across the *in vitro* perfused human placenta. Society for Gynecologic Investigation, 36th Annual Meeting, San Diego, CA, March 15–19, 1989 (abstract #3).

31. Little BB, Bawdon RE, Christmas JT, et al.: Pharmacokinetics of zidovudine (AZT) during late pregnancy in Long-Evans rats. Society of Perinatal Obstetricians, 9th Annual Meeting, New Orleans, LA, February 2–4, 1989 (abstract #239).

32. Christmas JT, Little BB, Bawdon RE, et al.: Teratogenic and embryocidal effects of zidovudine in Sprague-Dawley rats. Society of Perinatal Obstetricians, 9th Annual Meeting, New Orleans, LA, February 2–4, 1989 (abstract #155).

33. Centers for Disease Control: Recommendations for prevention of HIV transmission in health care settings. MMWR 36(2S):3–12, 1987.

34. Ziegler JB, Cooper DA, Johnson RO, et al.: Postnatal transmission of AIDS associated retrovirus from mothers to infant. Lancet 1:896–897, 1985.

19

Human Papillomavirus Infection During Pregnancy

Russell R. Snyder, M.D., and Gary D.V. Hankins, M.D.

Human papillomaviruses (HPV) have had a "back stage" entry into the arena of infectious diseases. This is remarkable considering that historically condylomata acuminata were recognized as having a venereal etiology by the ancient Greeks. Neither the experimental transmission of HPV to human volunteers at the turn of the century, the experimental induction of squamous carcinoma with the Shope rabbit papillomavirus in the 1930s, nor the 1949 demonstration of the actual virus particles by electron microscopy generated much scientific interest in this virus.[1] Research has been significantly hampered by the inability to culture the virus and by the lack of suitable animal models.

Renewed interest was kindled in the late 1970s when zur Hausen presented evidence of an association of benign condylomas, cervical intraepithelial neoplasia, and invasive cancer through progressive transformation.[2] The elucidation of the cellular events involved in the development of all types of tumors has grown massively with the recent explosion of sophisticated molecular biologic techniques. These have allowed identification of over 40 district HPV types and have provided insight into the host cell's suppression, regulation, or loss of control in response to oncogenic viruses.[3] The development of DNA probes has provided an avenue by which epidemiologic data can now be collected. Unfortunately, however, clinical research has lagged far behind these molecular techniques and the application of these tools to direct patient care remains undefined.[4]

EPIDEMIOLOGY

As the specific incidence of HPV infection in pregnancy is unknown, the more general consideration of the epidemiology of HPV in all reproductive age women is necessary. Although HPV infections are clearly becoming more common,[5] Gorthey and Krebs reported 22 cases of vulvar condyloma as early as 1954 and 14 of these patients were pregnant.[6] Precise calculations of trends are hampered because the majority of HPV infections in sexually active men and women are subclinical.[7,8] The prevalence of abnormal Papanicolaou smears (as an indicator of HPV infection) in the general population varies from 1 to 3% and almost all of these women are asymptomatic.[9-11] Examination of asymptomatic male partners of women with abnormal cervical cytologies has revealed that 64 to 75% have subclinical HPV infection.[12,13]

Infections in Pregnancy, pages 193–206
Published 1990 by Alan R. Liss, Inc.

TABLE 1. Common HPV Types Encountered in Women

Types 6, 11, 12
CIN I
CIN II
Flat warts
Anogenital infection
Juvenile/adult laryngeal papillomas
Types 16, 18, 31, 33, 39
CIN II
CIN III
Bowen's disease
Bowenoid papulosis
Cervical carcinoma
Laryngeal, esophageal carcinoma

Two studies using DNA probes on exfoliated cells from patients undergoing routine gynecologic exams revealed an incidence of HPV infection of 12 and 16%.[14,15] In another study, in which women were screened in the first trimester of pregnancy, the incidence of HPV infection was 11%.[16] Most recently, Waeckerlin et al. were able to demonstrate evidence of HPV infection in the cytologic specimens and immunohistochemically stained tissue specimens of 18% of patients presenting for a routine office visit,[17] while Reid and colleagues found HPV in 28% of women attending a sexually transmitted disease (STD) clinic in Detroit.[18] By comparison, genital herpes simplex virus (HSV) infections affect less than 5% of the population.[19,20]

Incidence figures are more confusing when the multifocality of genital HPV is taken into consideration. Cervical, vaginal, vulvar, anal, and urethral sites must be considered, as well as combinations of sites. Roy and associates found 20% of women with vulvar HPV to have concomitant cervical lesions.[21] Greenberg and colleagues reported a 68.6% incidence of coexisting cervical and/or vaginal disease in 169 women with vulvar condylomata.[22]

There are also general site predilections based on HPV type (Table I). The specific epithelial cell phenotype is a major determinant of HPV infection, controlling both morphological transformation and viral replication.[23] HPV 6 is very commonly associated with vulvar condylomata; HPV types 6, 11, and 42 frequently cause noncondylomatous cervical wart virus infections (flat warts); and HPV 16 and 18 are frequently associated with higher grades of cervical intraepithelial neoplasia (CIN).[7] Type 16 is also associated with vulvar intraepithelial neoplasia (VIN) and verrucous carcinoma of the larynx.[24,25]

The multicentricity of this disease is also manifested in other genital intraepithelial neoplasia. VIN can be demonstrated in at least 7% and vaginal intraepithelial neoplasia (VAIN) in 3% of women with CIN III.[1] This potential for involvement of the entire lower genital tract affects not only the diagnostic maneuvers but also planning for subsequent therapeutic maneuvers. HPV 6 and 11 are the most common viral types in recurrent respiratory papillomatosis, which is strong evidence for acquisition of fetal infection at parturition.[26,27]

The human papillomavirus is a potential oncogen. Evidence of an association between HPV and invasive cervical cancer and its precursors is accumulating rapidly.[14,26,28,29] Pfister reviewed the role of the human papillomavirus in the etiology of genital cancer and the reader is referred to his work for a more extensive discussion on this subject.[30] HPV DNA has been detected in more than 90% of anogenital cancers and precancers and the remainder likely represent unknown HPV DNA sequences.[30,31] It has not yet been determined whether the virus itself is necessary for induction, promotion, or both,[32] but it is likely that HPV infection alone is not sufficient to induce carcinoma in an immunocompetent host. Both spontaneous regression of HPV lesions and a long lag time for progression of some HPV lesions make the existence of cofactors such as tobacco metabolites or other chemical carcinogens, microbial infections such as HSV, or trauma and physical irritation necessary adjuncts in tumorigenesis.[33] Host factors are also important and will be considered below, especially in relation to the maternal physiologic changes of pregnancy.

The distribution of the specific HPV types among benign, premalignant, and malignant lesions is closely correlated with the specific virus/host cell interaction. As histopathologic abnormalities worsen in this continuum, so do abnormalities of nuclear DNA content, with diploidy giving way to polyploidy and then aneuploidy.[34] Specifically, types 6 and 11 are found in greater than 90% of condylomata acuminata. HPV 16 and 18 are detected in 70% of invasive cervical carcinomas, and types 31, 33, and 35 account for another 20% of cervical cancers.[14,35] The ability to screen patients for HPV DNA sequences and then type those who are HPV positive will soon allow clinicians to more specifically direct treatment based on whether patients have low-, intermediate-, or high-risk papillomaviral lesions.[35] Webb et al. employed a one-step DNA hybridization typing technique to analyze cervical scrapings of 66 women with a previous dysplastic cervical cytology. HPV DNA was identified in 96% of the patients and HPV 16 was found in 61% of CIN II-III lesions.[36] They also found HPV DNA in 7 of 12 women with normal or inflammatory changes in Pap smears who had a "history" of dysplasia. However, a word of caution is prudent. More mixed HPV infections are being reported from lesions in one anatomic site, and Reid et al. found that almost 25% of cases with multiple anatomic sites involved were related to multiple HPV types.[29] Just as all STDs are covariables of promiscuity, so are the various HPV types.

The recent finding by Kurman and associates of a significant deficit of HPV 18 in CIN (3%) compared to invasive cervical cancer (22%) is disconcerting. This is in contrast to HPV 16, which is present with equal frequency in CIN (37%) and invasive cancer (41%).[35] Their data suggest that HPV 18 may have the ability to rapidly progress through the precursor stages to frank carcinoma. This is a considerable deviation from the tradi-

tional view that the mean time for evolution of CIN III to cancer is 10 years.[37] However, this is a very important consideration when dealing with HPV in pregnancy. Rapid progression of neoplasia was evidenced by the report from our institution of six cases of CIN III and one early invasive vulvar carcinoma all in women less than 30 years old.[38] Indeed, Berkley et al. reported a series of women with a mean age of 32 years who presented with advanced-stage cervical invasive carcinoma and who had previously had normal screening cytologies within the preceding year.[39] Similar evidence of the existence of a subset of women with rapidly developing and highly aggressive tumors has been reported.[40,41]

This rapid transit time is even more frightening when one considers the frequency of false-negative Pap smears. To alter the terrible sequelae of HPV 18 infection, we would have to be able to screen all pregnant women for HPV infection and then be able to type those found positive. Fife and associates screened 234 inner-city women in the first trimester of pregnancy for HPV types 6, 11, 16, 18, and 31. Although 11% of the specimens were positive for HPV, only three patients had clinically evident condyloma (although 10 had a positive prior history).[16] Of significance was the fact that 46% of the positive women had no clinical or cytologic basis to suspect HPV infection. Types 16, 18, and 31 were present in 15 of the 26 specimens.

THE PREGNANT PATIENT

The precise physiologic alterations in the pregnant woman's immune system and the possible effects on the virus/host cell interaction have not been fully elucidated. The role of the increased vascularity of pregnancy with regard to HPV proliferation is also unclear. High estrogen levels may be another contributory factor. Because estrogen accelerates the process of squamous metaplasia at the squamocolumnar junction, it is possible that high levels of estrogen may stimulate a conversion of subclinical papillomavirus infection (SPI) to detectable CIN.[8,42] The physiologic eversion accompanying pregnancy also exposes a larger area of columnar epithelium to the vaginal flora and environs.

What is known is that pregnancy can be accompanied by rapid growth of existing HPV lesions or the macroscopic appearance of what was previously SPI.[43,44] Similarly, Woodruff and Peterson noted spontaneous regression of HPV lesions in 111 women in the postpartum period.[45]

Immunodeficient women are at increased risk for HPV infections, reinfections, extension of existing lesions, and progression to invasive cancer. This is well supported by studies dealing with organ transplant recipients on immunosuppressive therapy, patients on cytotoxic therapy, those with congenitally deficient cell-mediated immunity, women with the acquired immunodeficiency syndrome, and individuals on long-term corticosteroid therapy. These studies were recently reviewed by Sillman and Sedlis with regard to the possible role of HPV in the pathogenesis of neoplasia.[46] From a slightly different perspective, Marshburn and Trofatter presented evidence that the mere presence of recurrent condyloma in women over 40 years of age should be an indication for immunologic evaluation.[47] Further study of these women may provide insight into the immunological alterations that allow HPV to become activated and stimulated by the pregnant state. This enhanced susceptibility to HPV infection and its sequelae may ultimately be reason to expand current screening of new obstetrical patients from only gross physical examination and a cervical cytology specimen to use of quick DNA probes as they become available. Women testing positive would undergo serial colposcopic examinations throughout pregnancy. This information would also be beneficial in directing follow-up and/or therapy postpartum.

MANAGEMENT OF HPV INFECTION IN PREGNANCY

Although the scientific and medical communities are experiencing a logarithmic increase in literature regarding the human papillomaviruses and their treatment, there are no evolving concrete management protocols for any subset of women or men infected with HPV. This is certainly the case of HPV in pregnancy. There remain two basic issues that every clinician must face with their obstetrical patients: 1) determining whether treatment is indicated and 2) if necessary, how best to eradicate the problem.

Maternal Indications: Obstetrical

From a maternal standpoint, there is currently no firm scientific data that would support treatment of asymptomatic lesions in all pregnant women. Prospective studies are needed in order to ascertain whether treatment is indicated for fetal reasons, as discussed below, or to eliminate the more aggressive types of HPV such as 16 or 18. Treatment may only be necessary to eradicate specific types or grades of intraepithelial neoplasia.

Obviously, massive condylomata that occlude or obscure the vagina and cervix need to be addressed early in pregnancy if treatment is to be instituted. Benschine reported a maternal death following massive hemorrhage secondary to extensive genital condylomata at the time of vaginal delivery.[48] Young and colleagues treated seven patients with massive condyloma using electrocoagulation under general or regional anesthesia; the lesions were successfully eradicated in all patients. Although one patient had an estimated blood loss of 2,000 ml, vaginal delivery was accomplished in all seven. One patient, however, subsequently experienced dehiscence of her midline episiotomy and development of a rectovaginal fistula.[44] This case raises the question of HPV-induced poor wound healing, which we have observed in several patients with dehiscence of episiotomies.[49] Whether this represents sequelae of the actual HPV infection, secondary infection with other organisms (Fig. 1), or host factors predisposing to the growth of condy-

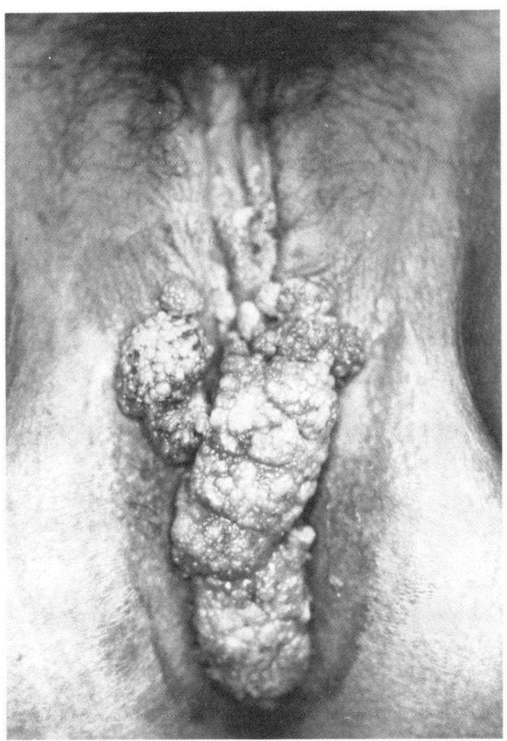

Fig. 1. Massive condyloma with secondary infection. (Photo courtesy of Dr. George Wendel, University of Texas Southwestern Medical Center, Dallas.)

lomata is purely speculative. In fact, condylomata along the future episiotomy site may become the principal maternal indication to treat patients antenatally.

If large lesions fail to respond to therapy or are diagnosed close to term, cesarean delivery may be inevitable to avoid dystocia or extensive maternal trauma and hemorrhage.[50] Condylomatous proliferation to the point of causing urinary retention, dyschezia, or extreme discomfort obviously needs to be treated. Coexisting STDs and superficial infections of the condylomata need to be eradicated prior to specific therapy directed at the condylomata.[43] Roberts advocated active treatment whenever HPV lesions are identified to avoid the possible development of "obstructed delivery."[51] Schwartz et al. also

profess the importance of active management, but they do so mainly for the potential fetal risks of exposure.[52]

A word of caution in dealing with massive condyloma is noteworthy. Miles et al. reported four cases of giant condylomas incorrectly interpreted histopathologically as invasive squamous cell carcinomas. This series included one pregnant patient with a lesion resembling the Buschke-Loewenstein giant condyloma.[53] There is also the potential to, in fact, be overlooking an exophytic, well-differentiated cervical carcinoma if histological sampling of "typical"-appearing condylomata acuminata in pregnancy is not performed. Clinical discretion and judgment must be invoked. A good tenet is to biopsy if any doubt exists.

Maternal Indications:Nonobstetrical

Until well-controlled prospective studies are available, the decision to treat a patient because of a certain type or subtype of HPV has no basis. In the future, it is conceivable, however, that the ability to identify an aggressive HPV, such as type 18, may by itself be reason to remove or destroy existing lesions in the vagina or on the cervix or vulva to avoid malignant progression.

Prompt evaluation of abnormal Pap smears in pregnancy is mandatory and is similar to that of the nonpregnant woman. Colposcopy is absolutely required in this evaluation.[54–58] Directed biopsy should not be delayed,[54,56,57,59] and conization should be performed as indicated.[57,59,60] Some authors have advocated the use of cervical wedge biopsies under anesthesia in lieu of conization, but convincing evidence of its enhanced benefits or reduced risks is lacking.[61] With proper evaluation and antenatal follow-up, the treatment of CIN can usually be postponed until after delivery.

A detailed discussion of the management of squamous cell carcinoma in pregnancy is beyond the scope of this chapter. Lee et al. reviewed their experiences with 41 women with invasive carcinoma of the cervix and found no difference in 5-year survival rates when compared to nonpregnant patients.[62] Hacker et al. reviewed the literature for the past 20 years and pointed out difficulties in interpreting definition, incidence, survival, and optimal management.[63] It is interesting, however, that the most common presenting symptom in those with invasive cancer was painless vaginal bleeding, the evaluation of which during pregnancy was frequently delayed because the bleeding was attributed to such conditions as threatened abortion. Only 20% of the invasive carcinomas were actually asymptomatic.[63]

Fetal Indications: Secondary Infections

The larger and more verruciform condylomata are prone to secondary infection by vaginal and/or colonic bacteria.[45] We encountered one giant cervical condyloma that contained numerous abscess pockets not clinically evident until laser vaporization was begun.[64] Such infection may serve as a reservoir for organisms for the possible development of chorioamnionitis and its attendant risk of fetal or maternal sepsis, premature labor, or intrauterine fetal demise. The woman referred to above developed chorioamnionitis with 8 hours of partial laser vaporization of a large cervical condyloma filling the upper one-third of the vagina. She spontaneously labored and was delivered abdominally secondary to birth canal obstruction by the remaining condyloma. The infant was septic and had a severe congenital pneumonia that was successfully treated.[64]

Prior to initiating specific therapy for condyloma, it is important to screen for and treat coexisting STDs. Even in the absence of overt infections, a risk of ascending infection exists (depending on lesion size and location).

Fetal Indications: Primary Infection (Respiratory Papillomatosis)

The literature is replete with articles implicating an association between juvenile onset recurrent respiratory papillomatosis (RRP)

and exposure of the fetus to a birth canal infected with HPV.[24,65–74] Although an association of maternal HPV infection to laryngeal papillomas was suggested as early as 1853,[75] to date no direct causal relationship has been proved.[76] The crucial point for obstetricians to remember is the low risk of RRP developing subsequent to any given exposure. This risk is somewhere between 1 in 80 to 1 in 1,500.[75] Very conservatively using an incidence of 5% of livebirths occurring in women with HPV infection and that 80% of these would have vaginal deliveries, the risk of papillomatosis developing in the offspring born to a mother with HPV genital infection would be approximately 1 in 400.[75]

Juvenile onset RRP, formerly called juvenile laryngeal papillomatosis (JLP), represents the most common neoplasia in infants and young children.[75] Symptomatology varies from painless hoarseness to complete upper airway obstruction. These children usually present by age 5 years and often require multiple endoscopic excisions, occasionally as often as weekly. There is also an adult form of the disease that behaves in a less aggressive manner, and it has been postulated that it may represent latent HPV acquired at birth.[76] Exposure through oral-genital sexual contact, however, is probably most likely.[69] It is well documented that the etiology of RRP is secondary to HPV, and multiple studies have implicated HPV types 6 and 11, commonly found in the female genital tract.[65,71] In addition, HPV-16-related DNA sequences have been found in verrucous carcinomas of the larynx.[24]

Quick et al. reported a positive maternal condyloma history in 21 of 31 RRP patients and raised not only the question of whether cesarean sections should be considered but also whether the minor trauma of suctioning meconium, etc. could increase the risk of HPV infection.[72] This question of trauma is intriguing since Gissman has hypothesized that traumatic activation of latent HPV may play an important role in the genesis of CIN in adult women.[26]

In a review of 28 women who delivered children who subsequently were diagnosed as having RRP, Hallden and Majmudar found a history of maternal vulvar condyloma in 54% of these women. They strongly advocated operative delivery in the setting of maternal vulvar condylomata at term.[69] Interestingly, they drew an analogy between maternal HPV and HSV infection and the subsequent need for abdominal delivery. But HSV clearly has a higher perinatal attack rate and much graver prognosis than HPV, and even the need for cesarean delivery in cases of known HSV infection in the absence of primary disease is questionable.[42,59,77–79]

In a larger review of 109 children with juvenile onset RRP, only one case was delivered by cesarean section, in contrast to an expected number of 10 cesarean sections based on the national cesarean section rate at that time.[73] The authors used this as prima facie evidence of acquisition of HPV at the time of vaginal delivery.

A well-controlled prospective study employing periodic laryngoscopic examinations of children at risk vs. those not at risk is lacking. Such a study will be difficult to perform. A 1988 study from Denmark examined by history the children, ages 4 to 9 years, of 77 mothers who had condylomata acuminata during pregnancy, and no laryngeal condylomata were reported.[70] These investigators also retrospectively looked at the maternal history of nine other infants with a diagnosis of RRP (8 weeks postpartum). Although their numbers were small, they found a less suggestive causal relationship of a maternal history of HPV and subsequent RRP. Numerous authors have also not considered the possibility of postnatal exposure.

It is confusing, however, that there are relatively few cases of HPV infection reported at sites other than the larynx. Why respiratory mucosa should be so inordinately susceptible during the birth process is not explainable.[73] A case of a newborn infant with perianal condyloma, born to a mother with genital condyloma, has been reported.[80]

Whether this was an ascending infection through an unknown defect in the fetal membranes or secondary to transplacental passage is unknown. The normal behavior of HPV, however, is local multiplication at the site of entry, which makes the former mechanism more likely.[73] No blood-borne infection has ever been documented.

Rock et al. reported five cases of genital HPV infection in children aged 2 to 8 years. Two cases were felt to be unrelated to child abuse and, therefore, presumably secondary to exposure at birth.[27] They also found HPV 6 or 11 in all five of their cases. A similar case of penile condyloma developing in a 14-month-old infant has also been reported.[81] The fact that anogenital warts in children have increased in frequency over the past several years[82] would be in concert with a similarly increasing incidence in adults and parturient mothers. It is obviously difficult, however, to sort out child abuse in any of these reports. The foreskins of 6 of 70 unselected infants were recently found to be positive for HPV DNA types 6, 11, 16, or 18. No correlation, however, could be identified with maternal history of condyloma or abnormal Pap smears on review.[83]

If congenital exposure becomes more common in the future, several large issues will appear. These children could become reservoirs for their future sexual partners.[82] The more aggressive HPV types would also be expected to lead to an increasing frequency of genital-tract neoplasia in adolescents. Vulvar carcinoma has been reported in a 14-year-old girl.[84]

TREATMENT MODALITIES

There is no single definitive treatment for condylomata acuminata; it is is dependent on the size, location, and number of lesions.[43] This is true regardless of pregnancy, although pregnancy poses some unique treatment problems. Various treatment modalities have been proposed, the most common of which are listed in Table 2.

TABLE 2. Common Treatment Modalities for HPV Infections

Topical chemical agents
Trichloroacetic acid
Podophyllum[a]
5-Fluorouracil[b]
Surgical
Excision
Electrocoagulation
Cryotherapy
Laser vaporization

[a]Should be used with caution during pregnancy (see text).
[b]Contraindicated during pregnancy.

Topical Chemical Compounds

Trichloroacetic acid (TCA) is a caustic and astringent agent that causes a superficial slough after topical application. It kills cells by precipitating proteins and its effect is local, thereby causing little reactive inflammation.[85] The meticulous application of 85% TCA solution gives excellent results with little patient discomfort and no worrisome systemic side effects.[86] However, it has a cure rate of only 20 to 30% after a single application, thereby necessitating at least weekly treatments.

Podophyllum has traditionally been the most commonly used treatment for external genital warts, but many clinicians feel that this antimitotic agent is absolutely contraindicated in pregnancy.[52,87] A case of maternal systemic toxicity and fetal demise (at 8 months' gestation) was reported following application of 25% podophyllum to a massive condyloma.[6] Chamberlain and associates also reported an intrauterine fetal demise at 32 weeks following topical application,[88] and Slater et al. reported a case of maternal flaccid paralysis, hypokalemia, coma, and death.[89] There has also been a case report of a possible teratogenic effect of podophyllum,[90] but there is little or no scientific data to substantiate this. There is also little data regarding the pharmacology of podophyllum during pregnancy. Although there are no controlled studies of its use in pregnancy, we feel that its judicious use after the first trimester of pregnancy on small external condylomas is associated with less risk than more aggressive therapies, especially if anesthesia would otherwise be necessary.

5-Fluorouracil (5-FU) is becoming a more and more attractive treatment for HPV infections in nonpregnant woman, not only because of its ability to be used intravaginally as well as externally, but also because of its ability to treat large geographic areas, thereby reducing recurrences related to subclinical disease.[91] This fluorinated pyrimidine, which is cytostatic and also inhibits cell division, is approximately 6% absorbed following intravaginal application. Although the patient is exposed to a small dose as compared to systemic chemotherapy, we agree with Schwartz et al. that its use in pregnancy is contraindicated at the present time.[52] Multiple fetal malformations in a patient treated with 5-FU at 11 to 12 weeks of gestation have been reported.[92] Two women who were inadvertently treated with a 5-day regimen of intravaginal topical 5% 5-FU cream during the first trimester of pregnancy were delivered of normal infants.[93] This report of normal outcome in only two cases is inadequate to make generalizations about the safety of topical 5-FU.

Surgical Excision/Electrocoagulation

Wide local excision of vulvar intraepithelial neoplasia and condylomata can be carried out at any time during pregnancy, but the presence of numerous or extensive lesions often makes this impractical. Pregnancy-enhanced vascularity increases surgical blood loss and postoperative edema.

As noted above, electrocoagulation was 100% successful in eradicating large condylomas in Young et al.'s series from 1973.[44] Today, however, the advantages of laser therapy, to be discussed below, make these other surgical therapies less attractive.[94]

Cryotherapy

One group of investigators has consistently reported good results with cryotherapy.[95–97]

Thirty-four patients were treated for vulvar, vaginal, and/or cervical condylomata acuminata in the second trimester (4 patients) and third trimester (30 patients) using nitrous oxide anesthesia and a small cryoprobe. No patients required general anesthesia, and all lesions were treated in one to three visits at 2-week intervals. They successfully eradicated the visible condylomata in 100% of women through the first postpartum visit but had no cases involving extensive disease.[95] No obstetric or neonatal complications were reported in this uncontrolled study.

Bergman et al. also reported the use of cervical cryotherapy in the second trimester (8 patients) and third trimester (20 patients) of pregnancy. Most patients had condylomata elsewhere in the genital tract that were also treated. Freeze time was short, usually 30–60 seconds. While one patient required four treatments, all lesions were successfully eradicated.[96] Advantages included no maternal or fetal complications and lack of need for general anesthesia. Although they have demonstrated the feasibility of this treatment modality, it is still unclear whether there is a need to treat cervical lesions.

Laser Vaporization

The CO_2 laser is a useful tool in the treatment of genital HPV lesions. The obvious advantages of precision, ability to remove large lesions, and ability to use in the upper vagina and cervix are enhanced by studies reporting reduced pain, reduced scarring, and reduced healing time.[85,86,94] The physical principles underlying expert control of the laser have been detailed by Reid.[98] Clinicians employing this technique should be familiar with these physical and surgical principles in order to achieve optimal results.

In 1981, Malfetano et al. reported the successful treatment of massive vulvar condyloma acuminata in a patient at 33 weeks gestation without complications.[87] The use of the laser in pregnant women, however, has lagged far behind the experience being gained in nonobstetrical patients. Fear of heavy blood loss because of increased vascularity and the long-held desire to avoid general or regional anesthesia antenatally are the major factors. The vascularity concern is not logical because all other modalities, especially local surgical excision, include the same physiologic change and risk but without the benefit of the laser's ability to thermally seal vessels up to 0.5–1.0 mm in size.[98,99] Moreover, regional anesthesia is both efficacious and relatively safe for use during pregnancy.

Ferenczy reported a 95% overall success rate in 43 pregnant women with extensive urogenital and anal condylomata who underwent simple laser vaporization.[99] All persistent lesions were in women who had multiple sites involved. He reported a 14% recurrence rate (lesions developing in areas not previously treated) that was inversely proportional to the gestational age of the patient when initially treated. The recurrence rate was 33% if treated in the first, 17% if treated in the second, and 0% if treated in the third trimester. He postulated a relative correction of the immunocompetence associated with pregnancy as the gestation advances.[99]

Schwartz et al. collected 32 patients treated with the CO_2 laser during pregnancy ranging from 9 to 37 weeks.[52] Spinal anesthesia was employed for all but one patient, who received a general anesthetic. There were three recurrences after initial treatments and in contrast to Ferenczy's series, they were all among the 25 women treated in the third trimester. Two of the recurrences were successfully managed with the use of TCA; however, the third proved refractory and ultimately required cesarean delivery because of massive lesions. Schwartz et al. included two control patients for each study subject to assess maternal and perinatal morbidity and found no significant differences between the groups. Among the treated women, one developed pyelonephritis, two required tocolysis to suppress uterine activity, and one experienced premature rupture of the membranes at 36 weeks, 4 days after the laser treatment.

We reported nine women who underwent laser vaporization in the second (6 patients) and third (3 patients) trimesters.[64] The only two antenatal recurrences were in patients initially treated at 17 and 21 weeks of gestation. An additional patient treated at 31 weeks was found to have recurrent lesions at her postpartum visit. There were no maternal or neonatal complications in seven patients. Of the other two women, one patient who had vaporization of cervical disease experienced significant postoperative bleeding requiring electrocautery to effect hemostasis. The other woman who presented with a massive 7 × 5 cm cervical condyloma deserves special consideration. At the time of the initial laser treatment at 36 weeks of gestation, only 60% of the lesion was vaporized over 2 1/2 hours and multiple unsuspected abscess pockets exuding frank pus were encountered. This patient subsequently entered premature labor 8 hours postoperatively with clinically evident chorioamnionitis and required operative delivery, which resulted in an infant with both hyaline membrane disease and congenital pneumonia. This case clearly demonstrates the need to consider the possibility of complications necessitating early delivery when planning therapy.

Early treatment minimizes the continued or accelerated proliferation of lesions but carries with it a greater chance of recurrent disease with the need for multiple treatments and anesthetics as well as posing a serious predicament if immediate delivery becomes necessary. Additional experience will allow more guidance in the timing of therapy for all types of lesions. The eradication of large cervical or vaginal fornix lesions should be delayed until the time of fetal viability or maybe even postpartum after cesarean delivery.

Posttreatment Follow-up

Irrespective of the treatment modality employed, adequate follow-up must be ensured antenatally to exclude residual disease or early recurrences. Most series have noted recurrences within 2 to 8 weeks of initial therapy.[43] Closer follow-up intervals in the majority of instances will detect recurrent lesions in a more manageable distribution.

Postpartum follow-up is crucial not only to check for recurrent disease but to also search for evidence of genital tract intraepithelial neoplasia. Colposcopy, in addition to cervical cytology, is prudent.

Postpartum regular follow-up for the offspring is probably warranted only on a historical basis.[43] To subject infants to repeated, indirect laryngoscopy for a risk of RRP of 1 in 400 or much less seems overly aggressive.

SUMMARY

Human papillomavirus infections are becoming an increasingly common and complex problem. Data collected through the use of DNA probes will hopefully provide us with a better understanding of not only the epidemiology of this viral infection but also the pathophysiologic consequences of each specific type of HPV. This basic and clinical research is needed before the specific effects on the host can be clearly elucidated.

The decision to treat women during pregnancy should be based on maternal indications and not on the unproven or low risk of recurrent respiratory papillomatosis in the infant. Abdominal delivery is indicated for massive genital lesions obstructing the birth canal. Otherwise the decision to begin treatment of lesser HPV lesions must be individualized. Vulvar and/or vaginal involvement at the site of anticipated episiotomy is the most common reason to initiate therapy. Prospective studies are needed to direct appropriate therapeutic goals of eradication of specific types of HPV or grades of intraepithelial neoplasia.

Outpatient therapeutic modalities have the advantage of few risks but disadvantage of poor success and necessity of frequent visits. If laser vaporization of cervical or upper vaginal lesions is deemed necessary, therapy should be delayed until fetal viability and performed only when the risks of possible complications culminating in delivery outweigh the risks of treatment. Laser vaporization of extensive vulvar disease in the second trimester may have a higher risk of later pregnancy recurrence. This must be weighed against massive enlargement occurring while a gestation advances if treatment in the third trimester is chosen.

REFERENCES

1. Campion MJ: Clinical manifestations and natural history of genital human papillomavirus infection. Obstet Gynecol Clin North Am 14:363–388, 1987.
2. zur Hausen H: Human papillomaviruses and their possible role in squamous cell carcinomas. Curr Top Microbiol Immunol 78:1–30, 1977.
3. Nowell PC: Molecular events in tumor development. N Engl J Med 319:575–577, 1988.
4. Reid R: Human papillomavirus. Obstet Gynecol Clin North Am 14:XIV, 1987.
5. Wilson J: Extensive vulval condylomata acuminata necessitating caesarean section. Aust NZ J Obstet Gynaecol 13:121–124, 1973.
6. Gorthey RL, Krebs MA: Vulvar condylomata acuminata complicating labor. Obstet Gynecol 4:67–74, 1954.
7. Broker TR: Structure and genetic expression of papillomaviruses. Obstet Gynecol Clin North Am 14:329–348, 1987.
8. Garry R, Jones R: Relationship between cervical condylomata, pregnancy and subclinical papillomavirus infection. J Reprod Med 30:393–399, 1985.
9. Grubb GS: Human papillomavirus and cervical neoplasia: Epidemiological considerations. Int J Epidemiol 15:1–7, 1986.
10. Meisels A, Roy M, Fortier M, et al.: Human papillomavirus infection of the cervix: The atypical condyloma. Acta Cytol 25:71–76, 1981.
11. Reid R, Laverty CR, Coppleson M, Insaragkul W, Hillis E: Noncondylomatous cervical wart-virus infection. Obstet Gynecol 55:476–483, 1980.
12. Barrasso R, DeBrux JD, Croissant O, Orth G: High prevalence of papillomavirus-associated penile intraepithelial neoplasia in sexual partners of women with cervical intraepithelial neoplasia. N Engl J Med 312:916–923, 1987.
13. Rosenberg SK, Reid R: Sexually transmitted papillomaviral infections in the male. I. Anatomic distribution and clinical features. Urology 29:488–492, 1987.
14. Lorincz AT, Temple GF, Patterson JA, Jensen AB, Kurman RJ, Lancaster WD: Correlation of cellular atypia and human papillomavirus deoxyribonucleic acid sequences in exfoliated cells of the uterine cavity. Obstet Gynecol 68:508–512, 1986.
15. Wickenden C, Steele A, Malcolm ADB, Coleman DV: Screening for women with virus infections in normal and abnormal cervices by DNA hybridization of cervical scrapes. Lancet 1:65–67, 1985.
16. Fife KH, Rogers RE, Zwickl BW: Symptomatic-asymptomatic cervical infections with human papillomavirus during pregnancy. J Infect Dis 156:904–911, 1987.
17. Waeckerlin RW, Potter NJ, Cheatham GR Jr: Correlation of cytologic, colposcopic, and histologic studies with immunohistochemical studies of human papillomavirus structural antigens in an unselected patient population. Am J Obstet Gynecol 158:1394–1402, 1988.
18. Reid R, Stanhope GR, Herschman BR, et al.: Genital warts and cervical cancer. I. Evidence of an association between subclinical papillomavirus infection and cervical malignancy. Cancer 50:377–387, 1982.
19. ACOG Technical Bulletin: Perinatal Herpes Simplex Virus Infections. No. 122, November 1988.
20. Bolognese RJ, Corson SL, Fuccilo DA, et al.: Herpes virus homins type II infection in asymptomatic pregnant women. Obstet Gynecol 48:507–510, 1976.
21. Roy M, Meisels A, Fortier M, et al.: Vaginal condylomata: A human papillomavirus infection. Clin Obstet Gynecol 24:461–483, 1981.
22. Greenberg H, Mann WJ, Chumes J, Zuna R, Patsner B, Loesch M, Baker D: Cervical and vaginal pathology in women with vulvar condylomata. J Reprod Med 32:801–804, 1987.
23. Kreider JW, Howett MK, Stoler MH, Zaino RJ, Welsh P: Susceptibility of various human tissues to transformation in vivo with human papillomavirus type II. Int J Cancer 39:459–465, 1987.
24. Brandsma JL, Steinberg BM, Abramson AL, Winkler B: Presence of human papillomavirus type 16 related sequences in verrucous carcinoma of the larynx. Cancer Res 46:2185–2188, 1986.
25. Karram M, Tabor M, Smotkin D, Wettstein F, Bhatia N, Micha J: Detection of human papillomavirus deoxyribonucleic acid from vulvar dystrophies and vulvar intraepithelial neoplastic lesions. Am J Obstet Gynecol 159:22–23, 1988.
26. Gissman L: Papillomaviruses and their association with cancer in animals and in man. Cancer Surv 3:161–181, 1984.
27. Rock B, Naghashfar Z, Barnett N, Buscema J, Woodruff JD, Shah K: Genital tract papillomavirus infection in children. Arch Dermatol 122:1129–1132, 1986.
28. Duerst M, Gissman L, Ikenberg H, zur Hausen H:

A papillomavirus from a cervical carcinoma and its prevalence in cancer biopsy samples from different geographic regions. Proc Natl Acad Sci USA 80:3812–3815, 1983.

29. Reid R, Greenberg M, Jensen AB, et al.: Sexually transmitted papillomaviral infections. I. The anatomic distribution and pathologic grade of neoplastic lesions associated with different viral types. Am J Obstet Gynecol 156:212–222, 1987.

30. Pfister H: Relationship of papillomavirus to anogenital cancer. Obstet Gynecol Clin North Am 14:349–361, 1987.

31. Sato S, Okagaki T, Clark BA, Twiggs LB, Fukushima M, Ostrow RS, Faras AJ: Sensitivity of koilocytosis, immunocytochemistry, and electron microscopy as compared to DNA hybridization in detecting human papillomavirus in cervical and vaginal condyloma and intraepithelial neoplasia. Int J Gynecol Pathol 5:297–307, 1987.

32. Pitot HC: The natural history of neoplastic development: The relation of experimental models to human cancer. Cancer 49:1206–1211, 1982.

33. Pfister H: Biology and biochemistry of papillomaviruses. Rev Physiol Biochem Pharmacol 99:111–181, 1984.

34. Reid R: Human papillomaviral infection: The key to rational triage of cervical neoplasia. Obstet Gynecol Clin North Am 14:407–429, 1987.

35. Kurman RJ, Schiffman MH, Lancaster WD, Reid R, Jenson AB, Temple GF, Lorincz AT: Analysis of individual human papillomavirus types in cervical neoplasia: A possible role for type 18 in rapid progression. Am J Obstet Gynecol 159:293–296, 1988.

36. Webb DH, Rogers RE, Fife KH: A one-step method for detecting and typing human papillomavirus DNA in cervical scrape specimens from women with cervical dysplasia. J Infect Dis 156:912–919, 1987.

37. Richart RM, Barron BA: A follow-up study of patients with cervical dysplasia. Am J Obstet Gynecol 105:386–393, 1969.

38. Hillard GD, Massey FM, O'Toole RVJ: Vulvar neoplasia in the young. Am J Obstet Gynecol 135:185–188, 1979.

39. Berkley AS, LiVols VA, Schwartz PE: Advanced squamous cell carcinoma of the cervix with recent normal Papanicolaou tests. Lancet 2:375–376, 1980.

40. Bain RW, Crocker DW: Rapid onset of cervical cancer in an upper socioeconomic group. Am J Obstet Gynecol 146:366–370, 1983.

41. Dunn JE, Schweitzer V: The relationship of cervical cytology to the incidence of cervical cancer and mortality in Alameda County, California, 1960 to 1974. Am J Obstet Gynecol 139:868–876, 1981.

42. Arvin AM, Hensleight PA, Prober CG, et al.: Failure of antepartum maternal cultures to predict the infant's risk of exposure to herpes simplex virus at delivery. N Engl J Med 315:796–800, 1986.

43. Schwartz DB, Greenberg MD, Daoud Y, Reid R: The management of genital condylomas in pregnant women. Obstet Gynecol Clin North Am 14:589–599, 1987.

44. Young RL, Acosta AA, Kaufmann RH: The treatment of large condylomata acuminata complicating pregnancy. Obstet Gynecol 41:65–73, 1973.

45. Woodruff JD, Peterson EF: Condylomata acuminata of the cervix. Am J Obstet Gynecol 75:1354–1362, 1958.

46. Sillman FH, Sedlis A: Anogenital papillomavirus infection and neoplasia in immunodeficient women. Obstet Gynecol Clin North Am 14:537–558, 1987.

47. Marshburn PB, Trofatter KF Jr: Recurrent condyloma acuminatum in women over age 40: Association with immunosuppression and malignant disease. Am J Obstet Gynecol 159:429–433, 1988.

48. Benschine FW: Massive condylomata acuminata of the vulva complicating labor. Am J Obstet Gynecol 42:338–340, 1941.

49. Snyder RR, Hammond TL, Hankins GDV: Human papilloma virus associated with poor healing of episiotomy repairs. Paper to be read at AFD ACOG ACM, Washington, D.C., November 1989.

50. Wilson J: Extensive vulval condylomata acuminata necessitating cesarean section. Aust NZ J Obstet Gynaecol 13:121–124, 1973.

51. Roberts JA: Management of gynecologic tumors during pregnancy. Clin Perinatol 10:369–382, 1983.

52. Schwartz DB, Greenberg MD, Daoud Y, Reid R: Genital condylomas in pregnancy: Use of trichloroacetic acid and laser therapy. Am J Obstet Gynecol 158:1407–1416, 1988.

53. Miles PA, Herrera GA, Greenberg H, Eckberg DJ: Condylomas of the uterine cervix initially interpreted as squamous carcinomas: A report of four cases including a lesion resembling the Bushke-Loewenstein giant condyloma. Gynecol Oncol 24:236–246, 1986.

54. Bertini-Oliveira AM, Keppler MM, Luisi A, Tarico S. Lopes VLD, Delascio D, Camano L: Comparative evaluation of abnormal cytology, colposcopy and histopathology in preclinical cervicalmalignancy during pregnancy. Acta Cytol 26:636–644, 1982.

55. Hellberg D, Axelsson O, Gad A, Nilsson S: Conservative management of the abnormal smear during pregnancy. Acta Obstet Gynecol Scand 66:195–199, 1987.

56. Kohan S, Beckman EM, Bigelow B, Klein SA, Douglas GW: The role of colposcopy in the management of cervical intraepithelial neoplasia during

pregnancy and postpartum. J Reprod Med 25:279–284, 1980.

57. LaPolla JP, O'Neill CO, Wetrich D: Colposcopic management of abnormal cervical cytology in pregnancy. J Reprod Med 33:301–306, 1988.

58. Ostergard DR, Nieberg RK: Evaluation of abnormal cervical cytology during pregnancy with colposcopy. Am J Obstet Gynecol 134:756–758, 1979.

59. Lurain JR, Gallup DG: Management of abnormal Papanicolaou smears in pregnancy. Obstet Gynecol 53:484–488, 1979.

60. Hannigan EV, Whitehouse HH II, Atkinson WD, Becker SN: Cone biopsy during pregnancy. Obstet Gynecol 60:450–455, 1982.

61. McDonnell JM, Mylotte MJ, Gustafson RC, Jordan JA: Colposcopy in pregnancy: A twelve year review. Br J Obstet Gynaecol 88:414–420, 1981.

62. Lee RB, Neglia W, Park RC: Cervical carcinoma in pregnancy. Obstet Gynecol 58:584–589, 1981.

63. Hacker NF, Berek JS, Lagasse LD, Charles EH, Savage EW, Moore JG: Carcinoma of the cervix associated with pregnancy. Obstet Gynecol 59:735–746, 1982.

64. Hankins GDV, Hammond TL, Snyder RR, Gilstrap LC: Management of extensive genital tract condyloma acuminata during pregnancy with laswer vaporization. J Infect Dis 159:1001–1002, 1989.

65. Bennett RS, Powell KR: Human papillomaviruses: Associations between laryngeal papillomas and genital warts. Pediatr Infec Dis J 6:229–232, 1987.

66. Cohen SR, Seltzer S, Geller KA, Thompson JW: Papilloma of the layrnx and tracheobronchial tree in children. A retrospective study. Ann Otol 89:497–503, 1980.

67. Cook TA, Cohn AM, Brunschwig JP, Butel JS, Rawls WE: Wart viruses and laryngeal papillomous. Lancet 1:782–783, 1973.

68. Cook TA, Cohn AM, Brunschwig JP, Goepfert H, Butel JS, Rawls WE: Laryngeal papilloma: Etiologic and therapeutic considerations. An Otol Rhinol Laryngol 82:649–655, 1973.

69. Hallden C, Majmudar B: The relationship between juvenile laryngeal papillomatosis and maternal condylomata acuminata. J Reprod Med 31:804–807, 1986.

70. Kjer JJ, Eldon K, Dreisler A: Maternal condylomata and juvenile laryngeal papillomas in their children. Zentral bl Gynakol 110:107–110, 1988.

71. Mounts P, Shah KV: Respiratory papillomatosis: Etiological relation to genital tract papillomaviruses. Prog Med Virol 29:90–114, 1984.

72. Quick CA, Krzyzek RA, Watts SL, Faras AJ: Relationship between condylomata and laryngeal papillomata: Clinical and molecular virological evidence. Ann Otol 89:467–471, 1980.

73. Shah K, Kashima H, Polk BF, Shah F, Abbey H, Abramson A: Rarity of cesarean delivery in cases of juvenile-onset respiratory papillomatosis. Obstet Gynecol 68:795–799, 1986.

74. Storrs FJ: Spread of condyloma acuminata to infants and children. Arch Dermatol 113:1294, 1977.

75. Kashima HK, Shah K: Recurrent respiratory papillomatosis: Clinical overview and management principles. Obstet Gynecol Clin North Am 14:581–588, 1987.

76. Healy GB, Gelber RD, Trowbridge AL, Grundfast KM, Ruben RJ, Price KN: Treatment of recurrent respiratory papillomatosis with human leukocyte interferon. Results of a multicenter randomized clinical trial. N Engl J Med 319:401–407, 1988.

77. Hankins GDV, Cunningham FG, Luby JP, Butler SL, Stroud J, Roark M: Asymptomatic genital excretion of herpes simples virus during early labor. Am J Obstet Gynecol 150:100–101, 1984.

78. Prober CG, Sullender WM, Hasukawa LL, et al.: Low risk of herpes simplex virus infections in neonates exposed to the virus at the time of vaginal delivery to mothers with recurrent genital herpes simplex virus infections. N Engl J Med 316:240–244, 1987.

79. Scher J, Bottone E, Desmond E, et al.: The incidence and outcome of asymptomatic herpes simplex genitalia in an obstetric population. Am J Obstet Gynecol 144:906–909, 1982.

80. Tang CK, Shermeta DW, Wood C: Congenital condylomata acuminata. Am J Obstet Gynecol 131:912–913, 1978.

81. Weiss JP, November S, Curtin CT: Recurrent penile condylomata acuminata in a 17-month-old boy. J Urol 136:468–469, 1986.

82. Bender ME: New concepts of condyloma acuminata in children. Arch Dermatol 122:1121–1124, 1986.

83. Roman A, Fife K: Human papillomavirus DNA associated with foreskins of normal newborns. J Infect Dis 153:855–861, 1986.

84. Lister VM, Akinla O: Carcinoma of the vulva in childhood. Br J Obstet Gynaecol 79:470–473, 1972.

85. Reid R: Superficial laser vulvectomy. III. A new surgical technique for appendage-conserving ablation of refractory condylomas and vulvar intraepithelial nepplasia. Am J Obstet Gynecol 152:504–509, 1985.

86. Reid R: Superficial laser vulvectomy. I. The efficacy of extended superficial ablation for refractory and very extensive condylomas. Am J Obstet Gynecol 151:1047–1052, 1985.

87. Malfetano JH, Marin AC, Malfetano JH Jr: Laser treatment of condylomata acuminata in pregnancy. J Reprod Med 26:574–576, 1981.

88. Chamberlain MJ, Reynolds AL, Yeomans WB: Toxic effect of podophyllum application in pregnancy. Br Med J 3:391–392, 1972.

89. Slater GE, Rumack BH, Peterson RG: Podophyllum poisoning: Systemic toxicity following cutaneous application. Obstet Gynecol 52:94–96, 1978.

90. Karol MD, Conner CS, Watanabe AS, Murphrey KJ: Podophyllum: Suspected teratogenicity from topical application. Clin Toxicol 16:283–286, 1980.

91. Krebs HB: The use of topical 5-fluorouracil in the treatment of genital condylomas. Obstet Gynecol Clin North Am 14:559–568, 1987.

92. Stephens JD, Golbus MS, Miller TR, Wilber RR, Epstein CJ: Multiple congenital anomalies in a fetus exposed to 5-fluorouracil during the first trimester. Am J Obstet Gynecol 137:747–749, 1980.

93. Kopelman JN, Miyazawa K: Topical 5-fluorouracil treatment in early pregnancy: A report of 2 cases. 27th Annual Meeting of the Armed Forces District ACOG, San Antonio, TX, November 1988 (abstract).

94. Reid R, Elfont EA, Zirkin RM: Superficial laser vulvectomy. II. The anatomic and biophysical principles permitting accurate control of the depth of dermal destruction with the carbon dioxide laser. Am J Obstet Gynecol 152:261–271, 1985.

95. Bergman A, Bhatia NN, Broen EM: Cryotherapy for treatment of genital condylomata during pregnancy. J Reprod Med 29:432–435, 1984.

96. Bergman A, Matsunaga J, Bhatia NN: Cervical cryotherapy for condylomata acuminata during pregnancy. Obstet Gynecol 69:47–50, 1987.

97. Matsunaga J, Bergman A, Bhatia NN: Genital condylomata acuminata in pregnancy: Effectiveness, safety and pregnancy outcome following cryotherapy. Br J Obstet Gynaecol 94:168–172, 1987.

98. Reid R: Physical and surgical principles governing expertise with the carbon dioxide laser. Obstet Gynecol Clin North Am 14:513–535, 1987.

99. Ferenczy A: Treating genital condyloma during pregnancy with the carbon dioxide laser. Am J Obstet Gynecol 148:9–12, 1984.

20

Other Viral Infections

Mark G. Martens, M.D.

With the development of vaccines decades ago, many of the viral infections that plagued millions of unfortunate individuals became preventable and, it was believed, were on their way to total eradication. Since then, generations of health-care personnel have trained with little, if any, experience with these diseases. However, recent adverse reactions with vaccines and waning enforcement of vaccination policies have allowed some of these viruses to rise again. Also, advances in the field of virology have permitted the accurate diagnosis of several of these viruses, and new viruses, viral types, and associated disease entities have also been uncovered. These changes necessitate that the effects of these infections in the pregnant patient and her fetus be reexamined. Several of these viruses are discussed in this chapter.

MUMPS

Mumps is an acute communicable disease that commonly involves the parotid and salivary glands. It is caused by an RNA virus from the paramyxovirus family. It is primarily a disease of childhood, with only 10 to 15% of cases occurring in adolescence or adulthood. Since the licensure of a mumps vaccine in 1967, the total number of mumps cases has declined, with 2.07 cases per 100,000 total population reported.[1] The incidence rate in pregnancy ranges from 0.8 to 10 cases of mumps per 10,000 pregnancies, making it a more frequent infection in pregnancy than either measles or chickenpox.

Mumps has a seasonal pattern, with the peak incidence in the winter and spring months. The disease is characterized by a prodrome of fever, malaise, myalgia, and anorexia, followed by development of parotitis within 24 hours. Disease is inapparent in approximately one-third of infected persons. When symptoms are present, they progress over 1 to 3 days and then slowly resolve during the next 3 to 7 days.[2]

The parotitis is usually bilateral, with the orifice of Stensen's duct erythematous and swollen. The submaxillary glands are sometimes involved, but almost always in conjunction with the parotid gland. The sublingual gland is rarely involved. Meningoencephalitis may be a serious manifestation, occurring approximately 10% of the cases. Fortunately, it is usually benign, with less than 15% of cases demonstrating meningeal symptoms.[3] Orchitis occurs in 20% of postpubertal males and may cause sterility. Mumps-related oophoritis is much less common in postpubertal women (approximately

Infections in Pregnancy, pages 207–220
© 1990 Alan R. Liss, Inc.

5%) and apparently does not lead to infertility.[4]

Other mumps-related complications are much more rare, with the most serious being deafness. It is usually unilateral and permanent, with an incidence rate of 0.5 to 5 per 100,000 cases of mumps. Other serious but rare complications include pancreatitis, thyroiditis, mastitis, nephritis, pericarditis, myocarditis, hepatitis, arthritis, and thrombocytopenia. Mortality due to these serious complications is estimated to be from 1 to 3.4 deaths per 10,000 reported mumps cases.[5]

The virus is transmitted through saliva or respiratory droplets, and it has been found in saliva from 7 days prior to 9 days after the onset of parotitis. Despite this extended period of infectivity and sometimes asymptomatic nature, the infectivity rate among susceptible exposed individuals in only 31%, less than the 76 and 61% rates for measles and chickenpox, respectively.[6]

Although mumps in pregnancy does not appear to occur more frequently or with increased severity than in nonpregnant patients,[7–9] there are reports of increased fetal mortality in women who contract the illness in the first trimester. Siegel et al. found a 27.3% rate of fetal wastage in women with mumps during the first trimester, as compared to a 13% rate in matched, non-ill controls.[10] Fetal loss, when it occurs, usually appears within 2 weeks of maternal infection. Histopathologic examination of the products of conception from mothers with mumps during pregnancy have demonstrated severe proliferative necrotic villitis and vasculitis in the placentas and viral inclusions consistent with mumps in the fetal tissues.[11] The mumps virus has been isolated as early as 10 weeks of gestation from a fetus that spontaneously aborted 4 days after onset of maternal symptoms.[12]

There does not appear, however, to be an association with mumps and prematurity, intrauterine growth retardation, or fetal mortality in maternal disease after the first trimester.[13]

The role of mumps in congenital disease remains controversial. Animal studies have demonstrated mumps-induced congenital malformations.[14,15] However, Siegel did not find an increased rate of congenital malformations in a controlled prospective study in humans.[15]

Prior concern had centered on the association of gestational mumps with endocardial fibroelastosis (EFE) in the neonate, which was demonstrated in a high number of children with positive mumps skin tests[16,17] and induced by St. Geme et al. in chicken embryo experiments.[18] However, subsequent studies did not demonstrate circulating humoral antibody in affected infants, nor did subsequent studies verify the association between positive mumps skin tests and EFE.[19–21] In either case, the rate of congenital malformations is low, less than 2% in infected or noninfected mothers, and therefore not a strong indication for pregnancy termination.

Mumps acquired in the immediate prenatal or postnatal period is an extremely rare occurrence and may result from transplacental acquisition[22]; no confirmed cases of mumps have been reported following exposure in the neonatal period.

Diagnosis is made by a history of recent exposure followed by the typical clinical presentation of the disease. However, if laboratory confirmation is required, serologic studies or viral isolation should be used. A fourfold rise in antibody titers with the convalescent specimen obtained 1 to 2 weeks after the onset of the illness will confirm the diagnosis. A third specimen at 3 weeks should be obtained if the first two are negative. The mumps skin test lacks sensitivity and specificity and should no longer be used.[23]

Treatment of mumps is symptomatic in pregnant patients, as in nonpregnant patients, and consists of analgesia, bed rest, and hot or cold therapy to affected areas. A live-attenuated mumps vaccine is available and is highly effective in preventing primary mumps. The duration of protection is not known. Immunization with the mumps vaccine is contraindicated in pregnancy based on the theoretical risks of exposure to a live-virus vaccine. However, no fetal infection or injury has ever been documented.

MEASLES

Measles (rubeola) is a paramyxovirus infection that results in an acute illness characterized by fever, coryza, conjunctivitis, cough, and a generalized maculopapular rash. It is the most communicable of the childhood exanthems, but fortunately, if contracted during pregnancy, it does not cause congenital malformations as does rubella (German measles).

Rubeola's morbidity and mortality are most prominent in adults and in infants less than 1 year of age and are usually the result of pneumonia and encephalitis.

While primarily a disease of childhood and adolescence prior to the advent of vaccination of school-age children, it is now being seen more frequently in preschool children and persons over 20 years of age.[24] Still, with recent emphasis in schools on vaccination programs, the incidence of measles should be reduced overall from the prevaccine era report incidence—6 to 40 cases per 100,000 pregnancies.[25]

The virus is spread chiefly by droplets aerosolized by coughing and is acquired by 75% of susceptible exposed individuals.[26] The incubation time is from 10 to 14 days, with a prodrome of fever and malaise starting approximately 10 to 11 days postexposure; this is followed in 24 hours by coryza, sneezing, conjunctivitis, and cough. Photophobia may occur over the next several days, with the pathognomonic Koplik's spots of the buccal mucosa appearing at the end of the prodrome.

The skin rash appears 12 to 14 days after exposure and begins on the head and neck, especially in the postauricular area. The rash subsequently spreads to the trunk and upper extremities, and then eventually to the lower extremities. It usually persists for 3 to 7 days, and disappears in the order of appearance.

Otitis media and croup occur frequently (7–9%), but secondary bacterial pneumonia is the cause of up to 60% of the mortality associated with measles.[27] The overall rate of pneumonia is 1.3 to 5.7% of all measles cases. Measles encephalitis occurs in 1 of every 2,000 reported measles cases, with a 15 to 33% mortality rate.[27] Subacute sclerosing periencephalitis (SSPE) is a rare but serious occurrence, found in 0.6 to 2.2 per 100,000 cases of measles. Its manifestation, though, is seen at an average of 7 years after the acute measles infection. Other rarely occurring complications include appendicitis, myocarditis, thrombocytopenia purpura, and reactivation of previously acquired tuberculosis.[28]

Atypical measles is a severe form of measles reinfection that affects young adults who had been previously vaccinated with a formalin-inactivated, killed measles vaccine, which had been used in the United States from 1963 to 1967.[29] These patients experience particularly high fevers (40–41°C) and develop severe pulmonary complications, including pneumonitis with pulmonary consolidation and pleural effusion. A coarse maculopapular, hemorrhagic, or urticarial rash that resembles Rocky Mountain spotted fever (RMSF) may also occur. A difference from typical measles is that the patient with atypical measles is not contagious to others. Treatment is supportive and the disease is usually self-limited, although hepatic, cardiac, or renal failure may rarely occur.

A modified measles may affect people who have received immune globulin during the incubation period or in infants who have received transplacentally acquired maternal antibody.[30] Modified measles usually is a milder illness, with lower peak temperatures and a rash reduced in intensity and extent.

Although it is unclear whether pregnant women are at greater risk for serious complications from measles than nonpregnant women, the disease in all adults can be quite severe and therefore requires immediate and intensive supportive care. Several studies of large measles epidemics have reported an increased mortality rate among pregnant women, of which pneumonia is the most common cause.[31–34]

Several investigations have suggested an increased rate of prematurity in pregnancies complicated by measles, especially when the disease occurs late in gestation.[33,35–41] However, the prematurity may be related to the severe maternal complications that sometimes necessitate delivery. Earlier reports of an increased risk of spontaneous abortion have not been substantiated.

Because measles is uncommon in pregnancy, it is unclear whether infection during pregnancy has teratogenic potential. Numerous cases of congenital malformations have been reported; however, no distinctive pattern of abnormalities such as that seen with congenital rubella syndrome has been demonstrated.[42] If congenital abnormalities due to measles do exist, they are small and almost always associated with infection in the first trimester.[36]

Measles that develops in an infant in the first 10 days of life is considered transplacental in origin, whereas disease occurring after 14 days was acquired postnatally. Postnatally acquired measles usually follows a milder course, presumably because of the benefit of passively acquired maternal antibodies, as mentioned earlier. Transplacentally acquired measles and postnatally acquired measles in children born to mothers without maternal antibody have a spectrum of illness from mild to rapidly progressing fatal disease. Pneumonia is the most common cause of death, as in adult disease. The mortality rate in infants with congenital measles is 32%, with a similar fatality rate regardless of the rash's presence at birth or subsequent appearance.[34,35,43,44] Premature infants with congenital measles appear to have a significantly higher increased mortality rate (56%) than do term infants (20%). However, these figures on mortality may be drastically reduced

as a result of ever-improving antimicrobial therapy for treatment of the secondary bacterial pneumonia, which often contributes to the cause of the infant mortality.

The diagnosis of measles can be made utilizing a clinical case definition in which there is a fever greater than or equal to 38.3°C, a rash lasting at least 3 days, and cough, coryza, or conjunctivitis. Other causes of rash, including rubella, scarlet fever, meningococcemia, roseola, RMSF, toxoplasmosis, enterovirus infection, and mononucleosis, should be excluded. Laboratory confirmation is available and consists of a fourfold rise or greater of measles antibody titers in acute and convalescent sera or detection of measles-specific IgM antibody.[45]

Uncomplicated measles is usually self-limited and requires only symptomatic care. Complications of otitis media should be treated with antibiotics, and pneumonia may require intensive supportive care and antibiotics for secondary bacterial infection. Aerosolized ribavirin therapy appears to be beneficial.[46] However, the drug is a potential animal teratogen,[47] and aerosolized ribavirin may represent a danger to pregnant health-care personnel; therefore, care should be taken in its administration in an attempt to limit the exposure to pregnant health-care workers.[48] However, its use is usually reserved for seriously ill patients, in whom the risk-benefit ratio is low compared to the significant mortality associated with complicated measles pneumonia and the poor documentation of the drug's teratogenic potential.

If a susceptible pregnant woman exposed to measles presents, immunoglobulin (Ig) at a dose of 0.25 mg/kg body weight should be administered. This may prevent or modify illness in the mother.[49] The benefit of Ig to the fetus is as yet unknown. Prematurity and spontaneous abortion risk should be explained to the patient; however, because of the low, if any, risk of congenital malformation from maternal measles infection, termination is not recommended. Children born to mothers who contracted measles in the week prior to or after delivery should be given Ig, also at a dose of 0.25 mg/kg.[49]

The currently available vaccine is a live, attenuated measles virus vaccine (LMV). It produces a mild or asymptomatic noncommunicable infection. Antibodies develop in at least 95% of susceptible persons, and although the levels are lower than in natural disease and are sometimes nondetectable after several years, it appears that protection is still afforded.[50]

Intrauterine transmission of LMV has not been reported. Every woman of childbearing age should be immune to measles. Immunity can be assumed if the patient has a physician-diagnosed measles infection, laboratory evidence of immunity, or had LVM administration after 1 year of age.[51] Most women born before 1957 have been infected naturally, but if the patient does not meet any of the above criteria, she may be vaccinated if desired. All women who lack evidence of immunity should be vaccinated, except for pregnant women. Women should be advised not to become pregnant for 3 months after vaccination because of the theoretical risk of a live virus; however, no reports of vaccine-related fetal infection have been documented.

Vaccines should not be given to patients who have received a dose of Ig in the last 3 months. Also, as the vaccine is prepared in chicken embryos, a history of anaphylactic reaction to egg products is also a contraindication. Persons with neomycin allergy or any immune altered state such as acquired immune deficiency syndrome (AIDS), malignancy, radiation, or high-dose corticosteroid therapy also should not receive the vaccine.

From 5 to 15% of persons receiving the vaccine have experienced a temperature rise greater than 39.4°C, usually 6 days postvaccination. Transient rashes occur in approximately 5% of vaccines, and encephalitis or encephalopathy have been reported in approximately one per million vaccines.

PARVOVIRUS B19 INFECTION

B19 parvovirus is a single-stranded DNA virus that only recently has been recognized as a cause of serious morbidity in the adult and fetus. B19 was first discovered in sera from healthy blood donors in 1975,[52] but it was not until 1981 that the serious complications of B19 infection were noted in humans.[53]

The virus belongs to the family Parvoviridae, of which there are two vertebrate and one invertebrate genera. B19 is in the genus *Parvovirus*, which was originally believed to comprise only animal parvoviruses such as the canine parvovirus and feline panleukopenia virus. These viruses still tend to be species specific, and human parvovirus infections are generally caused by B19.

B19 has been demonstrated to be the causative agent of erythema infectiousum (EI), or fifth disease,[54-56] and is the primary etiologic agent of transient aplastic crisis (TAC) in patients with chronic hemolytic anemias.[53,56,57] It is also associated with fetal death (both spontaneous abortions and stillbirths),[58-60] acute arthralgias and arthritis,[61,62] and chronic anemia in immunodeficient patients.[63-65]

EI, or fifth disease, usually presents as a mild childhood illness characterized by fever and a facial rash (slapped-face appearance) and a reticulated or lacelike rash on the trunk and extremities.[66]

In adults, the infection is more variable, and may even be absent. Other symptoms such as arthralgias and arthritis-like symptoms, pruritus, or rubella-like exanthems may be present.[66] Approximately 20% of B19 infections, confirmed serologically, may be asymptomatic.[56,67]

B19 transmission is believed to be through respiratory secretions.[56,67] In studies with human volunteers, serum and respiratory secretions become positive for B19 5 to 10 days after intranasal inoculation.[68,69] However, the rash does not occur until 17 to 18 days after inoculation and the confirmed disappearance of the virus from serum or respiratory secretions for at least 1 to 5 days.[68] Thus, the presence of B19 virus in serum or respiratory secretions correlates with infectiousness, and patients presenting with the symptoms of EI are probably past the period of infectiousness.

The transmissibility of the virus is found to be approximately 50 to 90% among susceptible household contacts.[56,67] In school outbreaks, 10 to 60% of students may develop EI, and 20 to 30% of susceptible staff develop serologic evidence of B19 infection.[19] If the infected staff members or any adult is pregnant, vertical transmission from mother to fetus can occur.[52,70] The virus can also be transmitted parenterally by transfusion of infected blood or blood products.[71,72]

Seroprevalence rates range from 2 to 15% in children aged 1 to 5 years, 15 to 60% in children 5–19 years, and 30 to 60% in adults.[66,73–75] Children and adults in confined areas such as schools, day-care centers, and hospitals are more likely to become exposed during outbreaks. These outbreaks often begin in late winter or early spring and may continue for several months.[70]

The risk of fetal death secondary to B19 infection is not exactly known, but preliminary results appear to place it as small. In one study, 174 pregnant women with IgM antibody to B19 were followed prospectively with a fetal loss rate of 17.2% overall.[70] Nineteen percent of 110 women infected during the first 12 weeks, 15% of 46 women infected during weeks 13–20, and 6% of 16 women infected after 20 weeks of pregnancy resulted in fetal death. As there was no control group, not all the fetal deaths can be attributed to B19 infection. Of those fetal deaths linked to B19 infection, tissues from 14 fetal deaths were examined for B19 DNA. Of these, six were positive, two were equivocal, and six were negative. Thus, by extrapolating these results to the remainder of the study populations, an estimated 10% of confirmed B19 infected fetuses will not survive. Antibody studies of the liveborn infants demonstrated

that less than a third of the infected women vertically transmitted the virus to their fetuses.[76]

In an ongoing study conducted by the Centers for Disease Control (CDC), following 95 pregnant women with IgM antibody, fetal loss occurred in 2 (4%) of 49 women delivered to date. One fetus was hydropic while the other was not described. No tissue was examined in either case.[70]

Rodis et al. recently reported the cases of four women who were exposed to B19 virus and who were positive for IgM to B19; three of the four developed hydropic fetuses with fetal loss.[60] In their review of 37 cases of IgM parvovirus-specific antibody-positive pregnant women, 38% had adverse outcomes, of which 11 of 14 (79%) had evidence of hydrops.[60]

Fetal hydrops is probably not a coincidental finding, as the virus has a well-known predilection for the hematopoietic system. B19-associated anemia in adults is often associated with chronic anemias, and Gray et al. have postulated that fetal blood and the blood of patients with chronic hemolytic anemia have similar red-cell kinetics.[77] Fetal blood sampling in an affected fetus demonstrated severe anemia and reticulocytopenia.[70] Conversely, in a review of 50 fetuses with nonimmunologic hydrops fetalis, 4 (8%) were positive for B19 DNA.[79]

Although some of the animal parvoviruses are teratogens,[80] there is little evidence to suggest that B19 infection results in congenital abnormalities. Only one fetus with multiple eye abnormalities[81] and one anacephalic fetus[60] have been reported in B19-infected women, thus the virus cannot be implicated as the causative agent for congenital abnormalities until larger studies are undertaken.

Diagnosis of recent B19 infection can be made by IgM-antibody assay. The B19 IgM antibody can be detected by capture-antibody radioimmunoassay or enzyme immunoassay by the 3rd day after symptoms of EI in 90% of patients.[82,83] Titers begin to decrease in 30 to 60 days after disease onset.

B19 IgG antibody usually becomes positive by day 7 of illness, and persists for years. Assays for B19 DNA are available, but at the present are feasible only for research purposes. Infection in tissue can be demonstrated by Southern or Western blot analysis of B19 DNA and nonstructural proteins.

There is no vaccine available to prevent B19 transmission, and thus the best method to avoid the complications of infection is still prevention. While isolation has been one of the cornerstones of prevention of other viral illnesses, it is usually ineffective and unnecessary with B19 infection, as patients exhibiting signs of EI are probably no longer infectious. However, virus may persist for up to 7 days in patients with TAC; thus isolation strategies are still helpful with this group.

Pregnant women and other people at risk for developing severe complications of B19 infection (i.e., those with chronic anemia or immunodeficient disorders) should be counseled regarding the effects of B19 infection to their fetus or themselves in the event of an outbreak in the workplace (day-care center, school, hospital, etc.). Susceptibility tests can be used to ascertain the risks of B19 acquisition by these patients and to follow up on recent exposures.

For pregnant women with documented recent infection, maternal serum α-fetoprotein levels and serial diagnostic ultrasound examinations should be performed. Fetal hydrops, as it appears to be associated with some severely affected infants, should be closely watched for.[60] If present, consideration of intrauterine blood transfusion may be considered, but there is as yet insufficient data to confirm its efficacy.[84]

ENTEROVIRUSES

Enteroviruses are small RNA viruses and are a subgroup of the picornaviruses. The enteroviruses are classified into three groups: polioviruses, coxsackieviruses, and the echo-viruses (enteric cytopathic human orphan viruses). Recent additions to the enterovirus group do not have specific names and are simply designated by "enterovirus" followed by a number, beginning with 68.[85]

Enterovirus infections show seasonality (June to November) in temperate climates, but are noted year-round in tropical regions. Transmission is predominantly by the fecal-oral route, except for transplacental acquisition and hand-to-eye contact resulting in acute hemorrhagic conjunctivitis.

Infection may occur in any age group; however, severe illness is more frequently seen in the fetus and newborn and in immunosuppressed adults.[86] The incubation period for enteroviruses is usually 3 to 5 days, but may vary from 2 to 20 days. Infectiousness is greatest the few days preceding and immediately following the onset of illness, but may persist for weeks. Infection is often asymptomatic and thus it may be difficult to ascertain the period of infectivity and initiate preventive measures. Reinfection can occur and also may be asymptomatic.[87]

Infection begins with viral replication in the lymphoid tissue of the oropharynx and gut. This phase lasts for 3 days and is symptom free. A viremia follows with spread of the virus to the reticuloendothelial system. In subclinical infection, the process ends here; however, continued viral dissemination to the skin, heart, liver, adrenals, pancreas, or central nervous system results in a subsequent clinically apparent infection. It is at this phase that transplacental infection may occur in pregnant patients.

Antibody formation begins within several days of viral exposure and effectively terminates the viremia. Circulating antibody confers lasting immunity to symptomatic disease, but repeated asymptomatic viral replication can still take place.

The enteroviruses can be isolated from the pharynx, face, cerebrospinal fluid, cord blood, skin vesicles, placenta, serum, and affected organs. They are fairly stable at room temperature and can survive several hours before transfer to the laboratory. Except for the coxsackie A group, most enteroviruses are easily isolated in cell culture and can be reported positive in as early as 18 hours.[85] Typing can be performed utilizing complement fixation (CF), immunofluorescence (EIA), and enzyme-linked immunosorbent assay (ELISA).[88–91]

The incidence of enterovirus infection in pregnancy is not known. However, prospective studies have found a prevalence of 0–9% of pregnant women with viral excretion near delivery.[92–94] However, none of the women with documented excretion developed any symptoms.

When symptoms do occur, a variety of presentations may occur. All the enteroviruses may cause a mild nonspecific illness lasting 2 to 5 days, and a nonexudative pharyngitis with or without lymphadenopathy often occurs. If severe disease follows, coxsackievirus infection in adults may manifest itself as herpangina, lymphomodular pharyngitis, hand-foot-and-mouth disease, rhinopharyngitis, pleurodynia, aseptic meningitis or encephalitis, myocarditis or pericarditis, pneumonia, hepatitis, gastroenteritis, or acute hemorrhagic conjunctivitis.

If continued symptomatology is present with echovirus infection, the clinical manifestations include a febrile illness with rash (Boston exanthem), gastroenteritis, pneumonitis, hepatitis, or aseptic meningitis. Polioviruses are well known to produce paralytic diseases. However, disease may subside after the initial febrile phase (abortive poliomyelitis), and this nonparalytic poliomyelitis is indistinguishable from the previously described coxsackie- and echovirus infections. Differentiation between these three enteroviruses can only be made by laboratory means, and virologic specimens of feces, serum, and CSF should be obtained as soon as possible.

If paralytic disease is to occur, early weakness, hyperesthesia, and muscular pain is followed by rapid loss of motor function, which is usually asymmetric. Weakness and paralysis without sensory loss differentiates poliomyelitis from Guillain-Barré syndrome. Life-threatening poliovirus infection occurs when the respiratory muscles or respiratory center becomes involved. One early report suggests that poliovirus infection may be more severe during pregnancy,[95] and pregnant women with poliovirus infection should be monitored closely.

Poliovirus infection in pregnancy has been demonstrated to cause intrauterine death.[96,97] Abortions and stillbirths following maternal infection with coxsackie- and echoviruses have been reported,[98–101] but the evidence is not as strong as that implicating the poliovirus. Even mild nonparalytic poliomyelitis has been associated with fetal loss; however, there is no evidence that oral polio vaccine received during pregnancy causes an increase in fetal death.

Although premature delivery has been associated with severe maternal enterovirus infection, it is probably related to the severe manifestations of the infection on maternal physiology and not to direct fetal involvement.

While it is difficult to ascertain the risk of congenital abnormalities associated with maternal enterovirus infections during pregnancy because of the small number of reported, documented infections, two studies observed an increased incidence of defects. A variety of defects were found more frequently in 48,000 Finnish mothers with coxsackie B5 infection,[102] as were urogenital anomalies (hypospadias, epispadias, and cryptorchidism), gastrointestinal defects, and cardiovascular lesions in the affected liveborn infants of 22,935 Michigan women with coxsackie B2, B4, and A9 infection respectively, when compared to 1,164 control mothers.[100,103–105] The risk of heart disease increased if the mother acquired more than one coxsackie B infection during pregnancy.[85] However, most of the echoviruses and the coxsackie A viruses have not been found to be associated with congenital abnormalities in several investigations.[106–110]

Severe coxsackievirus infection has been documented in newborns and may occur in coxsackie B, echo-, and poliovirus infections.[111–114] Classically, symptoms begin in the first week of life and presumably represent transplacental acquisition of the virus. Usually the mother will give a history of a recent mild febrile illness,[115] but this is not always present. The onset of the disease in the infant is manifested by a sudden loss of appetite, cough and vomiting, and abrupt development of dyspnea and cyanosis. Signs include marked tachypnea and pallor, followed by cardiac and hepatic enlargement. Electrocardiography often demonstrates evidence of severe myocardial damage. In cases that terminate in death, a grayish pallor and circulatory collapse occur. However, the disease is not uniformly fatal, and recovery may occur just as rapidly. If death does occur, pathologic findings include carditis, pulmonary and cerebral edema, subarachnoid hemorrhage, diffuse vascular congestion, and adrenal hemorrhage.[116,117]

Neonatal disease does not appear to be as severe if maternal infection occurs earlier in pregnancy,[118,119] presumably because of the transplacental passage of maternal antibody.[100,120–123] In four neonatal deaths attributed to echovirus II, delivery was immediately after maternal infection, and neither mother nor infant had type-specific antibody detected.[124]

Postnatal acquisition of enteroviruses by infants is also known to occur commonly, with manifestations similar to the prenatal infection described above.[110] Postnatal infection is believed to occur by maternal fecal contamination at birth, contact with infected hospital personnel or relatives, or nosocomial spread in the nursery.[125,126]

Outbreaks in nurseries are probably more common than reported, as the manifestations of the disease may often be mild, such as sneezing, occasional regurgitation of feeding, and loose stools. A prospective study of 587 infants found that 12.8% acquired enterovirus infection during the first month of life, of which 80% were asymptomatic.[93] Several factors may have modified the disease, such as breast-feeding and maternal serum antibody formation.[100] Thirty of 50 asymptomatic and none of the 13 symptomatic infants had significant type-specific neutralizing antibody titers in cord-blood specimens. Secretory immunoglobulin has also been found in breast milk[127] and may have a protective effect. As expected, premature infants appear to develop more serious enterovirus infection, presumably because of immunologic immaturity.[124] When severe illness occurs, it is often heralded by high fevers (40°C) and it follows the same course in fetal cases as described for prenatal infection.

Attenuated or killed poliovirus vaccines are the only enterovirus vaccines available, because the large number of coxsackie- and echovirus serotypes preclude effective vaccine development. Although no teratogenic or adverse effects have been associated with polio vaccine administration during pregnancy,[128] it is still prudent to delay immunization until after delivery as asymptomatic shedding has been documented after maternal vaccine administration.[129]

Pregnant women planning to travel to endemic areas of the world, however, may consider receiving the vaccine, as wild-virus infection may have serious maternal consequences. Previously unimmunized women should receive three monthly doses of killed vaccine if time permits, or a single dose of trivalent attenuated oral vaccine.[130] Susceptibility to the wild-type can be ascertained by testing for poliovirus antibodies by complement fixation CF.

If the infant is to receive the poliovirus vaccine, the mother needs to be questioned regarding breast-feeding, as breast milk from mothers with high antibody titers has been demonstrated to interfere with successful immunization by oral (live) vaccine in the immediate newborn period.[131]

With viral infections, isolation is often the standard of preventive measures; however, separation of an infected mother or infant is probably not necessary. Isolation from other susceptible neonates, though, may help to prevent outbreaks in nurseries. Enterovirus infections are probably very common in pregnancy and early neonatal life, but fortunately usually produce only mild infection. When severe neonatal disease does occur, mild non-specific maternal symptoms prior to delivery should alert the physician to the possibility of the enteroviral infection so proper testing can be performed and a correct diagnosis ascertained.

WESTERN EQUINE ENCEPHALITIS

Western equine encephalitis (WEE) infection was first recognized in 1930, is found predominantly in the west and southwest United States, and is endemic to the Central Valley of California. WEE is transmitted by mosquitoes and is epidemic in the summer months with cycles utilizing man, horses, and birds as hosts. It is a member of the large group of encephalitis-producing arboviruses and is a member of the togavirus subgroup, which are RNA viruses. WEE infection presents as an influenza-like disease or meningoencephalitis.

Transplacental transmission of WEE has been reported,[132,133] with mothers presenting with symptoms of headache, malaise, and lethargy 3 to 10 days prior to delivery. Infection was confirmed later by positive titers. The babies, apparently well at birth, develop evidence of meningitis at approximately day 5 of life. Although neonates with WEE infection may get severely ill, only one case of permanent neurologic damage has been reported.[134]

Because no vaccine is available and cases are so rare, specific strategies have not been developed, and therefore those mothers diagnosed with WEE infection in late pregnancy should be counseled regarding the early subtle signs and symptoms of neonatal meningitis so prompt symptomatic treatment can be effected.

VENEZUELAN EQUINE ENCEPHALITIS

Venezuelan equine encephalitis (VEE) was first recognized in horses in 1938, and while the majority of cases in humans occurs in Central and South America, cases have been reported in Florida and Texas.[135] VEE is a member of the togavirus group of the encephalitis-producing arboviruses and is transmitted by mosquitoes. Epidemics usually depend on horses and other small mammals as hosts; however, human infection is possible. When human infection does occur, presenting symptoms of an influenza-like disease or signs of encephalitis may be recognized. Maternal infection can result in abortion or congenital malformations, with the resultant damage found in fetal brain tissue.[136,137] Infection in the first trimester is associated with stillbirth, microcephaly, microophthalmia, and severe hypoplasia of the medulla. In two cases with maternal infection at 20 weeks of gestation, the resultant infants were born without a cerebellum and minimal cortical tissue.[134] Also, three cases of VEE infection in the third trimester have been reported, with resultant massive destruction of the neonates' cerebral and cerebellar tissue.[134]

Because no vaccine is available and little is known about the incidence of affected infants due to the rarity of VEE infection, the mother should be treated symptomatically and the patient counseled regarding the severity of the possible neonatal infection.

REFERENCES

1. Kim-Farley RJ: Mumps in pregnancy. In Amstey MS (ed): "Virus Infection in Pregnancy." Orlando, FL: Grune & Stratton, 1984, pp 169–177.
2. Drugman S, Katz SL: "Infectious Disease of Children," 7th edition. St. Louis: C.V. Mosby, 1981, pp 195–207.
3. Bang HO, Bang J: Involvement of the central nervous system in mumps. Bull Hyg 19:503–504, 1944.
4. Hopps HE, Parkman PD: Mumps virus. In: "Diagnostic Procedures for Viral, Rickettsial and Chlamydial Infections," 5th edition. Washington, DC:

American Public Health Association, 1979, pp 633–653.

5. Centers for Disease Control: Mumps Surveillance Report, January 1979–December 1981 (in press).

6. Hope-Simpson RE: Infectiousness of communicalbe diseases in the household. Lancet 549–554, 1952.

7. Bowers D: Mumps during pregnancy. West J Surg Obstet Gynecol 61:72, 1953.

8. Schwartz HA: Mumps in pregnancy. Am J Obstet Gynecol 60:875, 1950.

9. Hardy JB: Viral infection in pregnancy. A review. Am J Obstet Gynecol 93:1052, 1965.

10. Siegel M, Fuerst HT, Peress NS: Comparative fetal mortality in maternal virus disease. A prospective study on rubella, measles, mumps, chicken pox, and hepatitis. N Engl J Med 274:768, 1966.

11. Garcia AG, Periera JM, Vidigal N, et al.: Intrauterine infection with mumps virus. Obstet Gynecol 56:756–759, 1980.

12. Kurtz JB, Tomlinson AH, Pearson J: Mumps virus isolated from a fetus. Br Med J 284:471, 1982.

13. Siegel MS, Fuerst HT: Low birth weight and maternal virus diseases. A prospective study of rubella, measles, mumps, chickenpox, and hepatitis. JAMA 197:680–684, 1966.

14. Manson MM, Logan WPD, Loy RM: Rubella and other virus infections during pregnancy. In Ministry of Health: "Report on Public Health and Medical Subjects," No. 101. London: Her Majesty's Stationery Office, 1960, pp 1–101.

15. Siegel MS: Congenital malformations following chickenpox, measles, mumps and hepatitis: Results of a cohort study. JAMA 226:1521–1524, 1973.

16. Noren GR, Adams P Jr, Anderson RC: Positive skin reactivity to mumps virus antigen in endocardial fibroelastosis. J Pediatr 62:604, 1963.

17. St. Geme JW Jr, Noren GR, Adams P: Proposed embryopathic relation between mumps virus and primary endocardial fibroelastosis. N Engl J Med 275:339, 1966.

18. St. Geme JW Jr, Peralta H, Farias E, et al.: Experimental gestational mumps virus infection and anocardial fibroelastosis. Pediatrics 48:82, 1971.

19. Gersony WM, Katz SL, Nadas AS: Endocardial fibroelastosis and the mumps virus. Pediatrics 37:340, 1966.

20. Guneroth WG: Endocardial fibroelastosis and mumps. Pediatrics 38:309, 1966.

21. Nahmias AJ, Armstrong G: Mumps virus and endocardial fibroelastosis. N Engl J Med 275:1449, 1966.

22. Sever J, White LR: Intrauterine viral infections. Annu Rev Med 19:471–486, 1968.

23. Brunell PA: Mumps. In Wehrle PF, Top FH (eds): "Communicable and Infectious Diseases," 9th edition. St. Louis: C.V. Mosby, 1981, pp 439–443.

24. Amler RW, Bloch AB, Orenstein WA, et al.: Measles in the United States: Chains of transmission. In Campolucci RF (ed): "Proceedings of the 18th Immunization Conference," May 16–20, 1983. Atlanta: Centers for Disease Control, 1983 (in press).

25. Sever J, White LR: Intrauterine viral infections. Annu Rev Med 19:471–486, 1968.

26. Hope-Simpson RE: Infectiousness of communicable diseases in the household (measles, mumps, and chicken pox). Lancet 2:549, 1952.

27. Centers for Disease Control: Measles Surveillance Report No. 11, 1977–1981. Atlanta: Centers for Disease Control, 1982, pp 1–14.

28. Young NA: Chickenpox, measles and mumps. In Remington JS, Klein JO (eds): "Infectious Disease of the Fetus and Newborn Infant." Philadelphia: W.B. Saunders, 1976, pp 521–586.

29. Hinman AR, Koplan JP: Public Health policy toward atypical measles syndrome in the United States. Med Decision Making 2:71–77, 1982.

30. Krugman S, Giles JP, Friedman H, et al.: Studies with a further attenuated live measles-virus vaccine. Pediatrics 31:919–928, 1963.

31. Sweet RL, Gibbs R: "Infectious Diseases of the Female Genital Tract." Baltimore: Williams & Wilkins, 1985, pp 181–226.

32. Amler RW, Bloch AB, Orenstein WA, et al.: Imported measles in the United States. JAMA 248: 2129–2132, 1982.

33. Christensen PE, Schmidt H, Bang HO, et al.: An epidemic of measles in southern Greenland, 1951. Measles in virgin soil: II The epidemic proper. Acta Med Scand 144:430–449, 1953.

34. Dyer I: Measles complicating pregnancy. South Med J 33:601–604, 1940.

35. Kohn JL: Measles in newborn infants (maternal infection). J Pediatr 3:176–180, 1933.

36. Jespersen CS, Littauer J, Sagild U: Measles as a cause of fetal defects. A retrospective study of ten measles epidemics in Greenland. Acta Paediatr Scand 66:367–372, 1977.

37. Manson MM, Logan WPD, Loy RM: Rubella and other viruses during pregnancy. In Ministry of Health: "Report on Public Health and Medical Subjects," No. 101. London: Her Majesty's Stationary Office, 1960, pp 24–26, 75–91.

38. Packer AD: The influence of maternal measles (morbilli) on the unborn child. Med J Aust 1:835–838, 1950.

39. Siegel M, Fuerst HT: Low birth weight and maternal virus diseases. JAMA 197:680–684, 1966.

40. Young NA, Gershon AA: Chickenpox, measles and mumps. In Remington JS, Klein JO (eds): "Infectious Diseases of the Fetus and Newborn Infant." Philadelphia: W.B. Saunders, 1983, pp 375–427.

41. Sever JL, Larsen JW Jr, Grossman JH III: "Handbook of Perinatal Infections." Boston: Little, Brown, 1979, pp 63–64.

42. Siegel M: Congenital malformations following chickenpox, measles, mumps and hepatitis. Results of a cohort study. JAMA 226:1521–1524, 1973.

43. Nouvat JR: Rougeole et grossesse. Thesis 113, Bordeaux, 1904. [As described in Young NA, Gershon AA: Chickenpox, measles and mumps. In Remington JS, Klein JO (eds): "Infectious Diseases of the Fetus and Newborn Infant." Philadelphia: W.B. Saunders, 1983, pp 375–427.]

44. Richardson DL: Measles contracted in utero. RI Med 3:13, 1920.

45. Herrmann KL: Prospects for a more rapid and accurate test for measles. In Campolucci RF (ed): "Proceedings of the 16th Immunization Conference," May 18–21, 1981. Atlanta: Centers for Disease Control 1981, pp 53–54.

46. Sidwell RW: "Clinical Applications of Ribavarin." New York: Academic Press, 1984, p 19.

47. Virazol patent prescribing information. ICN Pharmaceuticals, Costa Mesa, CA, January 1986.

48. Rodriguez WJ, Dang Bui RHD, Connor JD, et al.: Study to assess the environmental exposure of primary personnel to ribavirin aerosol when supervising treatment of infants with RSV infection. Antimicrob Agents Chemother (in press).

49. American Academy of Pediatrics: "Report of the Committee on Infectious Diseases," 17th edition. Evanston, IL: AAP, 1974, pp 74–82.

50. Krugman S: Present status of measles and rubella immunization in the United States: A medical progress report. J Pediatr 90:1–12, 1977.

51. Centers for Disease Control, Immunization Practices Advisory Committee (ACIP): Measles prevention. MMWR 31:217–224, 229–231, 1982.

52. Cossart YE, Field AM, Cant B, Widdows D: Parvovirus-like particles in human sera. Lancet 1:72–73, 1975.

53. Pattison JR, Jones SE, Hodgson J, et al.: Parvovirus infections and hypoplastic crisis in sickle-cell anemia (letter). Lancet 1:664–665, 1981.

54. Anderson MJ, Jones SE, Fisher-Hoch SP, et al.: Human parvovirus, the cause of erythema infectiosum (fifth disease)? (letter). Lancet 1:1378, 1983.

55. Anderson MJ, Lewis E, Kidd IM, Hall SM, Cohen BJ: An outbreak of erythema infectiosum associated with human parvovirus infection. J Hyg (Lond) 93:85–93, 1984.

56. Plummer FA, Hammond GW, Forward K, et al.: An erythema infectiosum-like illness caused by human parvovirus infection. N Engl J Med 313:74–79, 1985.

57. Serjeant GR, Goldstein AR: B19 virus infection and the aplastic crisis. In: Pattison JR (ed): "Parvoviruses and Human Disease." Boca Raton, FL: CRC Press, 1988, pp 85–92.

58. Knott PD, Welply GAC, Anderson MJ: Serologically proved intrauterine infection with parvovirus. Br Med J 289:1660, 1984.

59. Brown T, Anand A, Ritchie LD, Clewley JP, Reid TMS: Intrauterine parvovirus infection associated with hydrops fetalis (letter). Lancet 2:133–134, 1984.

60. Rodis JF, Hovick TJ Jr, Quinn DL, Rosengren SS, Tattersall P: Human parvovirus infection in pregnancy. Obstet Gynecol 72:733–738, 1988.

61. White DG, Woolf AD, Mortimer PP, Cohen BJ, Blake DR, Bacon PA: Human parvovirus arthropathy. Lancet 1:419–421, 1985.

62. Reid DM, Reid TMS, Brown T, Rennie JAN, Eastmond CJ: Human parvovirus-associated arthritis: A clinical laboratory description. Lancet 1:422–425, 1985.

63. Kurtzman GJ, Ozawa K, Cohen B, Hanson G, Oseas R, Young NS: Chronic bone marrow failure due to persistent B19 parvovirus infection. N Engl J Med 317:287–294, 1987.

64. Smith MA, Shah NR, Lobel JS, Cera PJ, Gary GW, Anderson LJ: Severe anemia caused by human parvovirus in a leukemia patient on maintenance chemotherapy. Clin Pediatr 27:383–386, 1988.

65. Kurtzman GJ, Cohen B, Meyers P, Amunullah A, Young NS: Persistent B19 parvovirus infection as a cause of severe chronic anemia in children with acute lymphocytic leukaemia. Lancet 2:1159–1162, 1988.

66. Anderson LJ: Role of parvovirus B19 in human disease. Pediatr Infect Dis J 6:711–718, 1987.

67. Chorba T, Coccia P, Holman RC, et al.: The role of parvovirus B19 in aplastic crisis and erythema infectiosum (fifth disease). J Infect Dis 154:383–393, 1986.

68. Anderson MJ, Higgins PG, Davis LR, et al.: Experimental parvoviral infection in humans. J Infect Dis 152:257–265, 1985.

69. Potter CG, Potter AC, Hatton CSR, et al.: Variation of erythroid and myeloid precursors in the marrow and peripheral blood of volunteer subjects infected with human parvovirus (B19). J Clin Invest 79:1486–1492, 1987.

70. MMWR: 38(6):81–97. February 17, 1989.

71. Mortimer PP, Luban NLC, Kelleher JF, Cohen BJ: Transmission of serum parvovirus-like virus by clotting-factor concentrates. Lancet 2:482–484, 1983.

72. Bartolomei Corsi O, Assi A, Morfini M, Fanci R, Rossi Ferrini P: Human parvovirus infection in haemophiliacs first infused with treated clotting factor concentrates. J Med Virol 25:165–170, 1988.

73. Schwarz TF, Roggendorf M, Deinhardt F: Letter. Lancet 1:739, 1987.

74. Cohen BJ, Buckley MM: The prevalence of antibody to human parvovirus B19 in England and Wales. J Med Microbiol 25:151–153, 1988.

75. Mortimer PP, Cohen BJ, Buckley MM, et al.: Human parvovirus and the fetus (letter). Lancet 2: 1012, 1985.

76. Public Health Laboratory Service Working Party on Fifth Disease: Study of human parvovirus (B19) infection in pregnancy. Commun Dis Rep 87 20:3, 1987.

77. Gray ES, Davidson RJ, Ariand A: Human parvovirus and fetal anemia. Lancet i:1144, 1987.

78. Carrington D, Gilmore DH, Whittle MJ, et al.: Maternal serum alpha-fetoprotein—A marker of fetal aplastic crisis during intrauterine human parvovirus infection. Lancet 1:433–435, 1987.

79. Porter JH, Khong TY, Evans MF, Chan VT-W, Fleming KA: Parvovirus as a cause of hydrops fetalis: Detection by in-situ DNA hybridisation. J Clin Pathol 41:381–383, 1988.

80. Siegl G: Biology and pathogenicity of autonomous parvoviruses. In Berns KI (ed): "The Parvoviruses." New York: Plenum Press, 1984, pp 297–362.

81. Weiland HT, Vermey-Keers C, Salimans MMM, Fleuren GJ, Verwey RA, Anderson MJ: Parvovirus B19 associated with fetal abnormality (letter). Lancet 1:682–683, 1987.

82. Cohen BJ, Mortimer PP, Pereria MS: Diagnostic assays with monoclonal antibodies for the human serum parvovirus-like virus (SPLV). J Hyg (Lond) 91:113–130, 1983.

83. Anderson LJ, Tsou C, Parker RA, et al.: Detection of antibodies and antigens of human parvovirus B19 by enzyme-linked immunosorbent assay. J Clin Microbiol 24:522–526, 1986.

84. Schwarz TF, Roggendorf M, Hottentrager B, et al.: Human parvovirus B19 infection in pregnancy (letter). Lancet 2:566–567, 1988.

85. Jenista JA, Menegus MA: Enteroviruses: Coxsackie, ECHO, and poliovirus. In Amstey MS (ed): "Virus Infection in Pregnancy." Orlando, FL: Grune & Stratton, 1984, pp 1–17.

86. Townsend TR, Bolyard EA, Yolken RH, et al.: Outbreak of coxsackie A1 gastroenteritis: A complication of bone marrow transplantation. Lancet 1:820–823, 1982.

87. Melnick JL: Enteroviruses. In Evans AS (ed): "Viral Infections of Humans. Epidemiology and Control." New York: Plenum Press, 1976, pp 163–207.

88. French MLV, Schmidt NJ, Emmons RW, et al.: Immunofluorescence staining of group B coxsackieviruses. Appl Microbiol 23:54–61, 1972.

89. Yolken RH, Torsch V: Enzyme-linked immunosorbent assay for the detection and identification of coxsackie B antigen in tissue cultures and clinical specimens. J Med Virol 6:45–52, 1980.

90. Yolken RH, Torsch VM: Enzyme-linked immunosorbent assay for detection and identification of coxsackieviruses A. Infect Immun 31:742–750, 1981.

91. Gardner PS, McQuillin J, Grandien M: Picornaviruses. In Gardner PS, McQuillin J, Grandien M (eds): "Rapid Virus Diagnosis. Application of Immunofluorescence," 2nd edition. Boston: Butterworth, 1980, pp 164–173.

92. Jenista JA, Powell KR, Menegus MA: Epidemiology of neonatal enterovirus infection. J Pediatr 104(S):685–690, 1984.

93. Jenista JA, Menegus MA, Powell KR: Epidemiology of neonatal enterovirus infections. Pediatr Res 16:150, 1982 (abstract).

94. Modlin JF, Polk BF, Horton P, et al.: Perinatal echovirus infection: Risk of transmission during a community outbreak. N Engl J Med 305:368–371, 1981.

95. Aycock WL: The frequency of poliomyelitis in pregnancy. N Engl J Med 225:405–408, 1941.

96. Bates T: Poliomyelitis in pregnancy, fetus, and newborn. Am J Dis Child 90:189–195, 1955.

97. Wyatt HV: Poliomyelitis in the fetus and newborn. A comment on the new understanding of the pathogenesis. Clin Pediatr (Phila) 18:33–38, 1979.

98. Ogilvie MM, Tearne CF: Spontaneous abortion after hand-foot-mouth disease caused by coxsackie virus A16. Br Med J 281:1527–1528, 1980.

99. Skeels MR, Williams JJ, Ricker FM: Perinatal echovirus infection. N Engl J Med 305:1529, 1981.

100. Modlin JF: Perinatal echovirus and group B coxsackievirus infections. Clin Perinatol 15(2):233–246, 1988.

101. Horn P: Poliomyelitis in pregnancy. A twenty-year report from Los Angeles County, California. Obstet Gynecol 6:121–137, 1955.

102. Koskimies O, Lapinleimu K, Saxen L: Infections and other maternal factors as risk indicators for congenital malformations: A case-control study with paired serum samples. Pediatrics 61: 832–837, 1978.

103. Brown GC: Maternal virus infection and congenital anomalies. A prospective study. Arch Environ Health 21:362–365, 1970.

104. Brown GC, Evans TN: Serologic evidence of coxsackievirus etiology of congenital heart disease. JAMA 199:151–155, 1967.

105. Brown GC, Karunas RS: Relationship of congenital anomalies and maternal infection with selected enteroviruses. Am J Epidemiol 95:207–217, 1972.

106. Cherry JD: Enteroviruses. In Remington JS, Klein JO (eds): "Infectious Diseases of the Fetus and Newborn Infant." Philadelphia: W.B. Saunders, 1983, pp 290–344.

107. Elizan TS, Ajero-Froelich L, Fabiyi A, et al.: Viral infection in pregnancy and congenital CNS malformations in man. Arch Neurol 20:115–119, 1969.

108. Kurent JE, Sever JL: Perinatal infections and epidemiology of anecephaly and spina bifida. Teratology 8:359–362, 1973.

109. Heinonen OP, Shapiro S, Monson RR, et al.: Immunization during pregnancy against poliomyelitis and influenza in relation to childhood malignancy. Int J Epidemiol 2:229–235, 1973.

110. Moss PD, Heffernan CK, Thurston JG, et al.: Enteroviruses and congenital abnormalities. Br Med J 1:110–111, 1967.

111. Baker DA, Phillips CA: Maternal and neonatal infection with coxsackievirus. Obstet Gynecol 55(Suppl):12–15, 1980.

112. Berkovich S, Smithwick EM: Transplacental infection due to ECHO virus type 22. J Pediatr 72:94–96, 1968.

113. Eilard T, Kyllerman M, Wennerblom I, et al.: An outbreak of coxsackie virus type B2 among neonates in an obstetrical ward. Acta Paediatr Scand 63:103–107, 1974.

114. Rantakallio P, Lapinleimu K, Mantyjarvi R: Coxsackie B5 outbreak in a newborn nursery with 17 cases of serous meningitis. Scand J Infect Dis 2:17–23, 1970.

115. Lake AM, Lauer BA, Clark JC, et al.: Enterovirus infections in neonates. J Pediatr 89:787–791, 1976.

116. Bates JR Jr: Coxsackie virus B3 calcific pancarditis and hydrops fetalis. Am J Obstet Gynecol 106:629–630, 1970.

117. Skeels MR, Williams JJ, Ricker FM: Perinatal echovirus infection. N Engl J Med 305:1529, 1981.

118. Jenista JA, Prather S, Menegus MA: Determinants of severity of neonatal enterovirus infection. Am J Dis Child 137:532, 1983 (abstract).

119. Modlin JF, Polk BF, Horton P, et al.: Perinatal echovirus infection: Risk of transmission during a community outbreak. N Engl J Med 305:368–371, 1981.

120. Agarwal SC, Sehgal JNS, Gupta AN: Placental transmission of neutralizing antibodies to poliomyelitis virus. Indian J Med Res 59:1703–1707, 1971.

121. Arya SC: Poliomyelitis antibodies in normal immunoglobulin preparation from placental blood. J Commun Dis 12:100–101, 1980.

122. Evans HE, Millian SJ, Glass L: Antibody titers to measles, rubella, and poliomyelitis in umbilical cord serum. Obstet Gynecol 42:596–598, 1973.

123. Mukherjee P, Sengupta KP, Mukherjee KL: Passage of poliovirus antibodies across the placental barrier. Indian J Med Res 71:840–846, 1980.

124. Modlin JF: Fatal echovirus 11 disease in premature neonates. Pediatrics 66:775–780, 1980.

125. McDonald LL, St. Geme JW, Arnold BH: Nosocomial infection with ECHO virus type 31 in a neonatal intensive care unit. Pediatrics 47:995–999, 1971.

126. Brightman VJ, Scott TFM, Westphal M, et al.: An outbreak of coxsackie B-5 virus infection in a newborn nursery. J Pediatr 69:179–192, 1966.

127. Melnick JL, Clarke NA, Kraft LM: Immunological reactions of the coxsackie viruses: III. Cross-protection tests in infants born of vaccinated mothers. Transfer of immunity through the milk. J Exp Med 92:499–505, 1950.

128. Prem KA, Fergus JW, Mathers JE, et al.: Vaccination of pregnant women and young infants with trivalent oral attentuated live poliomyelitis vaccine. In: "Second International Conference on Live Poliovirus Vaccines." Washington, DC: Pan American Sanitary Bureau, 1960.

129. Plotkin SA, Katz M, Brown RE, et al.: Oral poliovirus vaccination in newborn African infants. Am J Dis Child 111:27–30, 1966.

130. Centers for Disease Control: Poliomyelitis prevention. MMWR 31:22–34, 1982.

131. Warren RJ, Lepow ML, Bartsch GE, et al.: The relationship of maternal antibody, breast feeding and age to the susceptibility of newborn infants to infection with attentuated polioviruses. Pediatrics 34:4–13, 1964.

132. Cops SC, Giddings LE: Transplacental transmission of western equine encephalitis. Report of a case. Pediatrics 24:31–33, 1959.

133. Shinefield HR, Townsend TE: Transplacental transmission of western equine encephalomyelitis. J Pediatr 43:21–25, 1953.

134. Sweet RL, Gibbs RS: "Infectious Diseases of the Female Genital Tract II." Baltimore: Williams & Wilkins, 1985, p 204.

135. Doherty RL: Viral encephalitis in infectious diseases. In Hoeprich PD (ed): "Infectious Diseases," 2nd edition. Hagerstown, MD: Harper and Row, 1977, pp 919–927.

136. Spertzel RO, Crabbs CL, Vaughn RE: Transplacental transmission of Venezuelan equine encephalomyelitis virus in mice. Infect Immun 6:339–343, 1972.

137. Wenger F: Venezuelan equine encephalitis. Teratology 16:369, 1977.

21

Protozoan Diseases in Pregnancy

Joseph G. Pastorek II, M.D.

The obstetrician practicing in the United States may feel that protozoan diseases are uncommon accompaniments of pregnancy. After all, this is a developed country, with fairly successful pest control, food processing, water purification, and personal hygiene. Of course, indigent patients in inner-city teaching hospitals may contract some of these diseases; this only improves the quality of the learning experiences of the students and house officers. Private practitioners, however, may believe that they will never see protozoan illnesses, especially complicating pregnancy. Nothing could be further from the truth.

Pathogenic protozoan organisms may appear in the "private" obstetric patient through a variety of mechanisms. Most commonly, one considers *Trichomonas vaginalis* in conjunction with other bacterial and fungal sources of vaginitis and cervicitis. In reality, however, it is a protozoan, and it is known to be widespread among private as well as public patients. The problematic microorganism *Toxoplasma gondii*, one of the so-called TORCH infectious agents, is also a protozoan. Endemic in areas of the Mississippi River valley, toxoplasmosis is a not-uncommon consideration in any pregnant woman with unexplained lymphadenopathy or neonate with the TORCH syndrome. *T. gondii* is usually thought of as an organism common to individuals living in rural areas; the rodent and feline vectors, though, are hardly strangers to the inner-city dweller. The more exotic of the protozoan microbes may be more of a surprise to the physician.

A pregnant woman in the middle trimester who has taken a recent excursion to Moscow (where she "drank the water" against the usual medical advice) presents with bloating and vague abdominal pains. A change in bowel habits stimulates her doctor to order a stool examination, basically as an afterthought. The identification of *Giardia lamblia* in the specimen precludes further investigation, such as ultrasonography of the gallbladder, for more mundane disorders. A colleague in a nearby city, meanwhile, is in the midst of a workup on a patient for hepatitis, nothing unsuspected in this immigrant from Southeast Asia who has family members positive for hepatitis B surface antigen. The picture changes when an alert hematology laboratory technician spots parasites of *Plasmodium vivax* in a peripheral smear during a routine white blood cell differential. Finally, a patient in the third trimester under-

Infections in Pregnancy, pages 221–245
© 1990 Alan R. Liss, Inc.

TABLE 1. Protozoan Diseases and Their Etiologic Agents

Disease entity	Microorganism
Amebiasis	*Entamoeba histolytica*
Babesiosis	*Babesia microti*
	B. divergens
	B. bovis
African sleeping sickness	*Trypanosoma brucei*
Chagas' disease	*Trypanosoma cruzi*
Cutaneous and mucocutaneous	*Leishmania tropica*
leishmaniasis	*L. braziliensis*
	L. mexicana
Visceral leishmaniasis	*Leishmania donovani*
(kala-azar)	
Giardiasis	*Giardia lamblia*
Malaria	*Plasmodium ovale*
	P. vivax
	P. malariae
	P. falciparum
Pneumocystis pneumonia	*Pneumocystis carinii*
Toxoplasmosis	*Toxoplasma gondii*
Trichomoniasis[a]	*Trichomonas vaginalis*

[a]Discussed in chapter 4.

goes cesarean delivery for a syndrome of intravascular hemolysis and fever. The delivery is effected with thoughts of HELLP syndrome, hemolytic-uremic syndrome, and thrombotic thrombocytopenic purpura. With little more than supportive care and some head scratching by the physicians of record, the patient slowly recovers. By serendipity, a new medical student on the service elicits the history of travel to Martha's Vineyard and environs in the month preceding the onset of the patient's illness. A retrospective review of Wright's stained thin blood smears in the hematology lab nails the diagnosis of *Babesia microti* infection.

These three hypothetical cases illustrate possible ways in which patients with protozoan diseases may present to the unsuspecting physician. It is therefore imperative that such organisms as listed in Table 1 and the diseases they cause be familiar to the obstetrician in the United States, and indeed in any developed country. It is not only the third world that experiences the disability and morbidity resulting from infection by these single-celled animals. This chapter is a short overview of the diseases listed in Table 1, with the ex-

ception of *Trichomonas vaginalis*, which is covered in chapter 4. Exhaustive coverage of each disease may be found in some of the cited references.

AMEBIASIS

The human intestinal tract may serve as home for a number of protozoan organisms. Examination of stool specimens from healthy individuals may reveal such microbes as *Entamoeba hartmanni*, *E. coli*, *E. polecki*, *Iodamoeba butschlii*, and *Endolimax nana*. Although the organism *Dientamoeba fragilis* is arguably a human pathogen (and will not be considered further in this discussion), the prime agent of human intestinal and extraintestinal amebiasis is the mobile ameba *Entamoeba histolytica*.[1]

E. histolytica is a member of the group of protozoa of the subphylum Sarcodina, organisms who form pseudopodia for motility (as opposed to flagella, common to the trichomonads and other similar organisms). As early as 1875, *E. histolytica* was documented to cause enteric lesions in an animal model,[2] while in 1886 it was shown to be the etiologic agent of intestinal and extraintestinal lesions in humans with diarrheal disease.[3] A primary reason that the organism is available to cause human disease to any great degree is the fact that up to 40% of individuals in tropical climes, and even 5% of persons in temperate areas, may be infected with the ameba, allowing overt disease to develop when the circumstances are favorable.

As with many other infectious diseases, certain high-risk groups exhibit the organism more frequently than the population in general. Patients in mental institutions, male homosexuals, immigrants from endemic areas (e.g., Mexico and Central America), and persons traveling to endemic areas all have been documented to have a variably higher prevalence of the organism.[4]

Pathophysiology

E. histolytica can live within the bowel lumen and large mucosal crypts of the colon

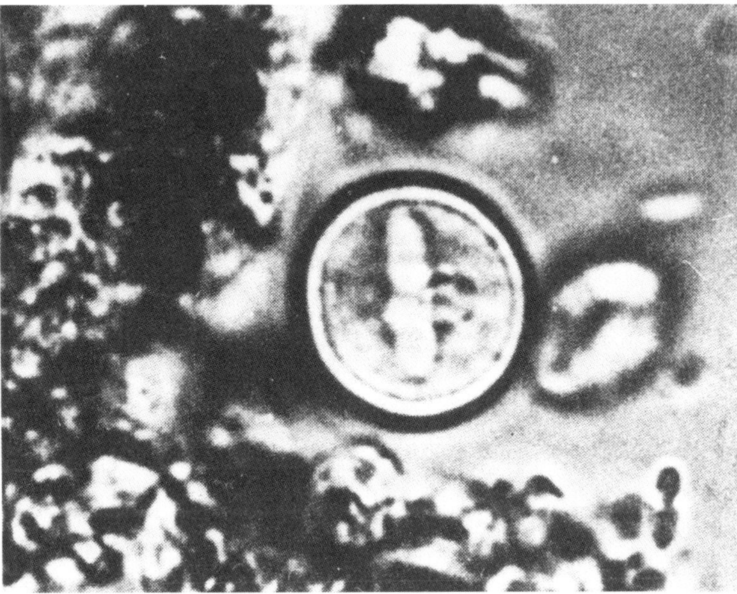

Fig. 1. Typical cyst of *Entamoeba histolytica* in a direct fecal smear. (From the Louisiana State University Medical Center.)

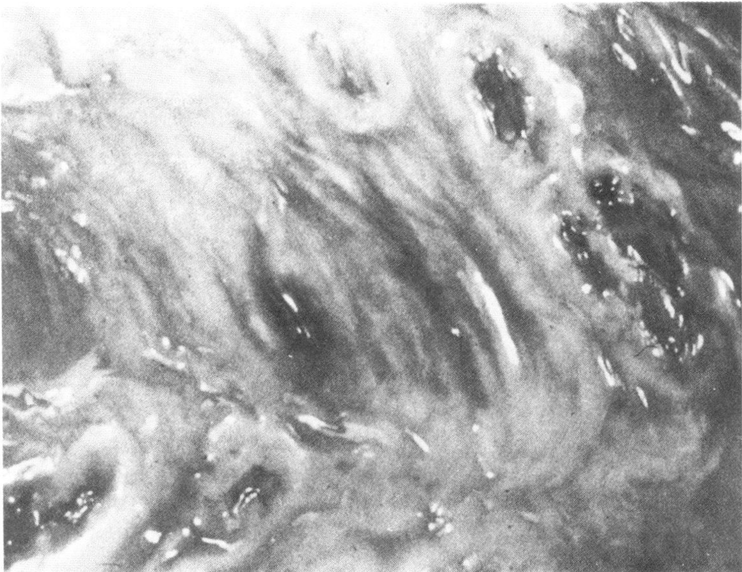

Fig. 2. Amebic ulcers of the large bowel. Note the characteristic raised margins. (From the Louisiana State University Medical Center.)

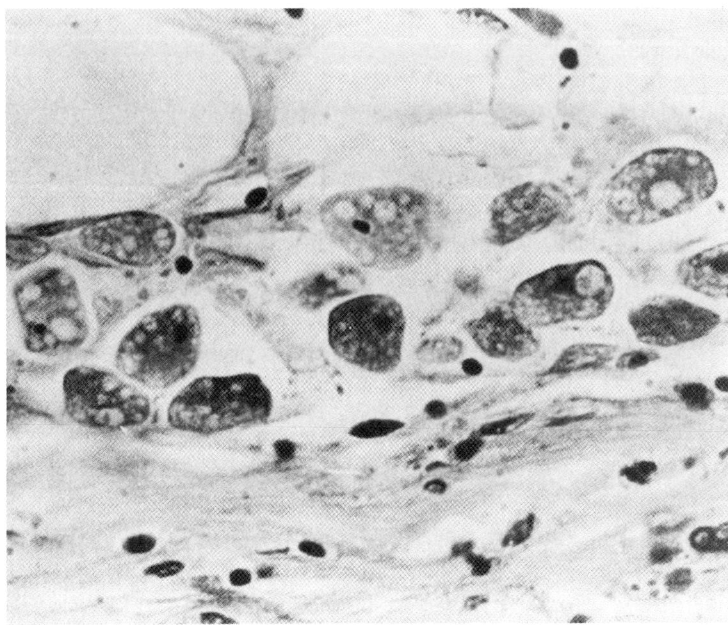

Fig. 3.   Trophozoites of *Entamoeba histolytica* invading the submucosa of the colon. (From the Louisiana State University Medical Center.)

without causing disease. The only evidence of the organism in such circumstances is the demonstration of the cyst form in fecal smears (Fig. 1). The cyst is the hardy form of the organism most resistant in unfavorable environments, usually forming in the bowel lumen for as-yet poorly understood reasons and subsequently being excreted to the outside of the body. However, if conditions are right, the cyst matures through three nuclear divisions and releases eight trophozoites, usually under the stimulus of passing through the small intestine of a new host. This form of the parasite is fragile, perishing rapidly under adverse conditions of low pH and enzymatic degradation in the small intestines.[4]

It is estimated that up to 75% of intestinal carriers of the organism are asymptomatic at any given instant, though an individual may shift over time from the asymptomatic carrier state to one of the invasive forms of the disease. The most common form of symptomatic disease, found in perhaps 20% of patients harboring *E. histolytica*, is chronic, or non-dysenteric, amebiasis. This syndrome consists of diarrhea of varying degree, abdominal cramping, flatulence, nausea, distension, and anorexia. There may be mucous stools, but no blood is present. Physical findings may include cecal tenderness and gaseous distension. The clinical signs and symptoms are the result of the invasion of the colonic mucosa by the amebas through their ameboid movement and secretion of proteolytic, cytopathic toxins. Classically, ulcers with raised margins may be seen in the large intestine (Fig. 2), which will histologically demonstrate trophozoites invading the submucosa (Fig. 3). If not adequately investigated for ameba, patients with this form of amebiasis are often misdiagnosed as having one of the common forms of inflammatory bowel disease.[5]

Preceding this chronic form of infection, or in some cases following it, is the syndrome of acute or dysenteric amebiasis, affecting approximately 5% of persons infected with the organism. This infection progresses over several days from abdominal cramping and loose stools to overt dysentery, i.e., marked diarrhea with stools composed of blood and mucus. Depending upon the severity of the colonic ulceration, necrotic debris may be present in the feces as well. If the disease progresses unchecked, the patient may suffer fever, dehydration, severe cramping (colic), and even gangrene of the colon; associated occurrences of hemorrhage, perforation, peritonitis in 3 to 4% of cases, and intraabdominal abscess are reported. Obviously, death is a possibility in severe cases. The severity and ultimate outcome of the illness and its sequelae may depend to a large degree upon the intrinsic health and constitution of the patient.[6]

If excessive production of granulation tissue follows ulceration in either form of infection mentioned above, a chronic inflammatory mass, or ameboma, which simulates intestinal neoplasm or paracolonic abscess but which is basically curable by antiamebic chemotherapy, may develop. These lesions may be single or multiple, usually involving the cecum and ascending colon.[4]

Extraintestinal amebiasis may affect the skin, especially about the anus in cases of intestinal disease, the lung, the brain, and most commonly the liver. Many patients presenting with amebic liver abscess have no history of diarrheal disease; indeed, the weight loss, abdominal findings, fever, and hepatomegaly suggest a neoplastic process, unless an antecedent or concurrent intestinal malady is appreciated. Usually in the right lobe, amebic liver abscesses are not commonly associated with massive changes in liver profile chemistries, but there is an anemia, leukocytosis, and shift to the left. In cases where the hepatic transaminases are markedly abnormal and the bilirubin level rises abruptly, multiple abscesses (Fig. 4) and more severe disease are generally noted. Rupture of the abscess into adjacent spaces (e.g., pleura, peritoneum) produces marked worsening of the patient's condition for obvious reasons. In fact, while uncomplicated amebic liver ab-

scess has a mortality rate of 0.7%, rupture into the chest, peritoneal cavity, or pericardium increases the mortality rate to 6.2, 18.4, or 29.6%, respectively.[4,7]

Pregnancy Considerations

Because ameba can defend themselves against antiamebic antibody, humoral immunity does not appear to be protective against infection.[8] However, cell-mediated immunity seems to be protective against amebic invasion. For this reason, depression of cell-mediated immunity by such factors as corticosteroid therapy or pregnancy favors more fulminant disease.[4] The adverse course of amebic colitis in pregnancy has been ascribed to the increase in circulating cholesterol, a known growth requirement of the organism, and/or a detrimental effect of increased cortisol.[9] On the other hand, amebic liver abscess appears to be less frequent during pregnancy, perhaps because of a protective effect of estrogen.[4]

In any event, women who present with amebiasis in pregnancy are at greater risk of fulminant disease than nonpregnant women and men. Transplacental infection is not reported; however, the dehydration and nutritional deprivation that may accompany invasive disease can theoretically lead to intrauterine growth retardation. In addition, acute febrile illnesses of any kind may, through a variety of pathways, lead to premature labor or premature rupture of the membranes.[10] Also, the infant may acquire the organism at the time of vaginal delivery or during the neonatal period by exposure to the mother and other infected family members.

Diagnosis

Cysts or trophozoites of *E. histolytica* demonstrated in stool specimens confirms the diagnosis of intestinal amebiasis. There is some controversy as to whether the degree of symptomatology in the patient correlates with the presence of cysts alone (asymptomatic) or cysts with trophozoites (symptomatic). In any case, multiple fecal specimens must be obtained. Approximately one-third

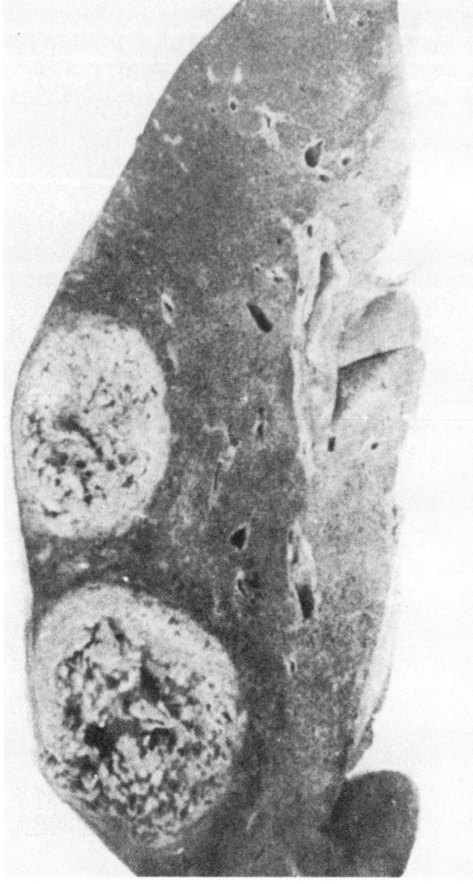

Fig. 4. Gross appearance of multiple amebic liver abscesses in an autopsy specimen. Note that the abscesses are relatively well localized, leaving distant hepatic parenchyma uninvolved. (From the Louisiana State University Medical Center.)

of cases will be detected by examination of one stool specimen, over 80% with three specimens, and over 90% with six, though this is not routinely practiced. Detection may be interfered with by previous antiamebic therapy, radiologic barium, oil enemas, or medications such as kaolin-pectin, bismuth, or magnesium hydroxide.[4] Fresh stool may also be inoculated in egg enrichment medium for culture of the parasites.

Specimens from proctoscopic, sigmoidoscopic, or colonoscopic examinations may be processed as scrapings for fresh examination or fixed in formalin for histologic preparation. It should be remembered that the cecum is a favorite site for the infestation, therefore anything less than colonoscopic is not necessarily definitive.

Serologic evaluation is occasionally helpful in the diagnosis of amebiasis. Patients with presumed inflammatory bowel disease should have amebic serology investigated, since over three-fourths of patients with invasive intestinal disease have positive serology.[11] However, it should be noted that most patients with noninvasive disease, i.e., asymptomatic cyst passers, have negative antibody titers. As well, antibody levels from one acute invasive episode of amebiasis may remain elevated for some time, obscuring the serological response to a second insult.

Therapy

The primary method of treatment of amebiasis is prevention. Because the organism usually gains access to the human gastrointestinal tract through fecal contamination of food and water, control of flies and other insects that frequent feces is paramount. The most common foods contaminated directly from soil, especially in areas where human excrement is used as fertilizer, are vegetables that are grown on the ground, such as lettuce. Vegetables of this type must be either boiled, as should suspect water, or treated with a strong detergent and subsequently soaked in vinegar (or acetic acid) for a quarter of an hour. Besides boiling, public water may be purified of ameba by sedimentation and filtration; chlorination at the usual commercial levels will not eliminate the cysts.[3,4]

Besides general supportive care, depending upon the severity of the fluid loss and other manifestations of amebiasis, therapy of infection with *E. histolytica* is based upon amebicidal antibiotics. Antiamebic therapy may be divided into two basic types of medications: intraluminal drugs, active only within the intestinal tract, and tissue drugs, active at achievable blood levels and useful for therapy of extraintestinal amebiasis, including ame-

TABLE 2. Therapy for Amebic Infections

Clinical disease	Efficacy (%)
Asymptomatic intestinal carriage	
Diloxanide furoate (500 mg t.i.d. for 10 days)	87–96
Tetracycline (250 mg q.i.d. for 10 days) then diiodohydroxyquin (650 mg t.i.d. for 20 days)	95
Metronidazole (750 mg t.i.d. for 10 days)	90
Paromomycin (30 mg/kg day, t.i.d. for 5–10 days)	—
Invasive amebic colitis	
Metronidazole (750 mg t.i.d. for 5–10 days)	>90
(2.4 g daily for 2–3 days)	>90
(50 mg/kg for one dose)	86
plus diloxanide or diiodohydroxyquin	
Tetracycline (250 mg q.i.d. for 15 days) plus chloroquin	94
Dehydroemetine (1.0–1.5 mg/kg/day for 5 days) plus diloxanide or diiodohydroxyquin	90
Amebic liver abscess	
Metronidazole (750 mg t.i.d. for 5–10 days or 2.4 g daily for 1–2 days) plus diloxanide or diiodohydroxyquin	95
Dehydroemitine (1.0–1.5 mg/kg/day for 5 days)	90
Chloroquine (base) (600 mg daily for 2 days, 300 mg daily for 2–3 weeks) (may be used in combination with other regimens)	60

Adapted from Ravdin and Jones.[4]

bic liver abscess. Importantly, no drug is active against the cyst form of the organism, only against the trophozoites.

Drugs useful against the various clinical presentations of amebiasis are listed in Table 2. Several points must be remembered, however, when dealing with these medications. The obstetrician must be aware that drugs relatively useful in pregnancy are paromomycin, chloroquine, and metronidazole. However, chloroquine is only active in the liver and hence cannot be relied upon in extrahepatic infection. Paromomycin is only active luminally. And some physicians are hesitant to use metronidazole in the first trimester, leading them to perhaps manage mild cases expectantly until later in pregnancy. However, the use of any drug for amebiasis in any trimester must be tempered with the knowledge that amebiasis may be severe, even lethal, to the pregnant woman.

BABESIOSIS

Infection in domestic animals with the various species of *Babesia* has been known for centuries. Some feel that the plague on the Egyptians' cattle, horses, and mules, which spared the animals of Israel and, in part, allowed the exodus out of Egypt, was babesiosis.[12] In a more modern vein, babesiosis was the first infection shown to be carried by arthropods, when Texas cattle fever, due to *Babesia bigemina*, was proved to be transmitted by ticks in 1893.[13] In any event, either because of an absolute increase in disease incidence or, more likely, a higher index of physician suspicion and hence reporting bias, babesiosis is being seen with increasing frequency in parts of the United States and Europe.

Pathophysiology

Babesia organisms are intraerythrocytic parasites of domesticated and wild animals. The organisms may be transmitted to humans by ticks. In Europe, the majority of cases, which occur sporadically and in quite varied geographical areas, are caused by *B. divergens*. This species is a parasite of cattle and is probably transmitted by the tick *Ixodes ricinus*. In the United States, *B. microti* is the usual cause of babesiosis. This protozoan is transmitted by the tick *I. dammini*, which feeds on rodents and deer.[14] Cases in the United States are generally acquired on the islands along the Atlantic coasts of Massachusetts and New York State, including Martha's Vineyard, Nantucket, Long Island, and Shelter Island. Besides tick-borne infection, babesiosis in the United States is also spread through blood transfusion.[15]

Babesia organisms gain access to the human bloodstream by way of an insect bite or infected blood transfusion. Once in the bloodstream, the parasite invades erythrocytes, maturing and reproducing by budding (without an extracellular sexual stage, as in *Plasmodium* infection). The erythrocytes ultimately rupture, releasing organisms to infect other red cells. As is the case with other blood-borne infections, the spleen plays an important role in the modification of the illness. In fact, the European form of the disease is found almost exclusively in asplenic patients. In addition, infection in older patients seems to be more severe. Even in the presence of a functional spleen, however, chronic parasitemia has been documented, even in the absence of clinical illness.[16]

Although many patients infected with *B. microti* remain asymptomatic throughout their infection, babesiosis, after an incubation period of 1 to 2 weeks, manifests as a febrile illness characterized by rigors, fatigue and malaise, diaphoresis, and myalgias. Hepatosplenomegaly is also common. Hemolysis and hemoglobinuria, even unto renal failure from acute tubular necrosis, may result from the destruction of red cells by the actively reproducing organisms. The white blood cell count may be normal or low, and elevated levels of liver enzymes and serum bilirubin are the rule. The hemolysis and quantitative parasitemia are generally worse in asplenic patients, though most patients recover eventually.[17] In contrast, infection with *B. divergens* is almost always fatal and, as stated above, is usually found in individuals who have undergone splenectomy. The clinical illness is not unlike the illness due to *B. microti*, only severe and fulminant.

Babesiosis has not been often described in pregnant women, so it is not certain whether the organism does or does not cross the placenta. Anecdotal reports indicate that the infant is unaffected,[18] although it is not unreasonable to expect that, given enough cases, transplacental spread will be encountered. This certainly happens in cases of malaria, and it is logical that minute transpla-cental hemorrhages, so common in the latter stages of pregnancy, would allow maternal parasites access to the fetal circulation. Since maternal infection may be relatively subclinical on the one hand, or maternal parasitemia may be fairly chronic, it would not be unexpected that cases of fetal disease may arise in endemic areas in apparently healthy pregnant women. Extrapolating from the pathophysiology of adult illness, it is tempting to predict that fetal babesiosis will present most dramatically as nonimmune hydrops, perhaps occurring in women with a history of travel to or residence in an endemic area or a history of blood transfusion. Fetal disease has been described in animals and resembles hemolytic disease of the newborn.[19]

Diagnosis

Babesiosis should be suspected in a patient presenting with the appropriate clinical illness, e.g., fever, hemolysis, and other manifestations mentioned above, who relates a history of travel to an endemic area, especially if a history of tick bite can be elicited. Thick or thin blood smears may be stained by the Giemsa method to demonstrate the intraerythrocytic parasites, which resemble young trophozoites of *Plasmodium falciparum*. The organisms may be grown in laboratory hamsters or gerbils for identification purposes. Serologic testing is possible, though not clinically useful, because the parasites may be directly viewed with relative ease, and cross reactions may occur between *Babesia* and *Plasmodium* organisms.[20]

Therapy

Aside from supportive care for the acute illness, therapies for babesiosis are few. Severe disease has been treated partially by exchange transfusion, presumably effective because of physical removal of the microorganisms from the patient's bloodstream by removal of the bloodstream itself.[15] Various antiprotozoal antibiotics, such as chloroquine[21] and pentamidine,[22] have been tried without definitive clinical success. However, the combination of clindamycin (600 mg t.i.d. for 1 week) and quinine (650 mg t.i.d. for 1 week) has shown some promise.[23] Clindamycin is relatively harmless in pregnancy; however, quinine is potentially ototoxic to the fetus, may incite uterine contractions, and has been associated with marked maternal hypoglycemia when used during pregnancy.[24]

In any event, babesiosis in the United States, due to *B. microti*, is rarely fatal and is apparently managed satisfactorily without antibiotics, whether during pregnancy or not.[18,25] European disease due to *B. divergens*, on the other hand, is almost uniformly fatal.

TRYPANOSOMIASIS

The flagellate protozoans of the genus *Trypanosoma* make up a large group of pathogenic organisms, only two of which infect man. In the New World, *T. cruzi* is the etiologic agent of Chagas' disease, or American trypanosomiasis, an acute and chronic illness found in tropical areas of Central and South America and Mexico.[26] In equatorial Africa, the *T. brucei* complex, consisting of *T. brucei gambiense* and *T. brucei rhodesiense*, are the causes of Gambian, or chronic, sleeping sickness (West African trypanosomiasis) and Rhodesian, or acute, sleeping sickness (East African trypanosomiasis).[27]

Organisms of this genus progress through different morphologic states—the amastigote, epimastigote, and trypomastigote—in the various animal hosts. However, not all forms are present in any given host. In Chagas' disease, *T. cruzi* lives in the human as an intracellular amastigote, often called the "leishmanial form" because it resembles *Leishmania* species. In sleeping sickness, *T. brucei* is present in the bloodstream in the trypomastigote stage.[26]

Trypanosomes are separated into two groups depending upon the location of the completion of their development. The Stercoraria group completes development in the

hindgut of their hematophagic insect vector, the triatomine Reduviidae bugs (also called the "kissing bug" because bites occur primarily about the lips and face while the victim sleeps). Infection occurs when insect feces containing the trypanosomes contaminate the bite sites.[28] The other group, the Salivaria, completes development in the salivary glands of tsetse flies (*Glossina* sp.). An infectious trypomastigote form is inoculated into the victim directly when the fly feeds.[29]

Pathophysiology

In Chagas' disease, clinical illness takes two distinct forms. The acute phase of the disease, which is most commonly seen in children, is only clinically evident in a very small percentage of persons infected by the organism and is characterized by a local inflammatory reaction, or chagoma, at the site of the initial insect bite, with swelling and enlargement of the regional lymph nodes draining that area. If there is significant conjunctivitis and edema of the eyelids and face, accompanied by lacrimal gland and related nodal enlargement, Romana's sign, or the oculoglandular complex, may be apparent (Fig. 5). Interstitial edema, parasitism of tissue macrophages, and lymphocytic infiltration are histologically demonstrated in the affected area. The organisms then disseminate, producing a clinical syndrome of fever, hepatosplenomegaly, and lymphadenopathy. During parasitemia, the protozoans may infect a variety of cell types; however, there is a marked tropism for smooth and cardiac muscle, as well as glial cells. The acute disease syndrome therefore often includes myocarditis, with attendant cardiac dilation and failure. Severe meningoencephalitis occurs in a small percentage of patients with acute disease. Severe myocarditis and CNS infection are the main causes of mortality with acute infection. Healing occurs without scarring or fibrosis over weeks or months. The lymphadenopathy and organomegaly may persist for weeks. Mortality from the acute

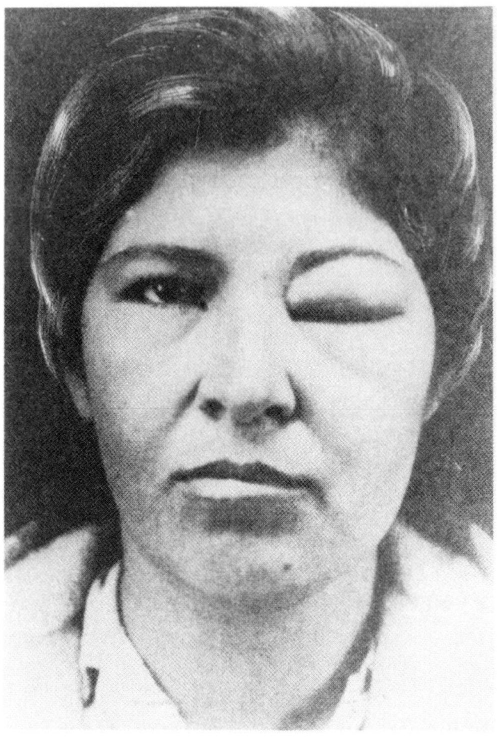

Fig. 5. Romana's sign—the ophthalmoglandular complex—in a patient with acute Chagas' disease. (From Strickland,[1] with permission of the publisher.)

infection is roughly 10%, especially in children.[26,28]

After survival from the acute infection, or an initial asymptomatic infestation, the blood is cleared of the trypanomastigotes as immunity rises. However, intracellular amastigotes remain viable, a source of intermittent parasitemia. This phase of the disease is called the indeterminate phase. After months or years of asymptomatic "carriage" of the organism, symptoms of chronic Chagas' disease arise. The cardiac muscle and smooth muscle of the gastrointestinal system, and occasionally the bladder, are usually involved. Cardiomegaly/cardiomyopathy may result in arrhythmias, failure, thrombi, and all the signs and symptoms appropriate for those circumstances. Effects on the intestinal smooth muscle lead to the so-called "me-

gasyndromes," such as megaesophagus and megacolon. Biopsy of these organs will demonstrate amastigotes forming psuedocysts within the smooth muscle bundles (Fig. 6).[28] Patients with megaesophagus develop carcinoma of the esophagus in roughly 7% of cases. Megacolon may be complicated by obstruction, volvulus, perforation, sepsis, and death.[26] If cardiac failure develops, nearly half of patients are dead within a year. The 5-year mortality rate for symptomatic Chagas' disease is on the order of 10 to 15%.[28]

Subjective symptoms of pregnancy may mimic symptoms of Chagas' disease; therefore, clinical clues may be confusing. Cardiac disease in the pregnant woman may be adversely affected by some medications, e.g., beta-agonists, used in pregnancy. Pregnant women with Chagas' disease are known to suffer pregnancy wastage, as well as congenital infection.[30] Infants born alive may exhibit hepatosplenomegaly, cardiac disease, nervous system damage, and cutaneous manifestations; signs of the disease depend upon the trimester of transplacental transmission. The placenta demonstrates necrosis and chronic inflammation, including amastigotes with placental macrophages. Transmission to the fetus is probably mediated by parasitemia and transplacental spread. Transmission through breast milk is also theoretically possible, having been documented in animals.[31]

The separation of African sleeping sickness into two separate diseases is not made solely on the basis of microbial etiology. Western, or Gambian, trypanosomiasis is a more chronic, lasting disease, whereas eastern, or Rhodesian, trypanosomiasis follows a stormy course. Ultimately, however, both illnesses are fatal.

Western sleeping sickness, much like Chagas' disease, begins with a characteristic skin lesion, the trypanoma or trypanosome chancre. This firm, tender papule, if it is noticed at all, generally appears roughly a week after the insect bite. The papule may ulcerate, may involve local lymph nodes, and usually resolves within a few weeks. Thereafter, the

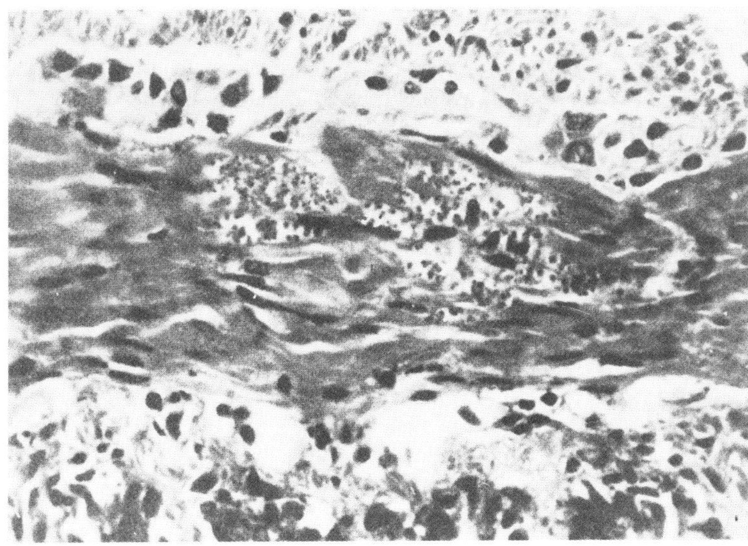

Fig. 6. Esophagus in a case of Chagas' disease, demonstrating *Trypanosoma cruzi* amastigotes forming a pseudocyst with the smooth muscles. (From the Louisiana State University Medical Center.)

disease is much more protean in its symptomatology, initially becoming manifest as high fever, severe headache, malaise, arthralgias, and a relatively constant tachycardia, the so-called hemolymphatic stage or early stage. Generalized parasitemia is responsible for these findings, as well as for papular skin eruptions (trypanids), dizziness, and pruritis. All of the above are mediated by way of a small-vessel vasculitis, with perivascular infiltrates of mostly mononuclear cells and edema. In roughly three-quarters of patients, the posterior cervical nodes are enlarged, nontender, and of the consistency of ripe plums or child's testicles, called "Winterbottom's sign."[27,29]

After months to years, the organisms pass through the blood-brain barrier into the CNS, where a generalized meningoencephalitis ensues. As in the circulation elsewhere, perivascular cuffing and edema are the histologic findings (Fig. 7). Initially, sleep disorders are seen in persons with late disease. As further brain damage occurs, appetite disturbances are noted, motor and tonus abnormalities arise, including frank epilepsy, hyperre-

flexia and abnormal reflexes are seen, and hyperesthesias and loss of proprioception occur. Ultimately, patients lapse into coma and die from respiratory embarrassment, cardiac failure, starvation/wasting, accidents, or infection.

Eastern trypanosomiasis follows a course similar to Gambian disease, only much more fulminant. High fever and rash, with tachycardia and arrhythmia, are common early. Winterbottom's sign is often obscured, becoming only part of a generalized lymphadenopathy/hepatosplenomegaly/edema syndrome. Polyserositis is found, even with overt ascites. CNS involvement occurs early, with rapid deterioration and death within weeks or months. Often the disease is so rapid that a hemolymphatic stage cannot be differentiated from a meningoencephalitis stage.

Pregnancy is not often a complicating factor in Eastern sleeping sickness, as most patients die before a pregnancy can be achieved or carried for any length of time. Occasional reports, however, do describe transplacental spread of *T. brucei rhodesiense*, with some small rate of neonatal survival after

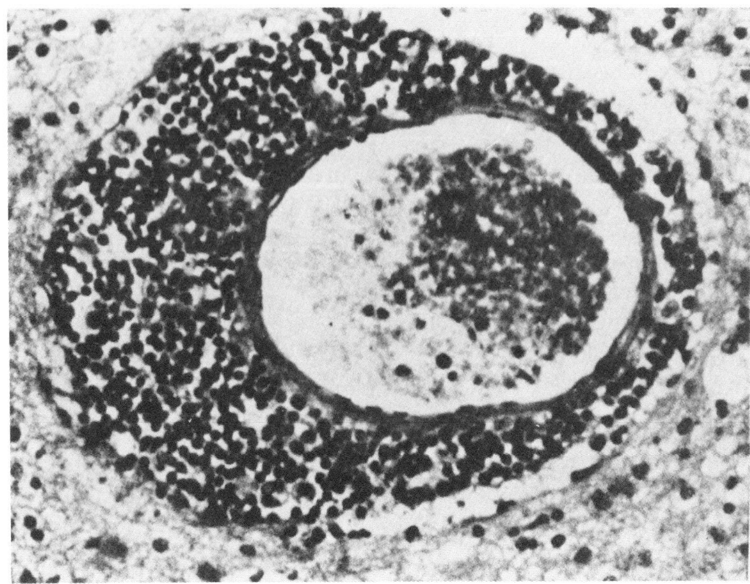

Fig. 7. Histologic picture of perivascular infiltration (cuffing) with mononuclear cells, and interstitial edema in the brain in African sleeping sickness. (From Strickland,[1] with permission of the publisher.)

therapy.[32] Most commonly in the western form of the illness, abortion and prematurity are reported in affected pregnancies. As with American trypanosomiasis, the placenta is parasitized, leading to IUGR and fetal infection. At birth, the infants may exhibit fever, anemia, and CNS disease.[31]

Diagnosis

The definitive diagnosis of any form of trypanosomiasis involves demonstration of the parasite. Blood, CSF, lymph node biopsy, or other tissue may yield results. In sleeping sickness or acute Chagas' disease, the protozoans may be demonstrated in thin or thick blood smears (Figs. 8, 9). Chronic Chagas' disease, however, is often diagnosed by the finding of *T. cruzi* antibody in a patient with the appropriate clinical presentation (e.g., megacolon). In any event, it is recommended that an exact diagnosis be made, since the various therapeutic regimens available are rather toxic.

Therapy

Antiprotozoal treatment for Chagas' disease is problematic. Only two drugs have a reasonable effect on the organism: nifurtimox, a nitrofuran, and benznidazole, a nitroimidazole. Neither of these drugs completely sterilizes the body of parasites, though parasitemia and symptoms are reduced, as is mortality from cardiac and CNS infection. Of course, organ damage already sustained is not reversed. Nifurtimox (8–16 mg/kg/day in three divided doses) is given for 50 to 120 days. Side effects include weight loss, anorexia, CNS symptoms (nervousness, insomnia, occasional hallucinations), and peripheral neuritis. Benznidazole (5–6 mg/kg/day) is given for 60 days. Abdominal and neurological side effects are very common. Although both of these drugs are possibly dangerous in pregnancy, treatment of acute Chagas' disease in the gravida is recommended. In chronic or indeterminate disease, it is perhaps best to wait until after de-

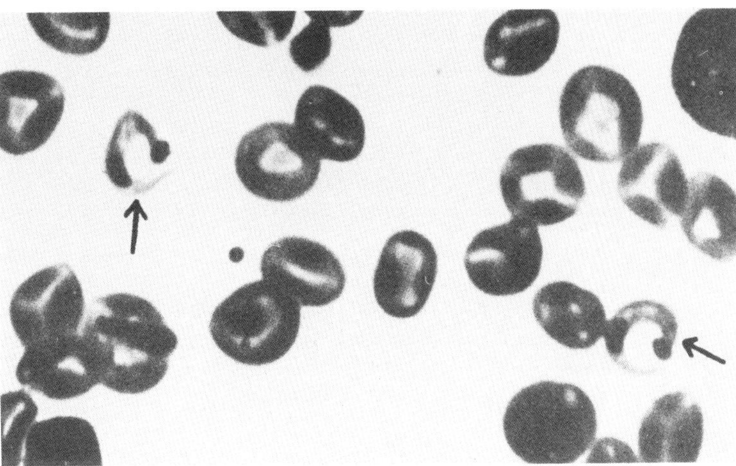

Fig. 8. *Trypanosoma cruzi* in stained blood film. (From Strickland,[1] with permission of the publisher.)

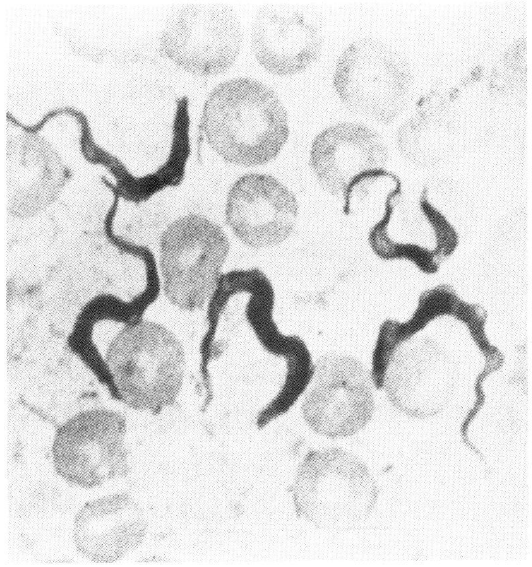

Fig. 9. *Trypanosoma brucei gambiense* in stained blood film. (From Strickland,[1] with permission of the publisher.)

livery, at which point the infant will need to be treated as well.

The forms of sleeping sickness are treated differently, depending whether or not there is CNS involvement (i.e., a positive lumbar puncture). Gambian trypanosomiasis in the hemolymphatic stage may be treated with seven to ten injections of pentamidine (4 mg/kg IM daily or every other day). Side effects include pain at the site, vomiting, hypotension, syncopy, hypoglycemia, and neuritis. Occasional reports of resistance have been encountered. For the early form of both types of sleeping sickness, five to seven injections of suramin (20 mg/kg—maximum dose 1 g—at 5- to 7-day intervals) may be given. Very rarely, there is an idiosyncratic reaction of vomiting, seizures, and shock, with occasional mortality. Therefore, a test dose of 5 mg/kg is given initially. Preexisting renal disease is a contraindication, since suramin may cause renal tubular damage. No resistance to suramin has been reported.[28,29]

Central nervous system trypanosomiasis is treated with the arsenical melarsoprol, after short pretreatment with one of the drugs above. Three or four daily injections (3.6 mg/kg, maximum 200–250 mg/injection) are given intravenously. Toxicity includes neurologic atrophy, rash, and an encephalitis-like picture (perhaps due to dying parasites in the brain).[27]

Again, these drugs may be toxic in pregnancy. In fact, pentamidine may cause uterine activity and subsequent abortion. However, the sequelae of *T. brucei* infection are so

TABLE 3. Geographic Distribution of Leishmaniasis

Disease entity	Local name	Species name	Geographic range
Visceral leishmaniasis	Kala-azar	*L. donovani*	Near East, Middle East, Asia, Africa
		L. chagasi	South and Central America
Cutaneous leishmaniasis	Oriental sore (Old World cutaneous leishmaniasis)	*L. tropica*	Mediterranean, Near and Middle East, West and Northeast Africa
	Chiclero ulcer	*L. mexicana*	Central America
	Espundia, forest yaws	*L. braziliensis*	Amazonia
	Uta	*L. peruviana*	Western Andes

Adapted from Lee.[31]

severe that pregnant women should be treated expeditiously as soon as the proper diagnosis is made. Of course, suramin may be used in lieu of pentamidine.

LEISHMANIASIS

Like the trypanosomes, the *Leishmania* species are polymorphic protozoans that take a different form, depending upon their location. In the mammalian host, the organism lives as an amastigote intracellularly in cells of the reticuloendothelial system. In the gut of the insect vector, the sandfly, the parasite exists in the promastigote stage. When the flies feed on infected animals (or man), the amastigote is ingested with the blood meal and converted to promastigotes, which replicate. When the fly bites a human thereafter, promastigotes are inoculated into the wound. Reservoirs include rodents, canines, sloths, and humans, depending upon the species of *Leishmania*.

Most *Leishmania* species, including *L. tropica*, *L. braziliensis*, and *L. mexicana*, cause cutaneous and mucocutaneous disease, the extension of the infection being modified by host immunity. However, *L. donovani* causes infection of the reticuloendothelial cells systemically, the disease termed "kala-azar." The geographic distribution of the various species is given in Table 3.

Pathophysiology

Visceral leishmaniasis, or kala-azar, is caused by infection with *L. donovani*. It is a chronic disease characterized by fever, he-patosplenomegaly, pancytopenia, and wasting. The vector is the sandfly, which feeds on infected canines in most endemic regions of the world, though humans are the reservoirs in India. The initial, minor lesion is a granuloma filled with mononuclear cells that contain amastigotes. After an incubation period of several months, the organisms disseminate throughout the reticuloendothelial system, causing fever and inciting proliferation of monocytes in the liver and spleen (hence, the massive organomegaly). Replacement of marrow leads to the anemia, as well as thrombocytopenia and a tendency to bleed freely. The skin progressively darkens, especially about the hands and feet—hence the name kala-azar (black sickness). Death is common in the untreated susceptible patient, often secondary to infection in the debilitated, cachectic victim. However, in some endemic areas, apparent subclinical disease seems to be common, indicating a high level of immunity in some populations.[33,34]

Pregnancy in a patient with established kala-azar is unusual, because of the wasting effect of the disease. Pregnancy does occur, however, and appears to accelerate the course of the illness, perhaps by affecting the cellular immune response.[31] Congenital infection has been described.[35,36]

Cutaneous and mucocutaneous leishmaniasis are clinically separated into Old World disease, or Oriental sore, due to *L. tropica*, and New World disease, due to *L. braziliensis* and *L. mexicana*. Both forms of the disease are spread in their respective ranges by sandflies that have fed on infected animal reser-

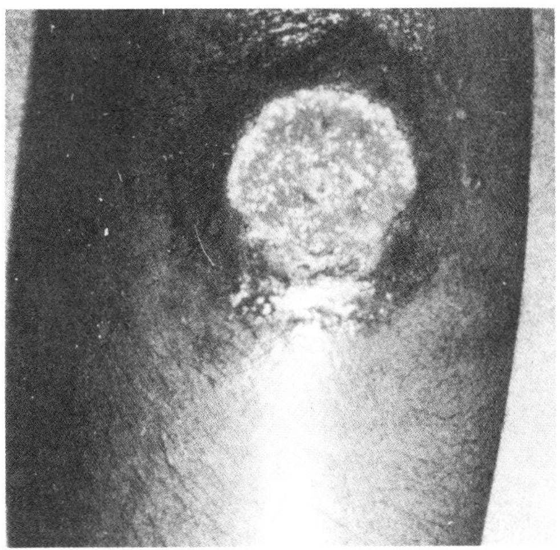

Fig. 10. Typical lesion of New World cutaneous leishmaniasis on the forearm of a patient. (From the Louisiana State University Medical Center.)

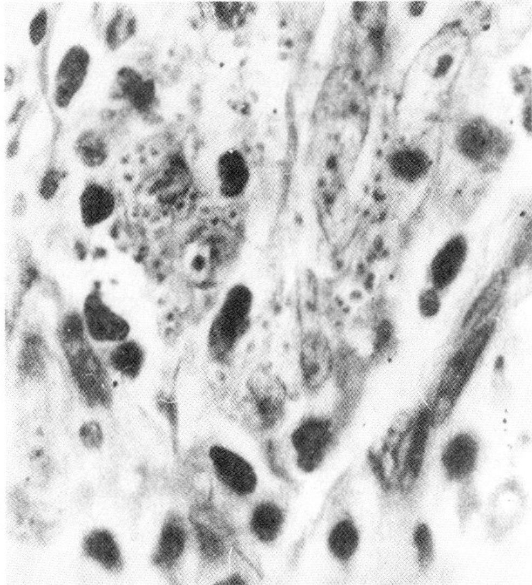

Fig. 11. Biopsy specimen through the edge of an Oriental sore, demonstrating cellular infiltration and heavily parasitized reticuloendothelial cells. (From the Louisiana State University Medical Center.)

voirs, much the same as in visceral disease. However, it is apparently the cooler temperatures of the skin that allow these parasites to persist and infect.

Oriental sore is composed of a granulomatous inflammatory reaction about the area of inoculation. A papule, formed by an influx of mononuclear cells in response to the amastigotes, enlarges and eventually ulcerates. As immunity develops, parasites disappear and an atrophic scar finally remains. If the patient remains anergic to the organism, diffuse cutaneous disease may result, disseminating organisms throughout the skin without ulceration.

New World cutaneous and mucocutaneous leishmaniasis, though spread by sandflies similarly to the Old World disease, present different clinical pictures in different geographical areas. A single cutaneous ulcer (Fig. 10) and diffuse, life-threatening mucocutaneous disease (known as espundia) are the two ends of the clinical spectrum. While the disease caused by *L. mexicana* appears to be similar to that from *L. tropica,* disease due to *L. braziliensis* often, if untreated, attacks the nasal and oral cartilaginous areas, presumably because the cooler tissues and lack of

effective cell-mediated immunity in these areas. This mucocutaneous disease, arising months or years after the usual cutaneous lesions are healed, may cause such facial destruction that the patient can no longer eat. These mucocutaneous lesions do not spontaneously heal, as do skin ulcers.[33]

Cutaneous and mucocutaneous leishmaniasis are occasionally found in pregnant women. The organisms are not known to spread transplacentally, apparently because of the higher temperatures of the deeper tissues of the body. However, the lessened cell-mediated immunity of pregnancy seems to predispose to more invasive disease, leading some to advocate termination of pregnancy to avert more serious sequelae.[31]

Diagnosis

Cutaneous disease may be definitively diagnosed by demonstration of the organisms in scrapings or biopsies of the skin or mucous membrane lesions (Fig. 11). Older, healing lesions may be problematic in that they may

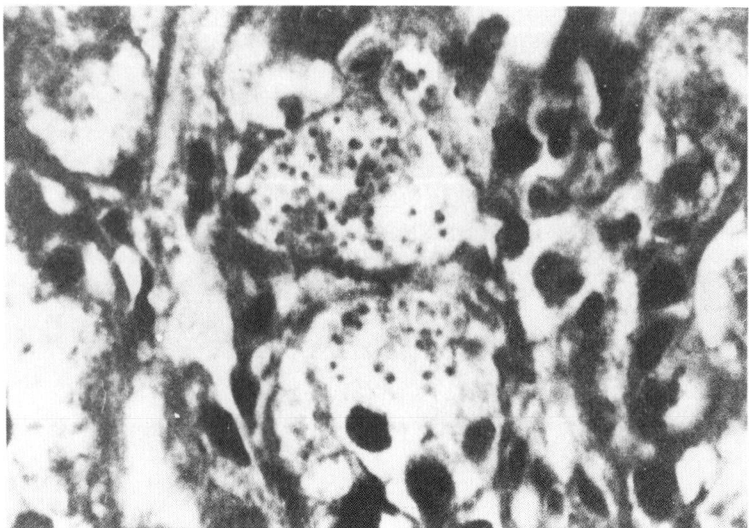

Fig. 12.   *Leishmania donovani* in the liver of a patient with kala-azar.

have very few amastigotes left because of the immune response. In such situations, antibody levels may be tested and combined with the clinical impression for the appropriate diagnosis. If the lesion is healed, of course, the diagnosis may be academic.

Visceral leishmaniasis is identified when amastigotes are visualized in hepatic or splenic tissue (Figs. 12, 13) or in aspirates of lymph nodes or bone marrow. *L. donovani*, as well as the other *Leishmania* organisms, may also be grown on special semisolid media, though culture may take weeks to be definitive.

Therapy

Simple cutaneous disease due to *L. mexicana* or *L. tropica* is usually self-limiting, though scarring. Local heat may hasten recovery. Although disease may be more invasive during pregnancy, gravidas with cutaneous disease may be managed expectantly and treated only if their condition appears to be worsening instead of spontaneously resolving. Alternatively, therapy may be withheld until after delivery.

Treatment for all other forms of leishma-niasis is pentavalent antimony (Sb^{5+}).[37] The recommended regimen is 10 mg Sb^{5+}/kg daily (maximum of 850 mg/day) either IM or slow IV, continuing therapy until cure is obvious, though at least for 4 weeks. Relapses are treated for twice the original durations of therapy. Commercially available antimony preparations include sodium stibogluconate, commonly used in the New World and available from the CDC, and N-methylglucamine antimoniate, used in the Old World. Individual dosing is based upon the actual antimony content of the compound and not upon the weight/volume of the individual preparation.

Side effects of stibogluconate are infrequent at doses of 20 mg/kg/day or less. Gastrointestinal and constitutional symptoms (e.g., nausea, fever, headache) are uncommon. Very rarely, shock, urticaria, and dyspnea may arise, which may require treatment with epinephrine. The safety of stibogluconate in pregnancy is not established, although treatment of a pregnant woman is carried out regardless if the disease is progressive.

Alternate drugs in cases of failure or severe

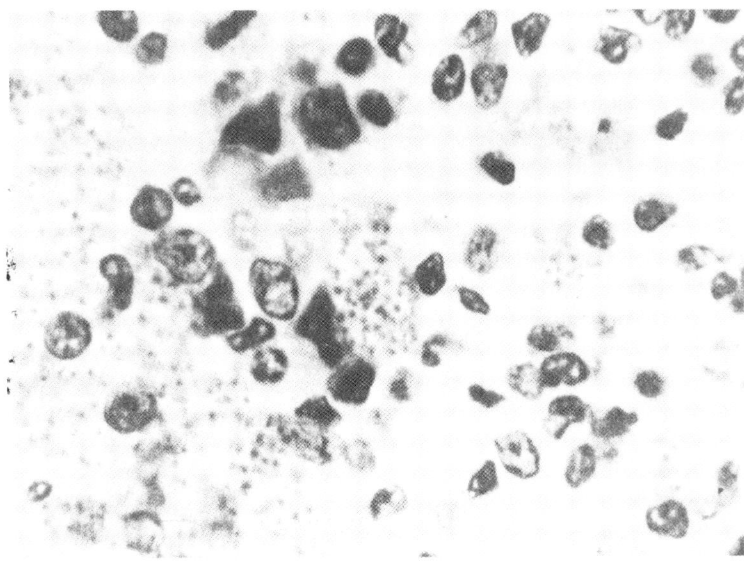

Fig. 13. *Leishmania donovani* parasitized in the reticuloendothelial cells of the spleen of a patient with kala-azar.

adverse reactions with antimonials are pentamidine and amphotericin B.

GIARDIASIS

The flagellated protozoan *Giardia lamblia* is the most commonly identified intestinal parasite in the United States, demonstrated in perhaps 5% of stool specimens. The organism has been implicated in symptomatic diarrhea, pediatric malabsorption, and traveler's diarrhea.[38–40] The organism exists in two stages, the cyst and the trophozoite, much like *Entamoeba histolytica.* Of course, the trophozoite is the active, free-living form that reproduces in the intestinal tract of the host.

Pathophysiology

After the cyst is ingested by the host animal, either by person-to-person fecal-oral contact or by the drinking of infected water, the organism is converted to the trophozoite form, which multiplies in the upper small bowel. By some poorly understood mechanism that does not seem to include invasion of the bowel wall to any great extent, the parasite induces a malabsorbtive phenomenon at the enzymatic level in the gut epithelium, leading to the clinical syndrome.

Commonly, infestation with *G. lamblia* leads to a syndrome of explosive, foul-smelling diarrhea accompanied by abdominal pain and cramping beginning about a week or two after ingestion of the cysts. Most persons will spontaneously heal over several weeks or so, though some will develop chronic diarrhea and clinical malabsorption. The chronic illness may wax and wane over some months, leading to substantial weight loss, as abdominal findings may be aggravated or brought on by eating.

The fetus is not directly involved in cases of maternal giardiasis. However, the malabsorption and nutritional deprivation, especially in chronic cases, may have a general deleterious effect on the pregnancy and fetal growth. As well, the myriad of seemingly vague gastrointestinal complaints that mimic pregnancy symptoms may confuse the patient and obstetrician as to the correct diagnosis during pregnancy.

TABLE 4. Antimicrobials for the Treatment of Giardiasis

Initial therapy	Paromomycin (30 mg/kg/day, t.i.d.) for 5–10 days
Alternative drugs	Metronidazole (250 mg t.i.d.) for 5–10 days
	or
	Quinacrine (100 mg t.i.d.) for 3–10 days

Adapted from Lee.[31]

Diagnosis

Giardiasis is appropriately sought in patients with chronic diarrhea and/or malabsorption. The cysts or trophozoites are readily seen in fresh stool samples, though occasionally semiformed stools will not yield the parasites. The duodenum may be targeted with either endoscopic sampling or by the "string test," whereby a string weighted with a gelatin capsule is swallowed, left in situ for 6 hours or so, and then pulled back out of the mouth for examination for fresh organisms.[41]

Therapy

A number of antiprotozoal drugs are effective against *G. lamblia*.[42] Metronidazole, quinacrine, and paromomycin in the doses shown in Table 4 are all effective. For reasons of "possible" teratogenicity, some authors prefer paromomycin for treatment of giardiasis in pregnancy.[43] However, especially after the first trimester, there appears to be no risk in the use of metronidazole in the pregnant woman or her fetus.

MALARIA

Mal'aria, or "bad air" as the Italians called it in the seventeenth century, is caused by infection with protozoan parasites of the genus *Plasmodium*. These organisms reproduce sexually within anopheline mosquitoes and are transmitted to humans by the bite of an infected female mosquito. Asexual reproduction occurs in the human host. Four species of *Plasmodium* infect man: *P. falciparum*, *P. vivax*, *P. ovale*, and *P. malariae*.[44]

Malaria is generally considered to be a disease of the tropical third world. While the more than 100 million cases each year are concentrated in Africa, South and Central America, Asia, and Oceania, recent increased travel and immigration trends have stimulated an increase in cases in the United States[45] and Europe.[46]

Pathophysiology

After the bite of the infected mosquito introduces infective sporozoites into the victim's bloodstream, the organisms circulate to the liver, where the hepatocytes are then invaded. The parasites then evolve into hepatic schizonts, which, after a couple of weeks of development, rupture, releasing thousands of merozoites that enter the peripheral circulation to invade erythrocytes. In malaria with *P. falciparum* and *P. malariae*, all of the schizonts rupture simultaneously. In the other species, forms called hypnozoites may remain in the liver for months before rupture, leading to relapses of the systemic infection. Erythrocytic forms, by the way, do not reinvade the liver; hence transfusion malaria has no liver phase.[47]

Schizont rupture is associated with the classic malarial paroxysm of high fever, chills, and rigors. The exact physiologic mechanism for the fever is obscure, but the vasodilation resulting from it may cause orthostatic changes, diaphoresis, vomiting, and eventually hyponatremia.[48] Rupture of parasite-laden red blood cells, as well as sequestration in the liver, leads to anemia that is roughly proportional to the parasitic load. If severe hemolysis and hemoglobinuria occur, the clinical syndrome is known as blackwater fever. Further, because of decreased tissue oxygenation from anemia and sludging in the vascular beds, other end organs may be affected, including the brain, kidney, and lungs.[49]

The pregnant woman and her fetus are at unusually high risk for contracting malaria. Because of an apparent decrease in immunity, the gravida is many times more likely to

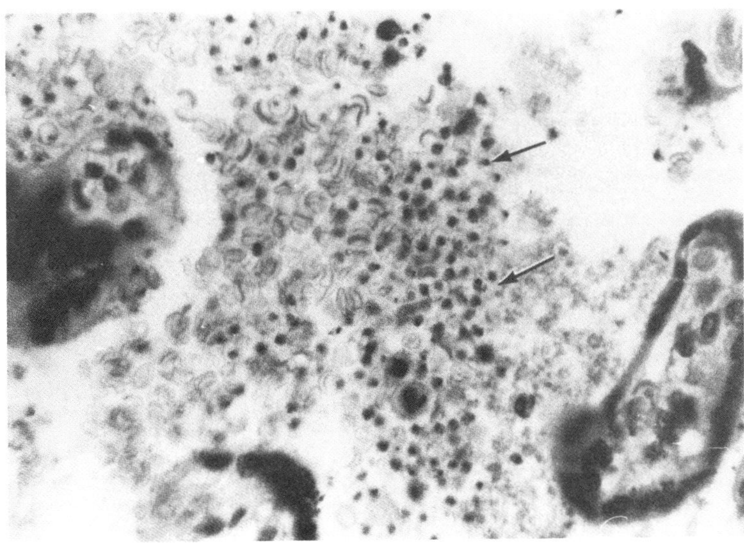

Fig. 14. Placental section from a patient with *Plasmodium falciparum* malaria demonstrating numerous red blood cells within the intervillous space parasitized with protozoans (arrows), while the fetal cells within the villus itself are not. (From Strickland,[1] with permission of the publisher.)

become infected than the nonpregnant woman. Anemia may become severe, especially in the middle trimester.[50] The fetus may die or suffer intrauterine growth retardation because of effects on the placenta.[51] In fact, even when the mother is adequately treated for acute disease, the products of conception appear to be a favorite spot for the parasites to elude chemotherapy and persist (Fig. 14).[52]

Diagnosis

Malaria should be suspected in any individual who presents with the characteristic high spiking fever and a history of having visited, even for a short time, a malaria endemic country. In addition, recipients of blood transfusions and intravenous drug abusers may contract the disease directly from another human, without a mosquito go-between. Malaria may mimic other febrile illnesses, as well as diseases that cause hepatomegaly, arthritis, and other various symptoms, making the use of ancillary methods prudent.

As is the case with babesiosis, the definitive diagnosis of malaria rests with the demonstration of the parasites in a thin or thick blood smear. Smears should be obtained several times over the day to ensure visualization of the organisms during one of their sporadic showerings. The morphology of the intraerythrocytic forms usually enables the pathologist to identify the species of *Plasmodium*.

Therapy

Except for resistant strains of *P. falciparum*, all malarial organisms are sensitive to chloroquine. Although this drug may have the potential to cause retinal and ototoxicity in women and their fetuses, oral chloroquine in the usual doses may be given fairly safely during pregnancy. The usual dose is 600 mg of base followed by 300 mg of base in 6 hours, then 300 mg of base per day for 2 days. A parenteral formulation is also available for persons unable to take oral drug. Normally, relapses from *P. ovale* and *P. vivax* are treated with primaquine. The pregnant woman, however, should only be treated for each recurrence with chloroquine and the primaquine reserved until after delivery.[53]

Chloroquine-resistant *P. falciparum* infection is problematic in the pregnant woman. First and foremost, it is prudent for pregnant women to stay out of areas where this organism is endemic. In the nonpregnant patient, quinine, tetracyclines, pyrimethamine, sulfadiazine, or sulfisoxazole may be used. However, quinine may produce uterine contractions and severe maternal hypoglycemia, and tetracyclines may damage the fetal teeth and bones. Therefore, as in toxoplasmosis, the combination of pyramethamine (25 mg b.i.d. for 3 days) and sulfisoxazole (500 mg q.i.d. for 5 days), perhaps with folinic acid, has been advocated.[54] It should be remembered, however, that sulfonamides may aggravate hyperbilirubinemia in newborns, and they therefore should not be given to a mother near term or otherwise near delivery. As well, pyramethamine is a folate antagonist and theoretically should not be administered in the first trimester.

PNEUMOCYSTIS CARINII

Pneumocystis carinii is an interesting organism that almost exclusively attacks immunocompromised hosts. In fact, the organism is found in the lungs (without causing disease) of almost every type of mammal throughout every part of the world. The majority of normal children have antibody to *P. carinii* by age 2 to 4 years.[55]

The organism exists in two forms: a thick-walled cyst form containing eight sporozoites and the trophozoite or extracystic form (which has a thin wall). The organism is not visualized in tissue with H&E stain; special stains, especially methenamine-silver nitrate, are necessary for demonstration of infection in tissue.

Classically, the pneumonitis caused by the organism was restricted to patients on immunosuppressive drugs, premature infants, and debilitated persons in nursing homes and the like. However, since the epidemic of HIV infection in the 1980s, *P. carinii* pneumonia (PCP) is a frequent finding in the general hospital.

Pathophysiology

P. carinii is apparently transmitted from person to person by way of respiratory droplets. In the appropriate host, the initial infectious event is formation of the cyst in the wall of the alveolus. If extensive infection occurs, some mild inflammatory changes arise with some desquamation of alveolar cells. Clinical signs and symptoms arise when there is finally marked desquamative alveolitis. Histologically, the alveoli are filled with organisms and macrophages (Fig. 15). Signs and symptoms, as well as the characteristic diffuse bilateral alveolar pattern on chest roentgenogram, are present at this point.[56]

Clinical disease, except in neonates, typically includes fever, cough, tachypnea, and coryza. There are usually no rales, even when the chest x-ray shows infiltrates and air bronchograms. Cyanosis may occur later in the illness, as arterial oxygen pressure falls below 80 torr. Fever as high as 40°C occurs in most patients. The mortality of PCP is nearly universal if the disease is untreated. It is anticipated that as more pregnant women, for instance those with AIDS or other immunocompromising disease, are reported with PCP, their mortality rate will be as dismal as the literature suggests for the nonpregnant individual.

Diagnosis

The definitive diagnosis of PCP can be made only by demonstrating the organism in lung tissue. This may be obtained through open biopsy, brushings, or needle aspiration. In cases of non-AIDS PCP, however, brush techniques yield relatively poorer results. Additionally, antigen may be detected in the blood by counter-immunoelectrophoresis, although this technique yields a rather high false positivity rate among cancer patients.[57]

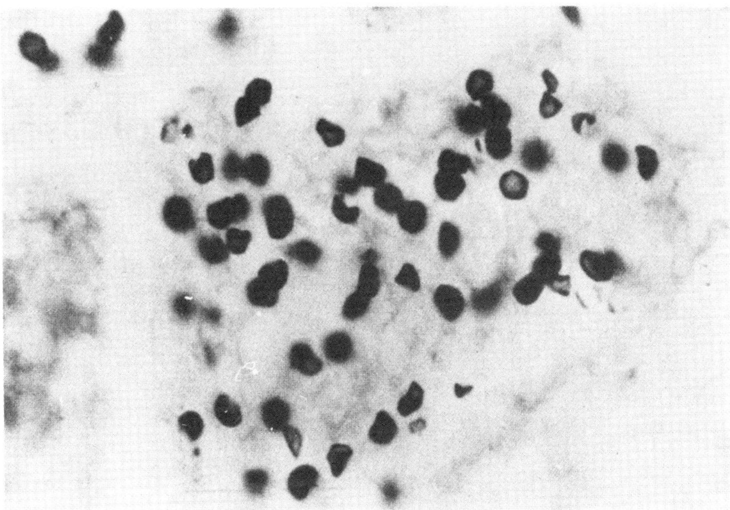

Fig. 15. Silver-methenamine stain of *Pneumocystis carinii* cysts in alveolar exudate in a case of *P. carinii* pneumonia.

Therapy

Besides oxygen therapy and supportive care, the mainstay of therapy for PCP has been antibiotics. Specifically, pentamidine (4 mg/kg/day for 2 weeks) shows good results despite significant toxicity. Pyrimethamine plus a sulfonamide is said to be effective in preliminary studies. More timely is the use of trimethoprim/sulfamethoxazole, which has worked well in all groups of infected persons, including those with AIDS. Because of the toxicity of pentamidine and the possible adverse fetal effect of pyrimethamine, it is probably prudent to treat the pregnant woman with trimethoprim/sulfamethoxazole. In fact, because the prognosis without treatment is so dismal, any efficacious drug must be used as necessary, in spite of any fetal effects.

TOXOPLASMOSIS

Toxoplasmosis, the illness caused by infection with the protozoan parasite *Toxoplasma gondii*, is a relatively uncommon disease, which is surprising, considering how universal the causative organism is. Asymptomatic carriage of *T. gondii* is widespread among animals as well as man. As many as one-third of adults have serologic markers for previous exposure to the organism.[58] In the reproductive age group, as many as 0.6% of women per year have a primary infection,[59] producing over 3,000 infants with congenital infection in the United States alone.

Pathophysiology

All infections with *T. gondii* ultimately come from cats. The organism is an obligate intracellular parasite, undergoing its reproductive cycle in the feline intestinal tract, from whence sheds oocysts that sporulate in the soil and remain infectious there for months, even in freezing temperatures. Contaminated soil causes rodent, avian, and grazing animal infection.

Human infection occurs by ingestion of poorly cooked meat containing tissue cysts, exposure to infectious cat feces, and transplacental spread during maternal parasitemia. The disease in humans most often arises from the first and third of these possibilities, as well as an occasional case of transfusion-related toxoplasmosis.[60]

Acute infection with *T. gondii* usually en-

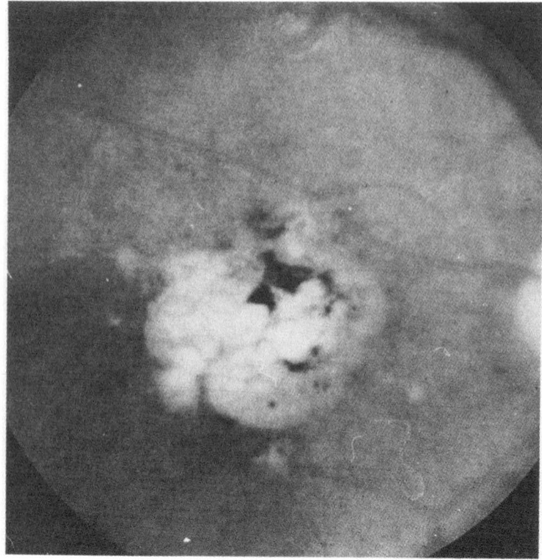

Fig. 16. Lesion of chorioretinitis in infection with *Toxoplasma gondii.* (From Strickland,[1] with permission of the publisher.)

TABLE 5. Neonatal Features of Severe Congenital Toxoplasmosis

Feature	Occurrence (%)
Splenomegaly	90
Jaundice	80
Fever	77
Anemia	77
Hepatomegaly	77
Adenopathy	68
Pneumonia	40
Rash	25

Modified from Eichenwald.[65]

tails parasitemia, although the patient with a competent immune system is generally asymptomatic. On occasion, a mononucleosis-like syndrome may be evident, though the most common syndrome is asymptomatic cervical lymphadenopathy. This infection will spontaneously clear in a few months in most normal patients. Rarely a chronic lymphadenopathy persists, and even more rarely does a healthy person develop disseminated disease (e.g., myocarditis, pneumonitis, hepatitis, chorioretinitis, etc.).[61]

The most serious infections occur in the fetus. Transplacentally acquired infection is generalized and persistent, on account of the relative immunologic immaturity of the infant. The fetal CNS is especially vulnerable, where progressive infection causes glial nodules, microinfarcts, and periventricular necrosis leading to calcifications.[60] The classic tetrad of congenital toxoplasmosis is chorioretinitis (Fig. 16), microcephaly or hydrocephaly, cerebral calcifications, and clinical cerebral damage.[62]

Transmission of the organism to the fetus occurs more often when parasitemia happens in the third trimester; however, these neonates are almost always free of clinical disease. If maternal infection occurs during the first trimester, fetal infection follows in perhaps 15% of neonates; second trimester infection effects 25% of neonates, and third trimester, 60%.[63] But although transmission to the fetus is less likely earlier in pregnancy, infection is more severe, including spontaneous abortion, stillbirth, or severe neurologic damage. A rule of thumb encompassing all trimesters is: If acute maternal infection is acquired during pregnancy, 40% of infants will be affected and 40% will be severely damaged.[64] Common clinical manifestations of severe fetal infection are detailed in Table 5.[65]

Diagnosis

The principal method of diagnosis of adult infection is antibody survey. A patient who demonstrates specific IgG antibody against *T. gondii* is protected against parasitemic infection, therefore protecting her fetus against intrauterine disease. (Rare exceptions are severely immunocompromised women.) A negative antibody assay implies susceptibility to acute infection, and thus to transplacental spread during pregnancy.

During acute infection, specific IgM antibody appears before IgG and persists for a shorter time. Recent acquisition of the organism may thus be inferred by measurement of antitoxoplasma IgM; this is now the standard method for documenting recent infection. ELISA methodology allows measurement of IgM for up to 8 months following acute disease. If no IgM is present, a low to

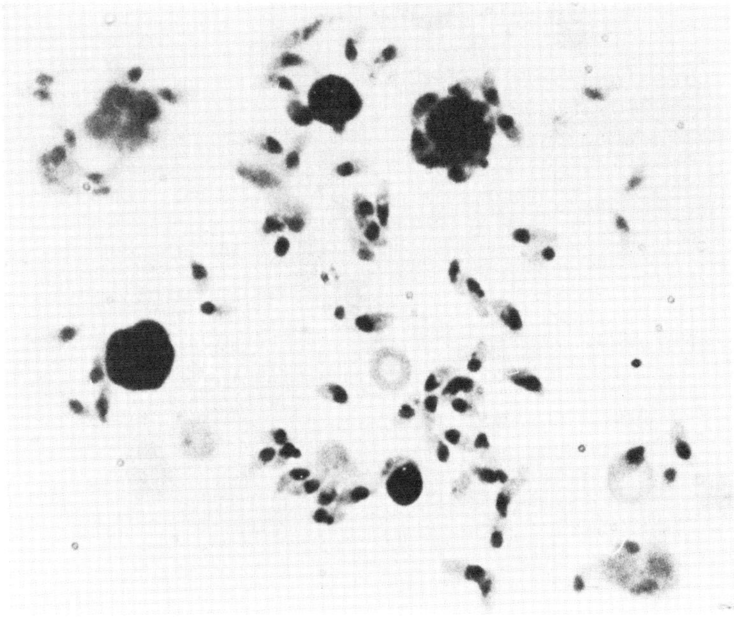

Fig. 17. Mouse peritoneal fluid demonstrating tachyzoites of *Toxoplasma gondii.* (From Strickland,[1] with permission of the publisher.)

moderate level of IgG indicates past disease. If IgM is present, acute infection is suggested, and a second sample is drawn for confirmation. A second positive titer of 1:500 or more is relatively conclusive.

Prenatal diagnosis of toxoplasmosis is by fetal blood sampling through fetoscopy or funipuncture.[66] Fetal blood is inoculated into mice (Fig. 17) or assayed for toxoplasma-specific IgM. An abnormal ultrasonographic finding, such as hydrocephaly, hydrops, or intracranial calcifications, in a patient with serologic evidence of infection will also help confirm the diagnosis of congenital infection.

Therapy

Antiparasitic therapy of acute toxoplasmosis can reduce but not eliminate the risk of congenital infection and fetal disease. Fetal lesions may also be modified.[67] Spiramycin has been used in Europe in the first trimester with no untoward effects. The drug crosses the placenta somewhat; its action may be due to placental treatment rather than fetal medication. The drug may be obtained by special request from the FDA in the United States.

The combination of pyrimethamine and sulfonamides, as mentioned under other infections above, is effective against acute toxoplasmosis.[60] As stated above, pyrimethamine should not be used in the first trimester, and sulfonamides should not be used near delivery. Because of the problematic nature of therapy with any of these drugs in pregnancy, accurate diagnosis is a must before treatment is initiated.

Medical opinion in the United States is currently shifting toward universal prenatal screening for toxoplasmosis in pregnancy.[68] Potentially, 3,000 affected infants could be saved annually. Practically speaking, however, specific hygienic measures to avoid acute infection during pregnancy may not be enforceable in a large population.[69]

REFERENCES

1. Protozoal diseases. In Strickland GT: "Hunter's Tropical Medicine," 6th edition. Philadelphia: W.B. Saunders, 1984, pp 474–477.

2. Losch FA: Massive development of amebas in the large intestine. Am J Trop Med Hyg 24:287–393, 1875.

3. Dean BH, Mott KE, Russel AJ: "Tropical Medicine and Parasitology: Classic Investigations." Ithaca, NY: Cornell University Press, 1978, p 79.

4. Ravdin JI, Jones TC: Entamoeba histolytica (amebiasis). In Mandell GL, Douglas RG, Bennett JE (eds): "Principles and Practice of Infectious Disease," 2nd edition. New York: John Wiley & Sons, 1985, pp 1506–1512.

5. Botero D: Amebiasis. In Goldsmith R, Heyneman D (eds): "Tropical Medicine and Parasitology." Norwalk, CT: Appleton & Lange, 1989, pp 224–236.

6. Adams EB, MacLeod IN: Invasive amebiasis. I. Amebic dysentery and its complications. Medicine 56:315–323, 1977.

7. Adams EB, MacLeod IN: Invasive amebiasis. II. Amebic liver abscess and its complications. Medicine 56:325–334, 1977.

8. Calderon J, de Lourdes-Munoz MA, Acosta HM: Surface redistribution and release of antibody-induced caps in *Entamoeba*. J Exp Med 151:184–190, 1980.

9. Armon PJ: Amoebiasis in pregnancy and the puerperium. Br J Obstet Gynaecol 85:264–269, 1978.

10. Miller JM, Pastorek JG: The microbiology of premature rupture of the membranes. Clin Obstet Gynecol 29:739–757, 1986.

11. Healy GR, Sumner CK: The indirect hemagglutination test for amebiasis in patients with inflammatory bowel disease. Am J Dig Dis 17:97–101, 1972.

12. Old Testament: Exodus 9:3.

13. Smith T, Kilbourne FL: Investigation into the nature, causation and prevention of Texas or south cattle fever. USDA Bureau Animal Ind Bull 1:1–10, 1893.

14. Spielman A: Human babesiosis on Nantucket Island: Transmission by nymphal *Ixodes* ticks. Am J Trop Med Hyg 25:784–798, 1976.

15. Jacoby GA, Hunt JV, Kosinski KS, et al.: Treatment of transfusion-transmitted babesiosis by exchange transfusion. N Engl J Med 303:1098–1100, 1980.

16. Ruebush TK: Babesia. In Mandell GL, Douglas RG, Bennett JE (eds): "Principles and Practice of Infectious Disease," 2nd edition. New York: John Wiley & Sons, 1985, pp 1559–1560.

17. Teutsch SM, Etkind P, Burwell EL, et al.: Babesiosis in postsplenectomy hosts. Am J Trop Med Hyg 29:738–741, 1980.

18. Raucher HS, Jaffin H, Glass JL: Babesiosis in pregnancy. Obstet Gynecol 63:7S–9S, 1984.

19. Erbsloh JK: Babesiosis in the newborn foal. J Reprod Fertil 23:725–728, 1975.

20. Ruebush TK: Babesiosis (Piroplasmosis). In Goldsmith R, Heyneman D (eds): "Tropical Medicine and Parasitology." Norwalk, CT: Appleton & Lange, 1989, pp 326–328.

21. Miller LH, Neva FA, Gill F: Failure of chloroquine in human babesiosis (*Babesia microti*): Case report and chemotherapeutic trials in hamsters. Ann Intern Med 88:200, 1978.

22. Francioli PB, Keithly JS, Jones TC, et al.: Response of babesiosis to pentamidine therapy. Ann Intern Med 94:326–330, 1981.

23. Wittner M, Rowin KS, Tanowitz HB, et al.: Successful chemotherapy of transfusion babesiosis. Ann Intern Med 96:601–604, 1982.

24. White NJ, Warrell DA, Chanthavanich P, et al.: Severe hypoglycemia and hyperinsulinemia in falciparum malaria. N Engl J Med 309:61–66, 1983.

25. Gombert ME, Goldstein EJC, Benach JL, et al.: Human babesiosis. Clinical and therapeutic considerations. JAMA 248:3005–3007, 1982.

26. Kirchhoff LV, Neva FA: Trypanosoma species (Chagas' disease). In Mandell GL, Douglas RG, Bennett JE (eds): "Principles and Practice of Infectious Disease," 2nd edition. New York: John Wiley & Sons, 1985, pp 1531–1537.

27. Eyckmans L: Trypanosoma species (African sleeping sickness). In Mandell GL, Douglas RG, Bennett JE (eds): "Principles and Practice of Infectious Disease," 2nd edition. New York: John Wiley & Sons, 1985, pp 1537–1540.

28. Prata A: American trypanosomiasis (Chagas' disease). In Goldsmith R, Heyneman D (eds): "Tropical Medicine and Parasitology." Norwalk, CT: Appleton & Lange, 1989, pp 265–275.

29. de Raadt P: African trypanosomiases (sleeping sickness). In Goldsmith R, Heyneman D (eds): "Tropical Medicine and Parasitology." Norwalk, CT: Appleton & Lange, 1989, pp 256–265.

30. Bittencourt AL: Congential Chagas' disease. Am J Dis Child 130:97–103, 1976.

31. Lee RV: Protozoan infections in pregnancy. In Gleicher N (ed): "Principles of Medical Therapy in Pregnancy." New York: Plenum Press, 1985, pp 603–623.

32. Traub N, Hira PR, Chintu C, et al.: Congenital trypanosomiasis: Report of a case due to *Trypanosoma brucei rhodesiense*. East Afr Med J 55:477–481, 1975.

33. Pearson RD, de Queiroz-Sousa A: Leishmania species (kala-azar, cutaneous and mucocutaneous leishmaniasis). In Mandell GL, Douglas RG, Bennett JE (eds): "Principles and Practice of Infectious

Disease," 2nd edition. New York: John Wiley & Sons, 1985, pp 1522–1531.

34. Lemma A, Kent DC: Visceral leishmaniasis (kala azar). In Goldsmith R, Heyneman D (eds): "Tropical Medicine and Parasitology." Norwalk, CT: Appleton & Lange, 1989, pp 295–302.

35. Low GC, Cooke WE: A congenital case of kala-azar. Lancet ii:1209, 1926.

36. Banerji D: Possible congenital infection of kala-azar. J Indian Med Assoc 24:433–437, 1955.

37. World Health Organization: "The Leischmaniases." WHO Technical Report Series No. 701. Geneva: WHO, 1984.

38. Peterson H: Giardiasis (lambliasis). Scand J Gastroenterol 7:1–8, 1972.

39. Burke JA: Giardiasis in childhood. Am J Dis Child 129:1304–1311, 1975.

40. Brandborg LL: Giardiasis and traveler's diarrhea. Gastroenterol 78:1602–1614, 1980.

41. Bezjak B: Evaluation of a new technique for sampling duodenal contents in parasitologic diagnosis. Dig Dis 17:848–850, 1972.

42. Lerman SJ, Walker RA: Treatment of giardiasis. Literature review and recommendations. Clin Pediatr 21:409–429, 1982.

43. Kreutner AK, Del Bene VE, Amstey MS: Giardiasis in pregnancy. Am J Obstet Gynecol 140:895–901, 1981.

44. Wyler DJ: Plasmodium species (malaria). In Mandell GL, Douglas RG, Bennett JE (eds): "Principles and Practice of Infectious Disease," 2nd edition. New York: John Wiley & Sons, 1985, pp 1514–1522.

45. Malaria surveillance: Annual summary 1980. Atlanta: Centers for Disease Control, January 1982.

46. Bruce-Chwatt LJ: Imported malaria: An uninvited guest. Br Med Bull 38:179–185, 1982.

47. Miller LH: Transfusion malaria. In Greenwalt TJ, Jamieson GA (eds): "Transmissible Disease and Blood Transfusion." New York: Grune and Stratton, 1975, pp 241–266.

48. Brooks MH, Malloy JP, Bartelloni PJ, et al.: Pathophysiology of acute falciparum malaria: I. Correlation of clinical and biochemical abnormalities. II. Fluid compartmentalization. Am J Med 43:735–741, 1967.

49. Aikawa M, Susuki M, Gutiervez Y: Pathology of malaria. In Drier JP (ed): "Malaria." New York: Academic Press, 1980, p 47.

50. Gilles HM, Lawson JB, Sibelas M, et al.: Malaria, anaemia, and pregnancy. Ann Trop Med Parasitol 63:245–263, 1969.

51. Bray RS, Sinder RE: The sequestration of *Plasmodium falciparum* infected erythrocytes in the placenta. Trans R Soc Trop Med Hyg 73:716–719, 1979.

52. Watkinson M, Rushton DI: Plasmodial pigmentation of placenta and outcome of pregnancy in West African mothers. Br Med J 287:251–252, 1983.

53. Wyler DJ: Malaria—Resurgence, resistance, and research. N Engl J Med 308:875–878, 1983.

54. Main EK, Main DM, Krogstad DJ: Treatment of chloroquine-resistent malaria during pregnancy. JAMA 249:3207–3209, 1983.

55. Pifer LL, Hughes WT, Stagno S, et al.: *Pneumocystis carinii* infection: Evidence for high prevalence in normal and immunosuppressed children. Pediatrics 61:35–39, 1978.

56. Price RA, Hughes WT: Histopathology of *Pneumocystis carinii* infestation and infection in malignant disease. Hum Pathol 5:737–741, 1974.

57. Hughes WT: Pneumocystis carinii. In Mandell GL, Douglas RG, Bennett JE (eds): "Principles and Practice of Infectious Disease," 2nd edition. New York: John Wiley & Sons, 1985, pp 1549–1552.

58. Sever JL: Infections in pregnancy: Highlights from the collaborative perinatal project. Teratology 25:227–235, 1982.

59. Hershey DW, McGregor JA: Case prevalence of toxoplasma infection in a Rocky Mountain prenatal population. Obstet Gynecol 70:900–902, 1987.

60. Frenkel JK: Toxoplasmosis: Mechanism of infection, laboratory diagnosis and management. Curr Top Pathol 54:28–35, 1971.

61. Remington JS: Toxoplasmosis in the adult. Bull NY Acad Med 50:211–227, 1974.

62. Sabin AB: Toxoplasmic encephalitis in children. JAMA 106:801–806, 1941.

63. Sever JL, Larsen JW, Grossman JH: Toxoplasmosis. In: "Handbook of Perianatal Infections." Boston: Little, Brown, 1979, pp 157–163.

64. Fuchs F, Kimball AC, Kean BH: The management of toxoplasmosis in pregnancy. Clin Perinatol 1:407–422, 1974.

65. Eichenwald HF: A study of congenital toxoplasmosis: In Siim JC (ed): "Human Toxoplasmosis." Copenhagen: Munksgaard, 1960, pp 41–49.

66. Daffos F, Forsetier JF, Capella-Pavlovsky J, et al.: Prenatal management of 746 pregnancies at risk of congenital toxoplasmosis. N Engl J Med 318:271–275, 1988.

67. Krick JA, Remington JS: Current concepts in parasitology: Toxoplasmosis in the adult—An overview. N Engl J Med 298:550–553, 1978.

68. Wilson CB, Remington JS: What can be done to prevent congenital toxoplasmosis? Am J Obstet Gynecol 138:357–363, 1980.

69. Foulon W, Naessens A, Lauwers S, et al.: Impact of primary prevention on the incidence of toxoplasmosis during pregnancy. Obstet Gynecol 72:363–366, 1988.

22

Infection-Induced Preterm Labor

Susan M. Cox, M.D.

One of the major health hazards in humans is an untimely birth. The optimal solution for the problem of preterm birth is its prevention, but regrettably an effective means for doing so has not been identified. The incidence of preterm birth in the United States ranges from 5 to 10%.[1,2] In spite of active therapeutic intervention, this incidence has not changed appreciably in the past three decades.[3,4] And notwithstanding the monumental strides that have been made in increasing survival rates and improving the well-being of premature newborns during the last decade, preterm birth still accounts for at least 70% of all perinatal deaths not associated with congenital anomalies.[5]

DEFINITION

The World Health Organization Expert Committee on Maternal & Child Health, in 1969, defined prematurity as those infants born at 37 weeks of gestation or less.[6] A distinction was made between "prematurity" (37 weeks of gestation or less) and "low birth weight" (2,500 g or less). This classification scheme is useful in delineating populations suffering from fetal growth retardation and pure prematurity. Although some ambigu-

ities exist, this distinction is important in terms of prognosis. The overall outcome is determined by the etiology of the low birth weight, both in terms of morbidity and survival.

ETIOLOGY

The cause of preterm labor remains largely unknown and is one of the most important unsolved problems of obstetrics. Risk factors associated with a higher incidence of preterm delivery are presented in Table 1. Categorically, these risk factors include demographic causes, environmental causes, past obstetrical performance, and obstetrical complications during the current pregnancy.[7]

PATHOGENESIS OF INFECTION-INDUCED PRETERM LABOR

Infectious conditions have long been associated with perterm birth. Any systemic infection, bacterial or viral, can potentially lead to the stimulation of uterine activity and subsequent preterm labor. The exact mechanism by which this occurs has not been clearly established. One mechanism, pro-

Infections in Pregnancy, pages 247–253

TABLE 1. Etiology of Preterm Labor

Demographic
  Non-Caucasians
  Lower socioeconomic status
  Singles
  Young age

Environmental
  Ethanol consumption
  Smoking
  Illicit drug use

Past obstetrical performances
  Previous preterm delivery
  Previous abortion (induced or spontaneous)

Obstetrical problems in current pregnancy
  Multiple fetuses
  Polyhydramnios
  Premature rupture of the membranes
  Uterine abnormalities
  Congenital malformations
  Cervical vaginal infection
  Antepartum hemorrhage

Adapted from Gravett.[7]

posed by Bejar and coworkers, is that genital microorganisms may release phospholipase A_2.[8] Additionally, McGregor and colleagues have shown that phospholipase-C from genital bacteria can cause local release of arachidonic acid.[9] These phospholipases may affect the release of arachidonic acid from the fetal membranes and glycerophospholipids. In this manner increased production of prostaglandins is obtained. Prostaglandins locally produced may be important in cervical ripening as well as labor.

A second potential mechanism involves bacterial production of immunoglobulin A, protease, neuraminadase, and mucinase enzymes, which can inhibit host immune response to organisms and facilitate passage of the organisms into the lower uterine segment of the decidua-chorion-amnion interface.[10] Bacteria that produce collagenases and other protease enzymes may focally weaken the amnion and chorion and predispose them to preterm rupture of membranes. In our population, if membranes rupture prematurely (less than 34 weeks of gestation), labor commences in less than 48 hours in 93%.[11]

Finally, the hypothesis proposed by Casey and MacDonald is that preterm labor is caused by bacterial toxin-mediated stimulation of cytokine and prostaglandin formation in the uterine decidua or the resident decidua macrophages.[12] We hypothesized that lipopolysaccharide (LPS), or bacterial endotoxin, and lipoteichoic acid (LTA) stimulation of the uterine decidua or macrophages would give rise to responses similar to those known to occur in LPS-stimulated macrophages. We know that the decidua is macrophage-like in that both tissues are 1) rich in arachidonic acid,[13–15] 2) sites of platelet-activating factor production,[16,17] 3) tissues that catalyze the 1α-hydroxylation of 25-OH vitamin D_3[18,19] 4) sites of β-endorphin formation,[20,21] 5) tissues that produce interleukin-1β and TNF-α in response to LPS,[22–26] and 7) tissues in which the messenger RNA for the protooncogene product C-*fms* is present.[27,28] The robust response characteristic of stimulative macrophages is elicited with LPS treatment of the uterine decidua.[29] Thus, an explanation is provided for the onset of preterm labor associated with infection and, in particular, silent infections.

ROLE OF INFECTION
Cervicovaginal Flora Studies

A growing body of evidence suggests that infection, particularly maternal genital infections, may be among important preventable causes of preterm delivery. Colonization of the genitourinary tract with selected microorganisms has been associated with prematurity, premature rupture of the membranes, and low birth weight. A limited number of studies have examined women in the early part of pregnancy and determined an association between colonization with pathogenic organisms and outcome. These include group B streptococcus, *Chlamydia trachomatis*, mycoplasma, herpes simplex infections, and *Neiserria gonorrhoeae*. For a critical and comprehensive review of these issues see Romero and Mazor.[30]

TABLE 2. Bacteriology in Preterm Labor

Year	Investigator	No. of patients	No. of positive cultures	% Positive cultures
1980	Miller et al.[32]	23	11	48
1981	Bobbitt et al.[33]	31	8	26
1981	Wallace and Herrick[34]	25	3	12
1984	Wahbeh et al.[35]	33	7	21
1984	Hameed et al.[36]	37	4	11
1985	Weible and Randal[37]	35	1	3
1986	Leigh and Garite[38]	59	7	12
1986	Gravett et al.[39]	54	13	24
1987	Duff and Kopelman[40]	24	1	4
1987	Iams et al.[41]	5	0	0
1988	Romero et al.[42]	41	4	10
1988	Cox et al.[43]	33	6	18
1988	Morales et al.[44]	150	16	11
Total		551	81	14.7

Intraamniotic Infection in Preterm Labor

Obstetricians have long suspected that infection was an important cause of preterm labor, yet this relationship is difficult to establish unless viable microorganisms are present in the amniotic fluid. The fact that unrecognized amnionitis, "silent infection," may be causally related to premature labor was first suggested by Bobbitt and Ledger in 1977.[31] Based on these observations, several investigators have performed amniocenteses to document intraamniotic infection in women with preterm labor and intact fetal membranes (Table 2).[32–44] By combining the available literature, there were 551 amniocenteses performed and 14.7% were positive by standard bacteriologic criteria.

Organisms recovered from the amniotic fluid of women in preterm labor with intact membranes are listed in Table 3. The most common single organism isolated is *Fusobacterium*.

Biomolecular Markers of Infection

Rarely do women in preterm labor have bacteriologic evidence of intraamniotic infection (~15%); therefore it has been proposed that infection involving the decidua, chorion laeve, or outer surface of fetal membranes could give rise to labor through the

TABLE 3. Organisms Isolated From Amniotic Fluid of Women in Preterm Labor With Intact Fetal Membranes

Type of organism	No. of organisms isolated
Aerobic organisms	
Staphylococcus sp.	4
Streptococcus agalactiae	5
Enterococcus	1
Listeria	2
Klebsiella	1
Pseudomonas	2
Providentia	1
Haemophilus influenzae	1
Gardnerella vaginalis	3
Anaerobic organisms	
Bacteroides sp.	14
Fusobacterium	14
Gram-negative rods	4
Gram-positive cocci	3
Veillonia	1
Other	
Mycoplasma/ureaplasma	7
Candida albicans	4

action of the bacterial products on the decidua or decidua macrophages.[23,29] Other methods, possibly more sensitive, have been used to evaluate amniotic fluids for the presence of bacterial products. In 1987, Iams and coworkers, using gas-liquid chromatography, identified short-chain organic fatty acids produced by microorganisms in the amniotic fluid of five of six patients with preterm labor and intact membranes.[41] Importantly, all six amniotic fluids were sterile by standard bacteriologic criteria. It was suggested that the bacteria and tissue adjacent to the amnion, namely the decidua and chorion laeve, produced the short-chain fatty acids, which easily traversed the amniotic membranes.

Recently, Romero and colleagues[42] as well as Cox, MacDonald, and Casy,[43,45] reported on the use of the *Limulus* amebocyte lysate assay to detect the presence of endotoxin in amniotic fluids from pregnancies complicated by preterm labor. In Romero's investigation, fetal membranes for the most part had ruptured spontaneously prior to the collection of the amniotic fluid and, therefore, whether postrupture colonization had occurred is not known. In the investigations by Cox et al.,[43,45] endotoxin was detected in amniotic fluids of pregnancies with intact fetal membranes and preterm labor. By using specially prepared syringes and glassware, amniotic fluid could be collected in a manner to avoid inadvertent contamination of the samples with LPS. Additionally, there was no evidence of an inhibitor of LPS in the amniotic fluid nor was the LPS a normal constituent of the amniotic fluid obtained at any stage of gestation prior to the commencement of labor. We found that LPS was present in approximately 40% of the amniotic fluids from pregnancies with preterm labor and intact fetal membranes.[43]

Interleukin-1β, a cytokine ordinarily produced by stimulated macrophages or monocytes, was present in the amniotic fluids of all subjects in preterm labor if bacterial toxins (LPS or LTA) were identified. The concentrations of interleukin-1β in these amniotic fluids ranged from 79 to >48,000 pg/ml. Importantly, none of the bacterial toxin-free amniotic fluid contained IL-1β.

TNF-α (cachectin), also produced by LPS-stimulated macrophages and decidua, accumulates in the amniotic fluid in some cases of preterm labor. In the LPS-positive fluids, TNF-α was identified in approximately 40%.

Significantly, TNF-α may promote preterm rupture of the fetal membranes by inhibiting amnion replication.[23]

Antibiotic Trials in Preterm Labor

Elder and colleagues were among the first investigators to report a decrease in the frequency of preterm birth with antibiotic therapy.[46] In a study of pregnant women with urinary tract infection, these authors reported a large incidence of preterm labor in control (noninfected) women treated with tetracycline.

To date, several investigators have conducted randomized clinical trials in which women with preterm labor and intact membranes were given antibiotic therapy as well as tocolytic therapy to inhibit preterm labor. In one study conducted by McGregor et al., prolongation of pregnancy for longer than 37 weeks occurred more commonly in the erythromycin-treated group than in the placebo-treated group ($P = .035$).[47] This was a small study: over 71% of the patients initially randomized were excluded and only 17 patients were utilized for analysis.

In a study by McCormack et al., women with vaginal cultures positive for mycoplasma or ureaplasma were randomized to receive either erythromycin, clindamycin, or placebo.[48] The incidence of low birth weight was similar in the clindamycin and erythromycin groups if the drugs were administered during the second trimester, but the group receiving erythromycin during the third trimester showed a decreased incidence of low birth weight from 11.9 to 3.1% ($P = .047$). If one takes into consideration the incidence of fetal growth retardation in these two groups, then one does not find a significant difference in the reduction of preterm birth in the erythromycin randomized group.

More recently, Morales et al. randomized 150 patients with preterm labor on tocolytics to three different antibiotic regimens: erythromycin orally vs. ampicillin orally vs. placebo.[49] In this investigation patients of similar gestational age and cervical dilatation, if randomized to receive antibiotics, had a statistically significant delay from admission to delivery (30 vs. 17 days). Importantly, in pregnancies in which the amniotic fluid cultures were positive, significantly less time was gained in utero after admission and there was a marked decrease in birth weight in the positive amniotic fluid group.

SUMMARY

Despite major advances in obstetrical care of the high-risk patient, the incidence of preterm labor has not changed appreciably in the last 30 years. Prematurity remains the greatest single cause of newborn morbidity and mortality. A majority of these pregnancies that end prematurely are complicated by infectious processes that involve the intrauterine tissue or extrauterine maternal tissues. Several investigators have long suspected and proposed that not only preterm labor but also premature rupture of the membranes may primarily be due to cervicovaginal microorganisms or other inflammatory reactions. An appreciable amount of information that evaluates the biomolecular processes involved in spontaneous preterm labor has been generated in the past 2 years. In these pregnancies, "silent infection" remains a major cause of the untimely birth. However, routine use of antimicrobials is not yet warranted in the absence of clinically apparent infection until well-designed, randomized, placebo-controlled investigations can be undertaken.

REFERENCES

1. Update incidence of low birthweight. MMWR 33: 1115, 1987.
2. Fuchs F: Prevention of prematurity. Am J Obstet Gynecol 126:809, 1976.
3. Leveno KJ, Little BB: National impact of ritodrine tocolysis. SPO (Society of Perinatal Obstetricians) 1989, abstract #357.
4. Institute of Medicine: "Preventing Low Birthweight." Washington, DC: National Academy Press, 1985.
5. Rush RW, Keirse MJ, Horvat P, et al.: Contribu-
tion of preterm delivery to prenatal mortality. Br Med J 2:965, 1976.
6. World Health Organization: Prevention of Perinatal Mortality and Morbidity. Public Health Papers 42, Geneva: WHO, 1969.
7. Gravett MG: Causes of preterm delivery. Semin Perinatol 8:246–257, 1984.
8. Bejar R, Curbello D, Davis C, Gluck L: Premature labor. II. Bacterial sources of phospholipase. Obstet Gynecol 57:479, 1981.
9. McGregor JA, Lawellin D, Franco-Buff A, et al.: Phospholipase C production by microorganisms associated with female upper genital tract infection. Proc Soc Gynecol Invest 32:208, 1985 (abstract).
10. McGregor JA: Prevention of preterm birth: New initiatives based on microbial-host interactions. Obstet Gynecol Surv 43:1–14, 1988.
11. Cox SM, Williams ML, Leveno KJ: The natural history of preterm ruptured membranes: *"What to Expect?"* of expectant management. Obstet Gynecol 71:558–562, 1988.
12. Casey ML, MacDonald PC: Decidua activation: The role of prostaglandins in labor. In MacNillas D, Challis J, MacDonald P, Nathanielsz P, Roberts J (eds): "The Onset of Labor, Cellular and Integrative Mechanism." Perinatology Press, pp 141–164.
13. Kunkel SL, Chensue SW: The role of arachidonic acid metabolites in mononuclear phagocytic cell interaction. Int J Dermatol 25:83–89, 1986.
14. Korte K, MacDonald PC, Johnston JM, Okita JR, Casey ML: Metabolism of arachidonic acid and prostanoids in human endometrial stromal cells in monolayer culture. Biochim Biophys Acta 752: 423–433, 1983.
15. Okita JR: Alterations in arachidonic acid content of specific glycerophospholipids of amnion and chorion laeve during human parturition. Doctorate dissertation, The University of Texas Southwestern Medical School, Dallas, 1981.
16. Albert DH, Snyder F: Biosynthesis of 1-alkyl-2-acetyl-sn-glycero-3-phosphocholine (platelet activating factor) from 1-alkyl-2-acyl-sn-glycero-3-phosphocholine by rat alveolar macrophages. Phospholipase A₂ and acetyl transferase activities during phagocytosis and ionophore stimulation. J Biol Chem 258:97–102, 1983.
17. Ban C, Billah MM, Truong CT, Johnston JM: Metabolism of platelet-activating factor (1-O-alkyl-2-acyl-sn-glycero-3-phosphocholine) in human fetal membranes and decidua vera. Arch Biochem Biophys 246:9–18, 1986.
18. Koeffler HP, Reichel H, Bishop FE, Norman AW: Gamma-interferon stimulates production of 1,25-dihydroxyvitamin D₃ by normal human macrophages. Biochem Biophys Res Commun 127:596–603, 1985.

19. Weisman Y, Harrell A, Edelstein S, David M, Spirer Z, Golander A: 1α,25-Dihydroxyvitamin D₃ and 24,25-dihydroxyvitamin D₃ *in vitro* synthesis by human decidua and placenta. Nature 281:317–319, 1979.

20. Lolait SJ, Clements JA, Markwick AJ, et al.: Pro-opiomelanocortin messenger ribonucleic acid and posttranslational processing of β-endorphin in spleen macrophages. J Clin Invest 77:1776, 1986.

21. Wahlstrom T, Laatikainen T, Salminen K, Leppaluoto J: Immunoreactive β-endorphin is demonstrable in the secretory but not in the proliferative endometrium. Life Sci 36:987–990, 1985.

22. Kunkel SL, Chensue SW: The role of arachidonic acid metabolites in mononuclear phagocytic cell interaction. Int J Dermatol 25:83–89, 1986.

23. Casey ML, Cox SM, Beutler B, Milewich L, MacDonald PC: Cachectin/tumor necrosis factor-α formation in human decidua. J Clin Invest 83:430–436, 1989.

24. Zahl PA, Bjerknes C: Induction of decidua-placental hemorrhage in mice by the endotoxins of certain gram-negative bacteria. Proc Soc Exp Biol Med 54:329–332, 1943.

25. Beutler B, Cerami A: Cachectin and tumor necrosis factor as two sides of the same biological coin. Nature 320:584–588, 1986.

26. Gery I, Gershon RK, Waksman BH: Potentiation of cultured mouse thymocyte responses by factors released by peritoneal leucocytes. J Exp Med 136:128–142, 1972.

27. Muller R, Tremblay JM, Adamson ED, Verma IM: Tissue and cell type-specific expression of two human c-*onc* genes. Nature 304:454–456, 1983.

28. Casey ML, Cox SM, Beutler B, MacDonald PC: The formation of cytokines in human decidua: The role of decidua in the initiation of both term and preterm labor. Proc Soc Gynecol Invest 35:219, 1988 (abstract).

29. Romero R, Wu YK, Brody DT, et al.: Human decidua: A source of interleukin-1. Obstet Gynecol 73:31–34, 1989.

30. Romero R, Mazor M: Infection in preterm labor. Clin Obstet Gynecol 31:553–584, 1988.

31. Bobbitt JR, Ledger WJ: Unrecognized amnionitis in prematurity: A preliminary report. J Reprod Med 19:8, 1977.

32. Miller JM, Pupkin MJ, Hill GB: Bacterial colonization of amniotic fluid from intact fetal membranes. Am J Obstet Gynecol 136:796, 1980.

33. Bobbitt JR, Hayslip CC, Damato JD: Amniotic fluid infection is determined by transabdominal amniocentesis in patients with intact membranes in premature labor. Am J Obstet Gynecol 140:947, 1981.

34. Wallace RL, Herrick CN: Amniocentesis in the evaluation of premature labor. Obstet Gynecol 57:483–486, 1981.

35. Wahbeh CJ, Hill GB, Eden RD, Stanley AG: Intra-amniotic bacterial colonization in premature labor. Am J Obstet Gynecol 148:739–743, 1984.

36. Hameed C, Tejani N, Verma UL, Archbald F: Silent chorioamnionitis as a cause of preterm labor refractory to tocolytic therapy. Am J Obstet Gynecol 149:726–730, 1984.

37. Weible DR, Randal HW Jr: Evaluation of amniotic fluid in preterm labor with intact membranes. J Reprod Med 30:777–780, 1985.

38. Leigh J, Garite TJ: Amniocentesis and the management of premature labor. Obstet Gynecol 67:500–506, 1986.

39. Gravett MG, Hummel D, Eschenbach DA, Holmes KK: Preterm labor associated with subclinical amniotic fluid infection and with bacterial vaginosis. Obstet Gynecol 67:229–237, 1986.

40. Duff P, Kopelman JN: Subclinical intra-amniotic infection in asymptomatic patients with refractory preterm labor. Obstet Gynecol 69:756–766, 1987.

41. Iams JD, Clapp DH, Contos DA, et al.: Does extra amniotic infection cause preterm labor? Gas-liquid chromatography studies of amniotic fluid in amnionitis, preterm labor, and normal controls. Obstet Gynecol 70:365–368, 1987.

42. Romero R, Emamian M, Quintero R, Wan M, Hobbins JC, Mazor M, Edberg S: The value and limitations of the Gram stain examination in the diagnosis of intraamniotic infection. Am J Obstet Gynecol 159:114–119, 1988.

43. Cox SM, MacDonald PC, Casey ML: Cytokines and prostaglandins in amniotic fluid of preterm labor pregnancies: Decidual origin in response to bacterial toxins [lipopolysaccharide (LPS) and lipoteichoic acid (LTA)]. Proc Soc Gynecol Invest 36:289, 1989 (abstract #413).

44. Morales WJ, Angel JL, O'Brien WF, Knuppel RA, Finazzo M: A randomized study of antibiotic therapy in idiopathic preterm labor. Obstet Gynecol 72:829–833, 1988.

45. Cox SM, MacDonald PC, Casey ML: Assay of bacterial endotoxin (lipopolysaccharide) in human amniotic fluid: Potential usefulness in diagnosis and management of preterm labor. Am J Obstet Gynecol 159:99–106, 1988.

46. Elder HA, Santamarine BAG, Smith S, et al.: The natural history of asymptomatic bacteriuria during pregnancy: The effects of tetracycline on the clinical cause and outcome of pregnancy. Am J Obstet Gynecol 111:441, 1971.

47. McGregor JA, French JI, Reller B, et al.: Adjunc-

tive erythromycin treatment for idiopathic preterm labor: Results of a randomized double-blinded placebo controlled trial. Am J Obstet Gynecol 154:98, 1986.

48. McCormack WM, Rosner D, Yhu-Hsiung L, et al.: Effect on birthweight of erythromycin treatment of pregnant women. Obstet Gynecol 69:202, 1987.

49. Morales WJ, Angel JL, O'Brien WF: A randomized study of antibiotic therapy in idiopathic preterm labor. Obstet Gynecol 72:829–833, 1988.

23

Pneumonia in Pregnancy

Maurizio L. Maccato, M.D.

The development of powerful antimicrobials and the refinement in the techniques of supportive care are responsible for the much-improved prognosis of pregnant patients with pneumonia, a disease that historically carried a 20% maternal mortality rate.[1] However, pneumonia, the inflammation of the lower respiratory tract, i.e., respiratory bronchioles and alveoli, is still responsible for significant morbidity and mortality.

Several infectious etiologic agents of pneumonia have been identified among all classes of microorganisms: bacteria, viruses, fungi, and parasites. An infectious disease of special significance, pulmonary tuberculosis, remains a serious health problem in high-risk groups, mainly recent immigrants and lower socioeconomic classes. Pregnancy remains a big risk factor in aspiration pneumonia, a condition whose prevention and treatment remains an area of much current investigation.

BACTERIAL PNEUMONIA

The response of the lung to an inoculum of pathogens varies depending on the interplay between the invading organisms and the host defense mechanisms. The alteration in cardiorespiratory physiology imposed by pregnancy, with the increased oxygen consumption of 15–25% and the decreased residual lung volume, makes the pregnant patient and her fetus less tolerant of impaired respiratory functions. Moreover, preterm labor is still reported in 8% of pregnancies complicated by pneumonia, a considerable improvement over the 70% rate reported before effective antibiotic development.[2] The different clinical picture elicited by the different microorganisms aids in the empiric choice of effective antimicrobials, whose prompt institution, prior to final microbiologic data, is of great importance in the outcome of the disease. Together with the history and physical examination, two rapid laboratory determinations that can be performed in the initial evaluation of the patient are the Gram stain of a properly collected sputum specimen and the chest radiograph. The chest radiograph, obtained in the pregnant patient with a shielded abdomen, poses a risk to the fetus that is probably too small to be measured.

The appearance of the chest x-ray in the patient with pneumonia depends on the pattern of increase in the intraalveolar and interstitial fluid resulting from the response of the lung to the invading pathogens. Both humoral and cellular immune responses are activated by the pathogens: IgG antibodies are active in the interstitium, while IgA antibod-

Infections in Pregnancy, pages 255–266
© 1990 Alan R. Liss, Inc.

ies are present in the secretion; alveolar macrophages and the reticuloendothelial cells are active in the clearing of the organisms, often after opsonization has taken place. Polymorphonuclear leukocytes are rapidly activated after the entry of the pathogens in the lower respiratory tree, contributing to the formation of an exudate that, if it spreads from alveolus to alveolus, with relative sparing of the bronchial tree, will give rise to a chest x-ray that reveals consolidation with air bronchograms, a pattern indicative of an airspace pneumonia. If the predominant site of inflammation and subsequent fluid collection is the interalveolar septum, then an interstitial pneumonia will result, with increased interstitial marking on the radiograph. If the bronchi themselves are affected, then, together with consolidation, atelectasis will be prominent and no air bronchograms will be seen, i.e., a bronchopneumonia. On the chest radiograph, pleural effusions, cavitation, and abscess formation are often recognized in association with certain types of pneumonia.

If the patient is not immunocompromised, relatively few bacteria are of such virulence as to be able to overcome the normal host defense mechanisms. Several factors, however, are responsible for lowering the host resistance to infections. The defense mechanisms and the factors affecting them can be broadly grouped into three categories: 1) mechanical barriers between the normally sterile lower respiratory tract and the colonized nasopharynx that may be bypassed by endotracheal tubes or made ineffective by suppression of the cough or gag reflex; 2) clearance of organisms that do gain access to the lower respiratory tract through ciliated epithelium and the activity of the pulmonary macrophages, with the activity of both being affected by smoking or viral infections; and 3) eradication of invading organisms by the immune system, affected by immunosuppressive drugs, immunodeficiencies or chronically debilitated states and anemia.

Based on a reported incidence of pneumo-

nia in the pregnant population of between 0.04 and 1%, it does not appear that the pregnant patient is at higher risk for the development of the disease.[1–3] However, once the infection is established, rapid and effective therapy is necessary to improve the patient's chances of recovery and of fetal salvage.

Evaluation

As stated above, for optimal results, the treatment of pneumonia in the pregnant woman must be initiated usually without the benefit of final culture and sensitivity data from the microbiology laboratory. Therefore, the initial evaluation of the patient is used to arrive at a decision on the most likely pathogens that may be responsible for the specific clinical case. This information, coupled with the general pattern of antibiotic resistance of the suspected pathogen in the particular community or hospital, will allow the selection of an appropriate initial therapeutic regimen. To this end, it is important to determine if the infection is community acquired or if it is nosocomial. Moreover, it is generally possible to divide the patients into two groups based on their symptoms pattern. Patients with a "classic" constellation of symptoms present with a disease of rapid onset, with fever and chills, productive sputum, and a chest x-ray pattern with lobar consolidation. Patients with "atypical" pneumonia have a slower onset of symptoms, usually over several days, with a low-grade fever and nonproductive cough. Headache and myalgia are common, and the chest x-ray often has a nonhomogenous appearance.

It is very important to secure an adequate sputum sample for Gram stain and culture prior to the administration of antibiotics. There is some controversy regarding the utility of the sputum Gram stain in the management of the patient.[4–7] It appears that for the specimen to be of use, it must be representative of lower bronchial secretions with as little contamination with saliva as possible. The presence of many polymorphonuclear leukocytes and rare epithelial cells suggest that the sample is suitable for isolation of a pathogen. However, some contamination with oropharyngeal secretion is inevitable. Therefore, the results of the sputum Gram stain and culture must be supported by the clinical findings to be considered valid. At times, a sputum sample may have to be induced with the help of nebulized saline. In certain circumstances, not even this technique will be sufficient for producing an acceptable sputum sample. The clinical situation will then dictate if more invasive methods for sputum collection will be needed, namely, transtracheal aspiration, bronchoscopy with bronchoalveolar lavage or biopsy, or open lung biopsy. If the patient has developed a pleural effusion, a thoracentesis with Gram stain and culture of the pleural fluid may yield the pathogenic organism. The clinician should inform the microbiology laboratory if unusual organisms are suspected, to ensure proper handling of the specimens and the use of appropriate culturing and identification techniques. Blood cultures should be obtained routinely as well, because when positive, they are highly specific. Again, the blood samples for culture should be collected prior to initiation of antimicrobial therapy. Serology may be of value in the selected patient: a high titer of cold agglutinins is suggestive of mycoplasma pneumonia,[8] but in about 25% of cases of mycoplasma pneumonia, the titer will be low. Conversely, a high titer has been described with other pneumonias. A fourfold rise in serum antibody titer against suspected pathogens, e.g., *Legionella*, may confirm the diagnosis. However, it is of little value in the initial evaluation of the patient. A promising technique under development is the use of monoclonal antibody stain to some pathogens to increase the sensitivity of a sputum smear.

In a pregnant patient with community-acquired pneumonia presenting with a classical syndrome, the organism most frequently isolated is *Streptococcus pneumoniae*. It was cultured from the sputum of 13 of 39 pregnant patients described by Benedetti et al. in a recent study.[2] This encapsulated gram-positive diplococcus resists phagocytosis, unless prior opsonization has taken place. The chest radiograph shows lobar consolidation and, usually, a pleural effusion. The sputum is often rusty in color, and pleuritic chest pain and leukocytosis is the rule. A significant increase in immature polymorphonuclear leukocytes is common. As a rule, the pneumococcal infection is not associated with tissue destruction, therefore healing occurs with no scarring or fibrosis.

Another rather common isolate is *Haemophilus influenzae*, found in four of the women in the series mentioned above.[2] Like *Streptococcus pneumoniae*, this is an encapsulated organism that requires opsonization for effective phagocytosis. On Gram stain it appears as a small gram-negative coccobacillus. Consolidation with air bronchograms is generally noted on x-rays. Abscess formation is rare.

Staphylococcus aureus was cultured in 2 of 23 cases collected in one series reported by Hopwood[3] and in 1 of 39 cases in the study by Benedetti et al.[2] The organism is a gram-positive coccus, responsible for a disease of abrupt onset, generally following a viral pneumonia. Its production of various exotoxins is partly responsible for the rapidly progressive course of the disease and extensive tissue destruction. Purulent sputum and pleuritic chest pain are the norm. The chest x-ray usually reveals a bronchopneumonia, frequently associated with a pleural effusion, and possibly cavitation.

Klebsiella pneumonia was isolated in 1 of 6 patients who had a bacterial isolate identified from a sputum culture in the series described by Hopwood.[3] This, too, is an organism that often results in lung tissue destruction, with frequent cavitation and fibrosis and scarring after resolution of the infection. In the general population, this encapsulated gram-negative rod has been associated with chronic alcoholism. The chest radiograph usually shows consolidation with air bronchograms, often in the upper lobes, commonly accompanied by a pleural effusion and with possible finding of abscess formation and cavitation.

A rare pneumonia of rapid onset with fever and chills and a nonproductive cough is caused by a small pleomorphic organism, *Francisella tularensis*. The pathogen is transmitted by tick bite or exposure to infected animals. Bronchopneumonia is the rule, with characteristic hilar lymphadenopathy.

In the general population, the most common organism responsible for "atypical" pneumonia is *Mycoplasma pneumoniae*. This small organism, lacking a rigid cell wall, produces a disease of slow onset, accompanied by low-grade temperature, nonproductive cough, and only mild leukocytosis. In the series by Benedetti et al., two patients had serologic evidence supporting this diagnosis.[2] The chest radiograph generally shows patchy alveolar infiltrates, often quite extensive, in spite of relatively mild symptoms. Among the general population, several associated conditions have been described, including bullous myringitis in up to 5% of cases, cervical lymphadenopathy, pharyngitis, and skin rash.[8] Recovery usually occurs in 2 to 3 weeks after onset of symptoms.

Legionella pneumophila is another organism responsible for a pneumonia with a gradual onset, associated with fever, chills, and a nonproductive cough. The symptoms are usually preceded by 3 to 4 days of an influenza-like illness, with headache and sore throat.[9] Healing occurs by fibrosis because of destruction of the interalveolar septa.

Two other organisms to be included in the differential of "atypical" pneumonia are *Coxiella burnettii* and *Chlamydia psittaci*. *Coxiella burnettii* is an obligate intracellular parasite responsible for Q fever. It resists drying well and this makes the organism quite stable outside the host cell. *Chlamydia psittaci*, another obligate intracellular parasite, may be acquired by inhalation of the contaminated fecal particles from infected birds.[10] The disease has an influenza-like prodrome, with nonproductive cough, and may be quite severe. A strain of *Chlamydia psittaci* (TWAR) has been shown to be transmitted from human to human and to cause a rather mild "atypical" pneumonia.[8]

In hospitalized patients, the upper airways are frequently colonized with organisms such as the Enterobacteriaceae, *Acinetobacter*, *Pseudomonas*, and *Serratia*, which are generally not recovered from that site. In patients with inefficient upper-airway protective mechanisms, these organisms alone or in conjunction with anaerobes may be responsible for the pneumonia. Pneumonias associated with anaerobic organisms usually follow an episode of aspiration. The pneumonia develops slowly and is associated with putrid sputum, frequent cavitation, and abscess formation. Pleural effusion is common. In a hospital setting, bacteria with unusual or multiple drug-resistance patterns may be found, thus making the isolation and sensitivity testing of the organisms responsible for the infection even more important.

Treatment

The two mainstays of treatment are supportive therapy and effective antibiotic coverage. Supportive therapy includes adequate hydration, oxygenation, and prompt treatment of ventilatory failure. Arterial blood gases are useful at the onset of therapy to obtain baseline oxygenation and ventilation values, which are useful in assessing the effectiveness of therapy. The pulse oximeter is a noninvasive method to follow oxygen saturation in the patient, and it is useful during the initial critical stage of evaluation and therapy. Based on the data provided by the arterial blood gases and the pulse oximeter, oxygen is administered so that the oxygen saturation remains above 95%. If, in spite of maximum inspired oxygen concentration, the arterial blood oxygen pressure remains at 60 mm Hg or below, or if the patient develops ventilatory failure with increasing blood PCO_2 and decreasing blood pH, then mechanical ventilation is needed. Invasive cardiovascular monitoring and evacuation of

TABLE 1. Initial Therapy of Pneumonia in Pregnancy

	Drug of choice	Alternative
Community acquired		
Classic	Ampicillin 1–2 g IV q 4–6 h	Erythromycin Cephalosporins Broad-spectrum penicillins
Atypical	Erythromycin 500 mg IV q 6 h	
Influenza	Amantadine 100 mg PO q 12 h Ribavirin inhalation	
Postinfluenza	Nafcillin 1–2 g IV q 6 h	Broad-spectrum penicillins with beta-lactamase inhibitors or cephalosporins
Varicella	Acyclovir 10 mg/kg IV q 8 h	
Nasocomial	Aminoglycoside plus 3rd-generation cephalosporin or broad-spectrum penicillin	
Aspiration	Clindamycin, 900 mg IV q 8 h plus aminoglycoside if gram-negative pathogens suspected	Penicillin G or cefoxitin plus aminoglycoside if gram-negative suspected

the uterus may be required in an effort to maximize cardiopulmonary function in the critically ill patient. Bronchodilators are useful if there is evidence of bronchospasm.

Of course, antibacterial therapy, or antiviral therapy when available, is of the utmost importance (Table 1). Empiric therapy should be started as soon as possible. However, it is important to try to obtain an adequate sputum sample and blood specimen for culture prior to antibiotic administration. For pregnant patients with community-acquired pneumonia presenting with "classical" symptoms, ampicillin is usually an adequate primary antibiotic. In the penicillin-allergic patient, erythromycin can be used. For patients with an "atypical" presentation of their pneumonia, erythromycin is recommended. If the infection follows a viral pneumonia, an antistaphylococcal agent should be used. If *Legionella* is the suspected pathogen, some studies suggest an improved outcome in the most seriously ill patients if rifampicin is added to erythromycin.[11] In

patients with nosocomial infections, a third-generation cephalosporin and an aminoglycoside may be used pending culture results.[12,13] In the general population, imipenem/cilastatin appears to be an effective alternative. If anaerobic infection is suspected, clindamycin has been demonstrated to be an effective agent.[14,15] The use of an aminoglycoside should be accompanied by monitoring of the blood levels achieved, in order to maximize efficacy and minimize side effects.[16]

Penicillins and cephalosporins are usually considered safe antibiotics in pregnancy, as are erythromycin base and clindamycin. Rifampin has been used in the treatment of tuberculosis in pregnancy and, except for one study that noted a small and not statistically significant increase in short-limb defects, no evidence of unexpected maternal or fetal toxicity has been reported.[17] Aminoglycosides have been linked to eighth nerve damage in fetuses, therefore their use in pregnancy should be cautious.[18]

VIRAL PNEUMONIA

Several viruses have been implicated as the etiologic agents of pneumonia in pregnancy. While they are usually part of the differential diagnosis of "atypical" pneumonia, in many cases pneumonia is a complication of an otherwise relatively benign viral disease, e.g., influenza, varicella, and measles.

Influenza A pneumonia usually develops 2 or 3 days after the onset of symptoms of influenza. The virus is responsible for intraalveolar hemorrhage, thickening of the interalveolar septa, and hyaline membrane formation.[19] The progression of the disease may be very rapid. In 1919, Harris reported a mortality rate of 50% in pregnant women with influenza pneumonia.[20] Pregnant women do not seem at higher risk of contracting influenza than the general population. However, women in their third trimester of pregnancy appear to be at higher risk of developing influenza pneumonia.[21] The virus generally can be cultured from the patient's nasopharynx, and it may be identified in secretion by immunofluorescence. Successful treatment has been reported using inhaled ribavirin and oral amantadine.[22] Ribavirin has demonstrated activity against both influenza A and B, and no teratogenicity was noted in nonhuman primates exposed to high doses of the compound.[22] Amantadine is effective against influenza A, and, in very high doses, it is embryotoxic to rats, but not to mice or rabbits.[21] It therefore should be used cautiously in pregnancy. Influenza vaccine is considered safe in pregnancy, and it is recommended that pregnant women with medical conditions putting them at high risk of complications be vaccinated.[23] Bacterial superinfection after influenza pneumonia is usually secondary to *Streptococcus pneumoniae* or *Staphylococcus aureus*. Of course, appropriate antibiotic treatment of this complication should be promptly instituted.

Varicella pneumonia is another uncommon but potentially devastating complication of an otherwise rather benign illness.

Vari[...]
more [...]
dren [...]
foun[...]
the [...]
opm[...]
with [...]
dysp[...]
mop[...]
deve[...]
disea[...]
failure. Several reports of successful treatment with acyclovir of pregnant women have been published.[24] Acyclovir seems effective, is well tolerated, and no evidence of fetal toxicity has been reported.[25–27]

Measles is associated with evidence of significant pulmonary involvement in about 50% of cases among the general population.[8] A study of a large epidemic of measles in Greenland in 1953 did not find a significant difference in the frequency of pneumonia between pregnant and nonpregnant women.[28] Pneumonia is the most common cause of death from measles, with autopsy findings of edema of the alveoli, coupled with mononuclear cell infiltration and hyaline membrane formation. Chest radiographs usually show a diffuse reticular infiltrate. Contrary to varicella pneumonia, measles pneumonia is frequently complicated by bacterial superinfection with *Streptococcus pneumoniae*, *Staphylococcus aureus* and, less commonly, other pathogens. Again, rapid treatment of the superinfection is necessary.

Adenovirus is responsible for pneumonia that is confined mainly to military recruits.[8] In adults, herpes simplex virus, Epstein-Barr virus, cytomegalovirus, and respiratory syncytial virus are responsible for pulmonary infections almost exclusively in the immunocompromised host.

FUNGAL AND PARASITIC PNEUMONIA

Pneumonia caused by fungi can present either as "atypical" pneumonia or as a slowly progressive disease, with constitutional and pulmonary symptoms.

Histoplasmosis is caused by *Histoplasma capsulatum,* a fungus that is frequent in the soil of large river valleys. The spores are inhaled and cause a granulomatous reaction in the lung. The infection may be asymptomatic or it may cause a mild influenza-like illness, associated with nonproductive cough, dyspnea, and pleuritic chest pain. The chest radiograph will show patchy infiltrates during the acute phase of the infection. In some patients, the granulomas will calcify and become evident in later chest radiographs. Disseminated disease is rare in patients who are not immunocompromised.[29] Treatment of disease confined to the lungs is generally not necessary. Amphotericin B is effective in disseminated disease.[30]

Coccidioidomycosis is caused by *Coccidioides immitis,* a fungus common in hot, arid regions. Like histoplasmosis, when spores from the soil are inhaled, a granulomatous reaction develops in the lungs. Pulmonary symptoms, when present, are mild, with an "atypical" pneumonia presentation. Arthralgias may develop. The chest radiograph will show patchy infiltrates, at times accompanied by pleural effusion. If the disease remains confined to the lungs, it usually will resolve with no significant risk to mother or fetus. In pregnancy, however, the infection has the propensity to disseminate, with a mortality rate approaching 100% if left untreated. Harris reported dissemination of the disease in 22 of 50 patients.[31] Therefore, in pregnancy, treatment with amphotericin B should be considered even if the disease is still confined to the lungs.

Other fungal infections have been described in pregnancy, but they appear to be of significance only in the immunocompromised host. Parasites, likewise, are of concern mainly in patients with impaired immune systems. *Pneumocystis carinii* is the most common opportunistic infection in patients with acquired immunodeficiency syndrome.[32,33] Symptoms may be quite mild at the onset,

thus a high degree of suspicion is necessary. Diagnosis may require bronchoscopy, with bronchoalveolar lavage or biopsy. Therapy requires pentamidine or trimethoprim-sulfamethoxazole. Recurrences are unfortunately common, and preventive and maintenance therapies are currently being investigated.[34]

Amphotericin B has been used in pregnancy with no reported fetal toxicity. Trimethoprim is a folate antagonist, and a theoretical concern about possible teratogenicity has been raised. There is very limited experience with pentamidine in pregnancy.

PULMONARY TUBERCULOSIS

In the United States, tuberculosis remains a serious health problem, mainly among recent immigrants and lower socioeconomic classes.[35]

Mycobacterium tuberculosis is an acid-fast, slow-growing pathogen that resists desiccation well, and therefore is easily transmitted from patient to patient through inhalation of sputum droplets. An uncommon mode of transmission is congenital acquisition by way of the placenta. Usually, the newborn is infected after birth from an infected caretaker.[36]

After the pathogen gains access to the lung, it elicits an inflammatory response that, in the majority of cases, confines the organisms with formation of a primary (Ghon) complex. This stage of the disease is asymptomatic. Uncommonly, this primary complex will progress to a clinical pneumonia, with caseation necrosis of the lung parenchyma, or even disseminated disease. Viable organisms may remain dormant in the primary complex for many years until a lowering of the effectiveness of the cell-mediated immunity of the host will allow for reactivation of the disease. The disease then progresses by direct extension. While the majority of cases of tuberculosis will be pulmonary, the disease may affect other organ systems. Pregnancy does not seem to affect the course of the disease.[37] Bjerkedal et al.

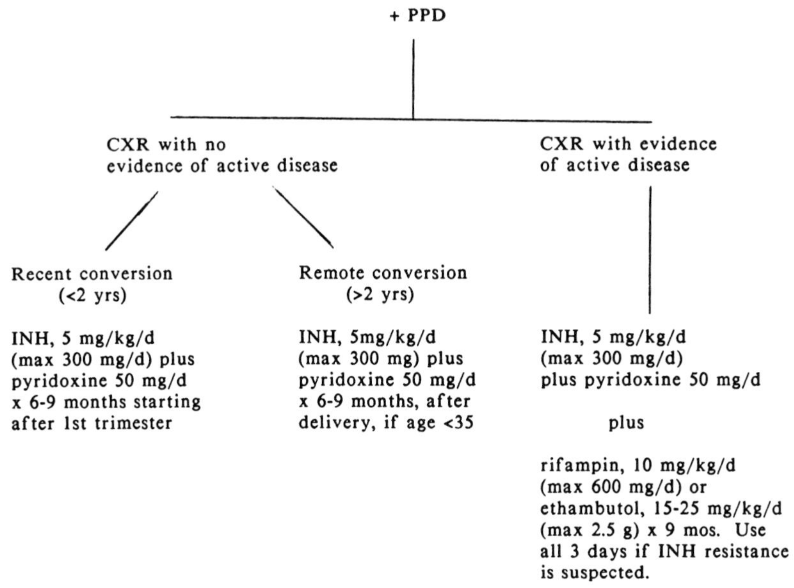

Fig. 1. Evaluation of asymptomatic patients with positive PPD.

reported 542 cases of pregnancy complicated by tuberculosis.[38] They noted a statistically significant increase in the frequency of pregnancy-induced hypertension, vaginal hemorrhage, and miscarriage among their affected patients.

Evaluation

The well-described signs and symptoms of pulmonary tuberculosis include cough, hemoptysis, fever and night sweats, weight loss, weakness, and anorexia. These symptoms are present both in the uncommon patient with primary tuberculosis pneumonitis and in the patient with reactivation of the disease. Most pregnant patients with active disease, however, will be asymptomatic. The chest radiograph will show patchy infiltrates, often with cavitary disease in the upper lobes. In pregnancy, findings on the chest x-ray may be more subtle than in the nonpregnant state because of the reduced vertical diameter of the chest. Sputum samples should be collected for three morn-

ings in a row to increase the likelihood of a positive acid-fast stain and successful culture of the organisms. Because the majority of affected patients will be asymptomatic, screening of all pregnant patients with purified protein derivative (PPD) has been suggested. Most centers around the country, however, routinely test only patients belonging to a high-risk group, e.g., recent immigrants or members of lower socioeconomic classes.[39] The PPD is safe and reliable in pregnancy, and, when positive, indicates that the patient has been exposed and has become sensitized to M. *tuberculosis*.[40] Thus, if a pregnant woman is asymptomatic and has a negative PPD test, she is assumed to be noninfected and no other diagnostic tests are recommended. If the PPD test is positive, then a chest radiograph with shielded abdomen is obtained to identify patients with active pulmonary disease (see Fig. 1). As noted above, the risk to the fetus from a chest radiograph with a shielded abdomen is considered too small to be measured. If active disease is present, treatment is immediately initiated. If there is no evidence of active disease and the patient has never been treated, isoniazid chemoprophylaxis is initiated as soon as the patient delivers, unless the conversion has occurred recently, in which case, because of the increased risk of developing the disease, chemoprophylaxis should be started immediately after the first trimester of pregnancy.[41] If the patient has signs or symptoms suggestive of tuberculosis, the chest radiograph should be obtained regardless of PPD status, because a significant portion of patients with active disease will have a negative PPD test. Of course, if extrapulmonary tuberculosis is suspected, appropriate cultures or biopsies should be obtained.

Treatment

Because of the slow-growing nature of *M. tuberculosis* culture and sensitivity results may not be available for several weeks. Empiric therapy, therefore, must be initiated. Isoniazid and rifampin or ethambutol should be started as soon as possible. Isoniazid should be administered with pyridoxine to prevent potential neurotoxicity. Isoniazid will cause an asymptomatic elevation of serum transaminases in 20% of adults and hepatitis in 0.3 to 1.5%, depending on the age of the patient. It is contraindicated in patients with active liver disease. Optic neuritis is a significant side effect of ethambutol. Baseline visual tests should therefore be obtained, and the patient instructed to report any visual symptoms such as blurred vision, decreased visual acuity, or red-green discrimination difficulties.[41] Patients should also be counseled that several unintended pregnancies have been reported with the concomitant use of rifampin and oral contraceptives, probably secondary to altered steroid metabolism in the liver.[42] These first-line drugs are considered relatively safe in pregnancy.

If results of sensitivity tests show the mycobacterium strain to be resistant to one or more of the primary drugs, than second-line drugs must be used. These drugs include streptomycin, pyrazinamide, cycloserine, para-amino salicylic acid, ethionamide, and capreomycin. Ethionamide is considered a teratogen, and streptomycin has been linked to eighth-nerve damage in the fetus. Cycloserine is rarely used because of significant central nervous system side effects. Little is known about the other second-line drugs in pregnancy.

Treatment of the disease requires the concomitant use of multiple drugs to which the organism is sensitive to avoid development of resistance. Treatment with two drugs, usually isoniazid and ethambutol or rifampin, is continued for 9 months. Isoniazid is also the drug of choice for chemoprophylaxis and is usually given for 6 to 9 months. Effective therapeutic regimens have been developed that allow for biweekly administration of the drugs after an initial period of daily administration of 1 to 2 months.

Vaccination with bacillus Calmette-Guérin (BCG) is in use in several countries. In the United States, vaccination was never used on a large scale because the data are discordant regarding its effectiveness, and the PPD test will become positive, thus eliminating a simple and effective screening method. In the United States, vaccination appears to have a role only in the newborn at high risk of infection in a situation where reliable administration of chemoprophylaxis and regular medical follow-up is not ensured.[43] The newborn should be carefully screened for congenital tuberculosis, and a PPD test performed. If the mother has active tuberculosis, isoniazid prophylaxis should be administered to the infant until the mother is acid-fast stain and culture negative, preferably for 3 months. If the infant, after 3 months, is still PPD negative with no evidence of disease on chest x-ray, the prophylaxis can be stopped. Breast-feeding is not contraindicated if adequate therapy of the infected mother and the infant can be achieved.

ASPIRATION PNEUMONIA

Aspiration pneumonia is a serious condition that carries with it a significant mortality rate.[44] In the obstetric patient, it frequently follows excessive sedation or induction and emergence from general anesthesia, often administered in emergency cases, when no adequate preoperative preparation was possible. This, coupled with the physiologic decrease in gastroesophageal sphincter tone and delayed gastric emptying, makes the pregnant patient particularly vulnerable.

The pulmonary injury in aspiration pneumonia depends on the aspirated material. Inert substances will mainly interfere mechanically with gas exchange at the level of the alveoli or cause obstruction of the airways, either mechanically or by triggering spasm and reflex closure of the bronchi. Partially digested food, nasogastric tube feedings, and irrigation solution are examples. If gastric acid is aspirated, a chemical pneumonitis will develop very rapidly, with damage to the alveolar capillary membrane.[45]

The onset of symptoms is rapid, with acute dyspnea, tachycardia, tachypnea, and usually marked bronchospasm. The chest radiograph will demonstrate an infiltrate in the affected lung segments. Bacterial superinfection is a feared complication of aspiration pneumonia. It appears that the bacteria involved are those colonizing the patient oropharynx. Thus, if the patient has spent time in the hospital, the presence of the Enterobacteriaceae, *Pseudomonas, Serratia,* or *Staphylococcus aureus,* together with the anaerobic flora of the mouth, should be suspected.

Treatment

Of course, the best treatment of aspiration pneumonia is prevention.[46] Therefore, when possible, careful preoperative preparation of the patient is important. In the patient in labor, neutralization of gastric acid and appropriate intubation and extubation technique have been demonstrated to be useful in decreasing the risk of aspiration or minimizing the damage to the lung if aspiration does occur.[47,48]

The treatment of aspiration pneumonia requires prompt ventilatory assistance, with mechanical ventilation and positive end expiratory pressure, if necessary, to maintain an oxygen saturation of 90% or better. Because bronchospasm is commonly present, bronchodilators can be of significant help.

Neither prophylactic use of antibiotics nor corticosteroids have been proved useful. Close attention must be paid, however, to the development of bacterial superinfection, with sudden deterioration of signs and symptoms, fever, and leukocytosis. Bynum and Pierce reported both gram-negative and gram-positive bacilli recovered from patients who developed bacterial superinfection.[45] Therefore, a combination of a broad-spectrum antibiotic with good anaerobic coverage, like a semisynthetic penicillin with a beta-lactamase inhibitor or some cephalosporins, with an aminoglycoside should be used until culture and sensitivity results are obtained.

REFERENCES

1. Oxorn H: The changing aspects of pneumonia complicating pregnancy. Am J Obstet Gynecol 70(5):1057–1063, 1955.
2. Benedetti TJ, Valle R, Ledger WJ: Antepartum pneumonia in pregnancy. Am J Obstet Gynecol 144(4):413–417, 1982.
3. Hopwood HG: Pneumonia in pregnancy. Obstet Gynecol 25(6):875–879, 1965.
4. Barrett-Connor E: The non-value of sputum culture in the diagnosis of pneumococcal pneumonia. Am Rev Respir Dis 103:845–848, 1971.
5. Perlino CH: Laboratory diagnosis of pneumonia due to *Streptococcus pneumoniae.* J Infect Dis 150:139–144, 1984.
6. Musher DM: Gram-stain and culture of sputum to diagnose bacterial pneumonia (letter). J Infect Dis 152(5):1096, 1985.
7. Kalin M: Accuracy of sputum examination for the diagnosis of pneumococcal pneumonia (letter). J Infect Dis 152(5):1097, 1985.
8. Luby JP: Southwestern Internal Medicine Conference: Pneumonia in adults due to Mycoplasma,

Chlamydia and viruses. Am J Med Sci 294(1):45–64, 1987.

9. Soper DE, Melone PJ, Conover WB: Legionnaire disease complicating pregnancy. Obstet Gynecol 67(Suppl):10S–12S, 1986.

10. Wainwright AP, Beaumont AC, Kox WJ: Psittacosis: Diagnosis and management of severe pneumonia and multiorgan failure. Intensive Care Med 13:419–421, 1987.

11. Fitzgeorge RB, Baskerville A, Featherstone ASR: Treatment of experimental Legionnaires disease by aerosol administration of rifampicin, ciprofloxacin, and erythromycin. Lancet 1:502–503:1986.

12. Quenzer RW: A perspective of cephalosporins in pneumonia. Chest 92(3):531–535, 1987.

13. Grassi GG: Respiratory infections: Established therapy and its limitations. Clin Ther 7(A Suppl):19–36, 1985.

14. MacFarlane JT: Treatment of lower respiratory infections. Lancet 2:1446–1449, 1987.

15. Bartlett JG, Gorbach SL: Treatment of aspiration pneumonia and primary lung abscess. Penicillin G vs. clindamycin. JAMA 234(9):935–937, 1975.

16. Lode H: Initial therapy in pneumonia. Clinical, radiographic, and laboratory data important for the choice. Am J Med 80(5C):70–74, 1986.

17. Snider DE, Layde P, Johnson MW, Lyle MA: Treatment of tuberculosis during pregnancy. Am Rev Respir Dis 122:65–79, 1980.

18. Chow AW, Jewesson PS: Pharmacokinetics and safety of antimicrobial agents during pregnancy. Rev Infect Dis 7:287–313, 1985.

19. Louria DB, Blumenfeld HL, Ellis JT, et al.: Studies on influenza in the pandemic of 1957–58. II. Pulmonary complications of influenza. J Clin Invest 38:213–265, 1959.

20. Harris JW: Influenza occurring in pregnant women. JAMA 72:978–980, 1919.

21. Kort BA, Cefalo RC, Baker VV: Fatal influenza A pneumonia in pregnancy. Am J Perinatol 3(3):179–182, 1986.

22. Kirshon B, Faro S, Zurawin RK, Samo TC, Carpenter RJ: Favorable outcome after treatment with amantadine and ribavirin in a pregnancy complicated by influenza pneumonia. A case report. J Reprod Med 33(4):399–401, 1988.

23. Centers for Disease Control: Prevention and control of influenza. MMWR 33:253, 1984.

24. Straus SE: The management of varicella and zoster infections. Infect Dis Clin North Am 1(2):367–382, 1987.

25. Hankins GDV, Gilstrap LC, Patterson AR: Acyclovir treatment of varicella pneumonia in pregnancy (letter). Crit Care Med 15(4):336–337, 1987.

26. Eder SE, Apuzzio JJ, Weiss G: Varicella pneumonia during pregnancy. Treatment of two cases with acyclovir. Am J Perinatol 5(1):16–18, 1988.

27. Landsberger EJ, Hager WD, Grossman JH III: Successful management of varicella pneumonia complicating pregnancy. A report of three cases. J Reprod Med 31(5):311–314, 1986.

28. Christensen PE, Schmidt H, Ban HO, et al.: An epidemic of measles in southern Greenland, 1951. Measles in virgin soil II. The epidemis proper. Acta Med Scand 144:431–440, 1953.

29. Goodwin RA, Loyd JE, DesPrez RM: Histoplasmosis in normal hosts. Medicine 60:231–266, 1981.

30. Sarosi GA: Management of fungal diseases. Am Rev Respir Dis 127:250–253, 1983.

31. Harris RE: Coccidioidomycosis complicating pregnancy. Report of 3 cases and review of the literature. Obstet Gynecol 28:401, 1966.

32. Minkoff H, DeRegt RH, Landesman S, Schwarz R: *Pneumocystis carinii* pneumonia associated with acquired immunodeficiency syndrome in pregnancy. A report of three maternal deaths. Obstet Gynecol 67(2):284–287, 1986.

33. Rogers MF, Ewing EP, Warfield D, Hardy AM, Emergy DR, Wolf GC: Virologic studies of HTLV-III/LAV in pregnancy. Case report of a woman with AIDS. Obstet Gynecol 68(3 Suppl):2S–6S, 1986.

34. Rankin JA, Collman R, Daniele RP: Acquired immunodeficiency syndrome and the lung. Chest 94(1):155–164, 1988.

35. Centers for Disease Control: Tuberculosis, final data—United States, 1986. MMWR 36:817–820, 1988.

36. Bate TWP, Sinclair RE, Robinson MJ: Neonatal tuberculosis. Arch Dis Child 61:512–514, 1986.

37. Nemir RL: Perspective in adolescent tuberculosis: Three decades of experience. Pediatrics 78(3):399–405, 1986.

38. Bjerkedal T, Bahna SL, Lehmann EH: Course and outcome of pregnancy in women with pulmonary tuberculosis. Scand J Resp Dis 56:245–250, 1975.

39. McIntyre PB, McCormack JG, Vacca A: Tuberculosis in pregnancy-implications for antenatal screening in Australia. Med J Aust 146:42–44, 1987.

40. Gillum MD, Maki DG: Brief report: Tuberculin testing, BCG in pregnancy. Infect Control Hosp Epidemiol 9(3):119–121, 1988.

41. American Thoracic Society: Treatment of tuberculosis and tuberculosis infection in adults and children. Am Rev Respir Dis 134:355–363, 1986.

42. Skolnick JL, Stolar BS, Katz DB, Anderson WH: Rifampin, oral contraceptives, and pregnancy. JAMA 236:1382, 1976.

43. Centers for Disease Control: Use of BCG vaccines in the control of tuberculosis: A joint statement by the ACIP and the Advisory Committee for Elimi-

nation of Tuberculosis. MMWR 37:663–675, 1988.

44. Morgan M: Anesthetic contribution to maternal mortality. Br J Anaesth 59(7):842–855, 1987.

45. Bynum LJ, Pierce AK: Pulmonary aspiration of gastric contents. Am Rev Respir Dis 114:1129–1136, 1976.

46. Power KJ: The prevention of the acid aspiration (Mendelson's) syndrome. A contribution to reduced maternal mortality. Midwifery 3(3):143–148, 1987.

47. Malinow AM, Ostheimer GW: Anesthesia for the high-risk parturient. Obstet Gynecol 69(6):951–964, 1987.

48. Kallos T, Lampe KF, Orkin FK: Pulmonary aspiration of gastric contents. In Orkin FK, Cooperman LK (eds): "Complications in Anesthesiology." Philadelphia: J.B. Lippincott, 1983.

Index